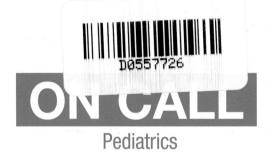

ON CALL

Pediatrics

ON CALL

Pediatrics

4th Edition

JAMES J. NOCTON, MD

Professor of Pediatrics
Section of Rheumatology,
Director, Pediatric Rheumatology Fellowship Training Program
Department of Pediatrics
Medical College of Wisconsin
and the Children's Hospital of Wisconsin
Milwaukee, Wisconsin

RAINER G. GEDEIT, MD

Professor of Pediatrics
Medical College of Wisconsin;
Clinical Director, Pediatric Intensive Care Unit
Children's Hospital of Wisconsin
Milwaukee, Wisconsin

*and the Pediatric Residents of Children's
Hospital of Wisconsin*

ELSEVIER

ELSEVIER

1600 John F. Kennedy Blvd.
Ste 1800
Philadelphia, PA 19103-2899

ON CALL PEDIATRICS, FOURTH EDITION   ISBN: 978-0-323-52905-1

Previous editions copyrighted 2006, 2001, and 1997.

Library of Congress Cataloging-in-Publication Data
Names: Nocton, James J., editor. | Gedeit, Rainer G., editor. | Children's
     Hospital of Wisconsin, issuing body.
Title: On call pediatrics / [edited by] James J. Nocton, Rainer G. Gedeit,
     and the pediatric residents of Children's Hospital of Wisconsin.
Other titles: Pediatrics | On call series.
Description: 4th edition. | Philadelphia, PA : Elsevier, [2019] | Series:
On call series | Includes bibliographical references and index.
Identifiers: LCCN 2017046943 | ISBN 9780323529051 (pbk. : alk. paper)
Subjects: | MESH: Pediatrics | Child | Emergencies | Infant | Handbooks
Classification: LCC RJ370 | NLM WS 39 | DDC 618.92–dc23 LC record available
     at https://lccn.loc.gov/2017046943

Content Strategist: James Merritt
Content Development Specialist: Katie DeFrancesco
Publishing Services Manager: Catherine Jackson
Senior Project Manager: Rachel E. McMullen
Design Direction: Amy Buxton

Printed in China
Last digit is the print number: 9   8   7   6   5   4   3   2   1

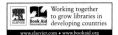

Working together
to grow libraries in
developing countries

www.elsevier.com • www.bookaid.org

To our children—
Amanda, Kay, Beth, and Claire Gedeit,
and Jeff and Sara Nocton—
who remain our greatest teachers.

Contributors

Laura Adams, MD
Resident
Department of Internal
　Medicine-Pediatrics
Medical College of Wisconsin
　and Children's Hospital of
　Wisconsin
Milwaukee, Wisconsin

Daniel Beacher, MD
Resident
Department of Pediatrics
Medical College of Wisconsin
　and Children's Hospital of
　Wisconsin
Milwaukee, Wisconsin

Alina G. Burek, MD
Resident
Department of Pediatrics
Medical College of Wisconsin
　and Children's Hospital of
　Wisconsin
Milwaukee, Wisconsin

Brian Carroll, MD
Resident
Department of Pediatrics
Medical College of Wisconsin
　and Children's Hospital of
　Wisconsin
Milwaukee, Wisconsin

Keli Coleman, MD
Resident
Department of Pediatrics
Medical College of Wisconsin
　and Children's Hospital of
　Wisconsin
Milwaukee, Wisconsin

Alison Coren, MD
Resident
Department of Pediatrics
Medical College of Wisconsin
　and Children's Hospital of
　Wisconsin
Milwaukee, Wisconsin

Rose Doolittle, MD
Resident
Department of Pediatrics
Medical College of Wisconsin
　and Children's Hospital of
　Wisconsin
Milwaukee, Wisconsin

Danielle DuMez, MD
Pediatric Resident
Department of Pediatrics
Medical College of Wisconsin
　and Children's Hospital of
　Wisconsin
Milwaukee, Wisconsin

Rainer G. Gedeit, MD
Professor of Pediatrics
Medical College of Wisconsin;
Clinical Director
Pediatric Intensive Care Unit
Children's Hospital of
    Wisconsin
Milwaukee, Wisconsin

Michael Girolami, MD
Resident
Department of Internal
    Medicine–Pediatrics
Medical College of Wisconsin
    and Children's Hospital of
    Wisconsin
Milwaukee, Wisconsin

Maja Z. Katusic
Resident
Department of Pediatrics
Medical College of Wisconsin
    and Children's Hospital of
    Wisconsin
Milwaukee, Wisconsin

Karlo Kovacic, MD
Resident
Department of Pediatrics
Medical College of Wisconsin
    and Children's Hospital of
    Wisconsin
Milwaukee, Wisconsin

Hema Krishna, MD
Resident
Department of Internal
    Medicine–Pediatrics
Medical College of Wisconsin
    and Children's Hospital of
    Wisconsin
Milwaukee, Wisconsin

Jennifer Lhost, MD
Resident
Department of Pediatrics
Medical College of Wisconsin
    and Children's Hospital of
    Wisconsin
Milwaukee, Wisconsin

Susan K. Light, MD
Resident
Department of Pediatrics
Medical College of Wisconsin
    and Children's Hospital of
    Wisconsin
Milwaukee, Wisconsin

Vanessa C. McFadden, MD, PhD
Resident
Department of Pediatrics
Medical College of Wisconsin
    and Children's Hospital of
    Wisconsin
Milwaukee, Wisconsin

James J. Nocton, MD
Professor of Pediatrics
Section of Rheumatology,
Director, Pediatric Rheumatology
    Fellowship Training Program
Department of Pediatrics
Medical College of Wisconsin and
    the Children's Hospital of
    Wisconsin
Milwaukee, Wisconsin

Julia Richards, MD
Resident Physician
Department of Pediatrics
Medical College of Wisconsin
    and Children's Hospital of
    Wisconsin
Milwaukee, Wisconsin

Kent Rosenwald, MD
Pediatrics Resident
Department of Pediatrics
Medical College of Wisconsin
 and Children's Hospital of
 Wisconsin
Milwaukee, Wisconsin

Kathryn M. Rubey, MD
Resident
Department of Pediatrics
Medical College of Wisconsin
 and Children's Hospital of
 Wisconsin
Milwaukee, Wisconsin

Anna Schmitz, MD
Resident
Department of Pediatrics
Medical College of Wisconsin
 and Children's Hospital of
 Wisconsin
Milwaukee, Wisconsin

Purabi Sonowal, MD
Resident
Department of Pediatrics
Medical College of Wisconsin
 and Children's Hospital of
 Wisconsin
Milwaukee, Wisconsin

Shela Sridhar, MD
Resident
Department of Internal
 Medicine/Pediatrics
Medical College of Wisconsin
 and Children's Hospital of
 Wisconsin
Milwaukee, Wisconsin

Lea Steffes, MD
Resident
Department of Pediatrics
Medical College of Wisconsin
 and Children's Hospital of
 Wisconsin
Milwaukee, Wisconsin

Rachel T. Sullivan, MD
Pediatric Resident
Department of Pediatrics
Medical College of Wisconsin
 and Children's Hospital of
 Wisconsin
Milwaukee, Wisconsin

Corinne Swearingen, MD
Resident
Department of Pediatrics
Medical College of Wisconsin
 and Children's Hospital of
 Wisconsin
Milwaukee, Wisconsin

Eric Velazquez, MD
Resident
Department of Pediatrics
Medical College of Wisconsin
 and Children's Hospital of
 Wisconsin
Milwaukee, Wisconsin

Rachel Weigert, MD
Resident Physician
Department of Pediatrics
Medical College of Wisconsin
 and Children's Hospital of
 Wisconsin
Milwaukee, Wisconsin

Amanda A. Wenzel, MD
Resident Physician
Department of Pediatrics
Medical College of Wisconsin
 and Children's Hospital of
 Wisconsin
Milwaukee, Wisconsin

Stephen E. Wilkinson, MD
Resident Physician
Department of Internal
 Medicine–Pediatrics
Medical College of Wisconsin
 and Children's Hospital of
 Wisconsin
Milwaukee, Wisconsin

Preface

We are very pleased to have the opportunity to write this revised and updated edition of *On Call Pediatrics*. Over the 11 years since the last edition was published, there have been considerable advances in diagnostics and management of many of the problems reviewed in this book. In addition, there have been significant changes in the way in which care is delivered to patients, including the staffing of residents and physicians within hospitals, the increasing number of non-physician advanced providers, and the growth of the electronic medical record. In fact, the entire concept of being "on call" in the hospital has been changing, with residents and staff moving away from intermittent long periods of being "on call" and responsible for patients that are "cross-covered" to systems of team-based care and scheduled night shifts or day shifts. Despite these trends, the concepts reviewed in this and previous versions of *On Call Pediatrics* remain very relevant, and the approach to patient problems discussed in this edition can continue to be applied effectively when evaluating hospitalized children. Therefore we believe that this edition will continue to serve as a valuable resource for all providers who care for children.

With this edition, we have included chapters on each of the problems reviewed in previous versions. We hope that this will permit this edition to remain most comprehensive and most helpful. With the development of multiple and easily accessed web-based resources, we decided to eliminate the formulary as well as several of the appendices that were included in earlier editions. We trust that the reader will not view this as an inconvenience.

We have again enlisted the assistance of the senior residents of the Children's Hospital of Wisconsin and the Medical College of Wisconsin Affiliated Hospitals to serve as contributors to nearly all of the chapters. These residents have been responding to calls exactly like those reviewed in this book for several years, and we believe that the knowledge and expertise that our residents are able to share will allow this edition to be most helpful.

It continues to be our intent that this book will remain a valuable and helpful resource to those who provide care to children, permitting the delivery of the best care to children, and contributing to the education of all providers in the process.

James J. Nocton, MD
Rainer G. Gedeit, MD

Acknowledgments

We are indebted to Robert M. Kliegman, MD, whose advice, support, and encouragement have made every edition of this book possible, and to Mr. Jim Merritt, Ms. Lauren Willis, Ms. Stacy Eastman, and Ms. Katie DeFrancesco of Elsevier, Inc., whose assistance and guidance were greatly appreciated during the preparation of this edition. We thank our colleagues at the Medical College of Wisconsin and Children's Hospital of Wisconsin for their support and wisdom, and the medical students and residents at these respective institutions, who challenge us to improve the care we provide to children, to become better teachers, and to continue to learn ourselves.

Structure of the Book

The book is divided into three main sections: I (Introduction), II (Patient-Related Problems), and III (Laboratory-Related Problems).

Section I covers introductory material in five chapters: The Diagnosis and Management of On-Call Problems, Communicating with Colleagues and Families, Common Mistakes, Remembering Your ABCs, and Teaching (and Learning) While On Call.

Section II discusses the common calls associated with patient-related problems. Each problem is approached from its inception, beginning with the relevant questions that should be asked over the phone, the temporary orders that should be given, and the major life-threatening problems to be considered as one approaches the bedside.

The setup of Section II is as follows.

PHONE CALL

Questions
Pertinent questions to assess the urgency of the situation.

Orders
Urgent orders to be carried out before the housestaff arrives at the bedside.

Inform RN
Nurse to be informed of the time the housestaff anticipates arrival at the bedside.

ELEVATOR THOUGHTS

The differential diagnosis to be considered by the housestaff while they are on their way to assess the patient (i.e., while they are in the elevator).

MAJOR THREAT TO LIFE

Identification of the major threat to life, which is essential in providing focus for the subsequent effective management of the patient.

BEDSIDE

Quick-Look Test

The quick-look test is a rapid visual assessment to place the patient into one of three categories: well, sick, or critical. This helps determine the necessity of immediate intervention.

Airway and Vital Signs
Selective History and Chart Review
Selective Physical Examination

MANAGEMENT

Section III contains the common calls associated with laboratory-related problems.

The Appendices consist of reference items that we have found useful in managing calls.

The On-Call Formulary is a compendium of commonly used medications that are likely to be prescribed by the student or resident on call. The formulary serves as a quick, alphabetically arranged reference for indications, drug dosages, routes of administration, side effects, contraindications, and modes of action.

Commonly Used Abbreviations

ABCs	Airway, breathing, and circulation
ABD	Abdomen
ABG	Arterial blood gas
AC	Before meals
ACE	Angiotensin-converting enzyme
ACLS	Advanced cardiac life support
AIDS	Acquired immunodeficiency syndrome
ANA	Antinuclear antibody
A/P	Anteroposterior
aPTT	Activated partial thromboplastin time
ARDS	Adult respiratory distress syndrome
ASD	Atrial septal defect
ASO	Antistreptolysin O
AV	Atrioventricular
BID	Twice a day
BP	Blood pressure
BPD	Bronchopulmonary dysplasia
BPM	Beats per minute
BSA	Body surface area
CBC	Complete blood count
CF	Cystic fibrosis
CHF	Congestive heart failure
CMV	Cytomegalovirus

CNS	Central nervous system
CO	Cardiac output
CO$_2$	Carbon dioxide
CPK	Creatine phosphokinase
CSF	Cerebrospinal fluid
CT	Computed tomography
CVAT	Costovertebral angle tenderness
CVS	Cardiovascular system
CXR	Chest x-ray
DDAVP	Desmopressin
DIC	Disseminated intravascular coagulation
DKA	Diabetic ketoacidosis
D$_5$NS	5% dextrose in normal saline solution
DOE	Dyspnea on exertion
DVT	Deep venous thrombosis
D$_5$W	5% dextrose in water
D$_{25}$W	25% dextrose in water
ECG	Electrocardiogram
EEG	Electroencephalogram
ELISA	Enzyme-linked immunosorbent assay
ENT	Ears, nose, and throat
ESR	Erythrocyte sedimentation rate
EXT	Extremities
F$_I$O$_2$	Fraction of inspired oxygen
Fr	French (unit of measurement for catheters and tubes)
FUO	Fever of unknown origin
GI	Gastrointestinal
G-6-PD	Glucose-6-phosphate dehydrogenase
GU	Genitourinary
Hb	Hemoglobin

HCT	Hematocrit
HEENT	Head, eyes, ears, nose, and throat
HIV	Human immunodeficiency virus
HPI	History of present illness
Hr	Hour
HR	Heart rate
HS	At bedtime
HSV	Herpes simplex virus
HUS	Hemolytic-uremic syndrome
ICP	Intracranial pressure
ICU	Intensive care unit
IDDM	Insulin-dependent diabetes mellitus
IgG	Immunoglobulin G
IM	Intramuscular
INR	International normalized ratio
ITP	Idiopathic thrombocytopenic purpura
IV	Intravenous
IVIG	Intravenous immunoglobulin
JRA	Juvenile rheumatoid arthritis
LDH	Lactate dehydrogenase
LOC	Loss of consciousness
LP	Lumbar puncture
LV	Left ventricle
LVH	Left ventricular hypertrophy
MAO	Monoamine oxidase
MCV	Mean corpuscular volume
mm Hg	Millimeters of mercury
MRI	Magnetic resonance imaging
NEC	Necrotizing enterocolitis
NEURO	Neurologic system

NG	Nasogastric
NIDDM	Non–insulin-dependent diabetes mellitus
NPH	Neutral protamine Hagedorn (insulin)
NPO	Nothing by mouth
NS	Normal saline
NSAID	Nonsteroidal anti-inflammatory drug
O$_2$	Oxygen
Osm	Osmolality
P/A	Posteroanterior
PAC	Premature atrial contraction
PALS	Pediatric Advanced Life Support
PC	After meals
PCA	Patient-controlled analgesia
P$_{CO_2}$	Partial pressure of carbon dioxide
PEEP	Positive end-expiratory pressure
PICU	Pediatric intensive care unit
PMI	Point of maximal intensity
PO	By mouth
P$_{O_2}$	Partial pressure of oxygen
PPD	Purified protein derivative
PPHN	Persistent pulmonary hypertension of the newborn
PR	Per rectum
PRBCs	Packed red blood cells
PRN	As necessary
PT	Prothrombin time
PTH	Parathyroid hormone
PTT	Partial thromboplastin time
PVC	Premature ventricular contraction
Q	Each
QHS	Each night at bedtime

QID	Four times a day
RBC	Red blood cell
RESP	Respiratory system
RN	Registered nurse
RR	Respiratory rate
RSV	Respiratory syncytial virus
RTA	Renal tubular acidosis
RV	Right ventricle
RVH	Right ventricular hypertrophy
SBE	Subacute bacterial endocarditis
SC	Subcutaneous
Sec	Second
SI	International System of Units
SIADH	Syndrome of inappropriate antidiuretic hormone
SL	Sublingual
SLE	Systemic lupus erythematosus
SOB	Shortness of breath
STAT	Immediately
SVT	Supraventricular tachycardia
T$_3$	Triiodothyronine
T$_4$	Thyroxine
TB	Tuberculosis
TCA	Tricyclic antidepressants
TKVO	To keep vein open
TORCH	Toxoplasmosis, other infections, rubella, cytomegalovirus, herpes (congenital infections)
TPN	Total parenteral nutrition
TSH	Thyroid-stimulating hormone
TTP	Thrombotic thrombocytopenic purpura
UAC	Umbilical arterial catheter
URI	Upper respiratory infection

UTI	Urinary tract infection
UVC	Umbilical venous catheter
V/Q	Ventilation/perfusion
VSD	Ventricular septal defect
VT	Ventricular tachycardia
WBC	White blood cell
WPW	Wolff-Parkinson-White syndrome

Contents

LABORATORY-RELATED PROBLEMS

APPENDICES

Introduction

The Diagnosis and Management of On-Call Problems

James J. Nocton, MD

The approach to the evaluation and management of problems that arise while on call is similar to that taken in other clinical situations. Initially, information about the patient and the specific problem must be collected. This information is acquired by obtaining a history, performing a physical examination, and potentially reviewing pertinent laboratory data or imaging studies. While collecting information, the physician is considering possible diagnoses. Eventually, a diagnostic impression is formulated, and appropriate management is undertaken. Although this general scheme is identical to that used when admitting a new patient or evaluating a patient in the ambulatory setting, the approach often needs to be modified when one is informed about a problem that arises in a patient already in the hospital.

The primary distinction between the approach to an on-call problem and a problem in a "new" patient is that the goals are different. In most cases, patients who are in the hospital have already undergone a complete history and physical examination, a diagnostic impression has already been formulated regarding their problems at the time of admission, and management of these problems has begun. It is not the goal of the physician on call to repeat this process. Instead, the physician on call is expected to evaluate and manage acute problems that either are causing discomfort or have the potential to lead to deterioration in the patient's condition. It is appropriate to ask the question, "What might happen today that may be causing this problem and may adversely affect the patient?" When one is admitting multiple patients and is responsible for many others, time is always a factor. Some problems need to be given priority over others. Rarely does one have time to deliberate extensively about problems that are not going to lead to immediate harm to the patient. These problems can and should be addressed at a later time. In some cases the cause of a problem may not be easily diagnosed, and specific management may therefore be deferred until the problem "declares itself." This approach may be acceptable if one keeps in mind that the goals are to maintain the comfort of the patient and exclude (or empirically treat) potential imminent causes of significant morbidity or mortality.

Because the goal of a physician on call is limited, the approach to a patient in whom a problem develops can be much more focused. One does not need to take a complete history or perform an exhaustive physical examination. Chart reviews may provide helpful information but should also be directed at answering specific questions. In many cases, historical information may have already been obtained during "sign-out." The sign-out process is the ideal time to enhance efficiency in managing on-call problems. Potential problems can often be anticipated by those who have been caring for a patient on a daily basis. Specific details about patients can be relayed to the on-call house officer, and management suggestions for anticipated problems can be discussed. Such a sign-out process can be extremely helpful, for example, when a problem is recurrent and previously successful or unsuccessful management strategies are known. The key to addressing on-call problems is efficiency. Being only as thorough as one needs to be and prioritizing appropriately allow one to be a successful physician on call.

The approach suggested in this book is designed to be efficient, yet appropriately thorough. For each problem, the sequence of thought processes that the physician should go through is discussed from the time that a problem is identified (usually with a phone call from a nurse) until the problem is managed. These thought processes are discussed in four separate parts for each chapter:

1. Phone call
2. Elevator thoughts
3. Major threat to life
4. Bedside

PHONE CALL

The phone call is usually how one first hears about a problem. The initial call should not simply be for notification but should also allow the physician to indirectly assess the severity of the problem, to begin developing a differential diagnosis, and, when necessary, to begin management. In this section of each chapter, questions that should be asked immediately, before hanging up the phone, are listed. If the severity of the problem can be determined, the physician can then appropriately decide how to prioritize the call. If the severity cannot be determined, the patient needs to be seen fairly quickly. Orders that may enhance efficient evaluation or management are also suggested in this section, and other information important for the nurse to know is discussed, such as when the physician will arrive at the bedside.

Not every call requires that the physician evaluate the patient directly. For quick, minor problems that pose no immediate threat to the patient, taking a history from the nurse may be sufficient to allow one to determine appropriate management. In these instances, it is reasonable to ask the nurse, "Do you think I need to see the patient?" If there is any doubt in either the nurse's or the physician's mind, the patient should be seen.

ELEVATOR THOUGHTS

After the physician has finished discussing the problem with the nurse, some time is usually required to travel to the patient's bedside. The time that it takes to walk or ride the elevator to see a patient can be used to reflect on the situation and to think about differential diagnoses. In this section of each chapter, the differential diagnosis for each problem is listed. The lists are not exhaustive but are intended to present the most common possibilities and those considered life threatening.

MAJOR THREAT TO LIFE

As part of the differential diagnosis, it is important for the physician on call to identify the possible diagnoses that are the most severe or potentially life threatening. One should ask, "What should I be considering that might be life threatening?" By asking this question, one ensures that even if definitive solutions are not found, the most serious possibilities have been considered and either excluded or empirically treated.

BEDSIDE

This section describes the steps that should be taken on arrival at the bedside. By this time, the chief complaint is known (the reason for the phone call from the nurse), possible diagnoses have been considered on the basis of the information available (elevator thoughts), and the major threat or threats to life have been identified (elevator thoughts). The steps to be taken at the bedside are presented in the following subsections in each chapter:

1. Quick-look test
2. Airway and vital signs
3. Selective history
4. Selective physical examination
5. Selective chart review
6. Management

The quick-look test and evaluation of the airway and vital signs should always be the first things done on arrival at the bedside, regardless of the complaint. The quick-look test involves an overall impression gained by observing the patient. The goal is to rapidly evaluate the patient's condition. The patient may appear comfortable and in no distress (e.g., sitting in bed having a conversation), mildly uncomfortable or distressed (e.g., crying, worried), or severely ill (e.g., comatose). Combined with evaluation of the airway and vital signs, the quick-look test enables the physician to determine the urgency of the situation and whether immediate intervention is necessary before obtaining a history and performing a physical examination. If the patient appears comfortable and has stable vital signs and an intact airway, the physician can proceed with less urgency. The sequence of the subsections describing the history, physical examination, chart review, and management varies among the chapters according to the problems presented. For some problems (e.g., hypotension and shock), some form of management probably needs to be undertaken before additional history is obtained or a selective chart review is performed. In other instances (e.g., constipation), the sequence is as expected, with management suggestions offered after suggestions regarding the history, physical examination, and chart review.

We believe that this approach to problems that may arise in a pediatric patient is helpful for the physician on call. As outlined here and presented in the individual chapters, this approach should provide an organized way for the physician to thoroughly and efficiently evaluate the common problems that arise in hospitalized pediatric patients.

CHAPTER 2

Communicating With Colleagues and Families

James J. Nocton, MD

As with all other clinical situations, appropriate communication is an essential component of the evaluation and management of a patient while one is on call. The results of the evaluation and management of the problem, if any, must be effectively communicated to the patient, the family, the nurse, and others responsible for care of the patient. Communicating while on call occurs in two ways: (1) discussions in person or by telephone and (2) documentation in the patient's chart. When one is busy admitting patients and evaluating patients with problems, taking the time for appropriate communication and documentation may often seem less important than the actual process of caring for the patients. However, the time spent talking with families, discussing the patient with the nurse, writing a note, or making the extra phone call is much appreciated by everyone, including your colleagues who will resume responsibility for the patient when you are no longer on call.

Communicating with the child, and usually the parents of the child, will begin as soon as you arrive at the bedside and will continue until you have addressed the problem and answered the family's questions. The family of a child in the hospital is under great stress. Their child's illness is a tremendous source of worry and anguish and causes a significant disruption in their daily lives. When a problem arises while unknown physicians are responsible for the care of their child, the family may feel lost without the physicians familiar to them. They may feel as though no one knows what is happening with their child and may not trust that the physician on call will know what to do. It will be up to you to evaluate and manage the problem and to communicate to the family in a manner that is comforting, gains their trust, and reassures them that their child will receive excellent care.

Once you arrive to evaluate the child, you need to formally introduce yourself to the family and the child and address the family by name, not as "Mom" or "Dad." This takes very little time, and it may make a difference in how the family reacts to you. Explain who you are, your role as part of the medical team, and why you have been called to see their child. Stating that you know why the child is in the hospital, the issues that are being evaluated or treated during this hospitalization, and that you have communicated with the physicians that may be more familiar to them will reassure the family that you do know something about their child and will hopefully build their trust in you. Then, proceed with your evaluation efficiently and thoroughly.

After you have finished your selective examination, history, and chart review and have developed an assessment and plan of action, this should be communicated directly to the family. The family will want to know whether their child is becoming "sicker" or is in danger of becoming critically ill as a result of the problem for which you have been called. You will need to address these issues and inform the family if there appears to have been a change in the child's status. When the findings of your evaluation imply a serious change in the child's condition, the family needs to be informed in a clear, understandable, and honest manner. Bad news is always difficult to deliver. The physician must never delegate this duty to a student or nurse. If the family is not present, the on-call physician should contact the family by telephone promptly, introduce himself or herself clearly, and truthfully explain the situation to the family.

One decision that will need to be made when managing problems on call is when to notify a supervising resident or attending physician. This is a process that must be individualized. The status of the patient, the severity of the problem, and your experience and degree of comfort are all factors that affect the decision to immediately notify others who are supervising care of the patient. Early in the first year of residency, nearly every problem is discussed immediately with a supervisor. As experience is gained, the physician on call is able to manage many of these problems independently, with discussion at a later time. In some cases, it is obvious that a supervisor must be notified, such as when a patient's condition changes significantly, transfer to an intensive care setting appears imminent, or diagnostic or therapeutic uncertainty exists. As a general rule, if there is any doubt regarding a problem that arises while one is on call, it is always best to discuss the problem with a supervisor. Knowing one's limitations is an extremely valuable asset that should not be forgotten while on call.

Discussing problems and their management with the nurse caring for the child is also essential. In many instances the nurse knows the patient well, may have more experience with specific problems, and has seen how others have managed similar problems

successfully. The nurse can be a great resource in these circumstances and may be able to offer very helpful suggestions. Listening
to the nurse, involving the nurse in the decision-making process,
and keeping the nurse informed of your plans will allow you to provide the best care to the patient and will keep everyone "on the
same page," thereby minimizing the potential for errors.

Regardless of whether a particular problem requires immediate
discussion or notification of others, documentation of the problem,
evaluation, and action taken is mandatory. With the exception of very
minor and inconsequential problems that can be resolved over the
phone without seeing the patient, all other problems require at least
some documentation. It is extremely helpful for those caring for the
patient on a daily basis to know what happened in the middle of the
night and to have access to such information via the patient's chart.
The written documentation of the evaluation and management of a
problem that arises while one is on call can take several forms. Simple
problems may require only a few sentences. For example:

> Called to see patient for sore throat. Patient afebrile, HR 84, RR 20,
> BP 120/75. Appeared comfortable. No complaints other than throat.
> Posterior pharynx slightly erythematous with patches of exudate on
> tonsils. Mild cervical adenopathy. Obtained rapid streptococcal test
> and throat culture. Will not administer antibiotics until results of
> tests known.

For other problems (e.g., new fever in an immunocompromised
patient), a more extensive note may be required, and the "SOAP"
format generally works well—listing the **S**ubjective complaint, **O**bjec-
tive findings, **A**ssessment, and **P**lan of management. One should be as
concise as possible, describing only as much historical, subjective
information as is essential and providing a brief summary of your
assessment and management plan. It is necessary to perform and
document only the pertinent parts of the physical examination.
The goal is to notify those who will be seeing the patient the following
day that a problem arose and that the problem was evaluated and
managed. As with all other types of documentation, notes should
be dated and timed. All procedures should be described. If the
problem was discussed with the family, attending physician, or
consultants, this should be documented along with the time that
the discussion took place. Finally, your name should be indicated,
followed by a phone or pager number. If someone has a question
regarding what happened, that person should be able to reach you
easily.

Discussing problems with colleagues and families and documenting the evaluation and management of problems are tasks that
are easy to ignore when one is on call and extremely busy. However,
maintaining communication should be a priority. Communicating

with the family promptly, honestly, and in person when possible is essential. Communicating with supervising colleagues in all situations in which there is any doubt is in the patient's best interest. By documenting problems, you are helping your colleagues and others caring for the patient. Through verbal communication and documentation, you can also remind yourself that you are never truly alone when you are on call.

CHAPTER 3

Common Mistakes

James J. Nocton, MD

Everyone makes mistakes. Although some mistakes are the result of fatigue and lack of sleep, the most common mistakes are made by physicians in a hurry. Therefore many mistakes are preventable. This chapter briefly discusses a few of the most common and most preventable errors made in the care of hospitalized children, including the following:

- Poorly entered orders
- Failure to communicate with the nurse
- Failure to communicate with a supervising physician
- Failure to listen to the family
- Failure to document in the chart while on call

The way you enter orders is important. An electronic health record is now used in most hospitals, and this helps to avoid legibility issues and some calculation errors; however, the potential for error remains, and one still needs to be compulsive about entering orders. Calls requesting clarification of confusing or incomplete orders will plague you and eat away at your time if you do not take this issue seriously. Enter every order as simply and as clearly as possible. Be meticulous. Specify the preparation of any medication, the dose, the route of administration, and the dosing frequency clearly. Be careful about decimal points! Always precede a decimal point by a 0 when prescribing less than a milligram (e.g., digoxin, 0.25 mg by mouth every day). Never follow the tenths or hundredths place with a 0; for example, captopril, 6.250 mg, could be misread easily as 6250 mg. Do not assume that an electronic system will autocorrect, and always double check the order you enter. Try to avoid abbreviations. Instead of writing (or typing) "qd" or "bid," write "once a day" or "twice a day." When ordering a liquid preparation, check that the concentration of the liquid is correct.

Another way to save yourself time is to communicate what you have ordered directly to the nurse. Having the nurse review the orders allows immediate clarification and prevents annoyingly time-consuming pages and clarification calls later. It also facilitates prompt and appropriate action on those orders by the nursing staff and other ancillary personnel.

As mentioned in Chapter 2, Communicating With Colleagues and Families, communication with supervising physicians should occur whenever there is any doubt regarding a problem or its management. Remember that notification does not always require a telephone conversation. Do not hesitate to text-page your analysis or plan of action. This allows supervising physicians to act at their convenience. Remember, if you think that the supervising physician might want to know, make the call, send a page, and communicate!

The same policy applies for the family. The more willing you are to communicate with the family, the more confident they will be having you care for their child. Families have many reasons for being present with their child in the hospital and equally many reasons why they sometimes cannot be with their child. Do not judge them. Involve them in their child's care and communicate freely, frequently, and honestly. A family would be very unlikely to complain because they were told too much or because providers in the hospital communicated too often with them.

Finally, as discussed in Chapter 2, Communicating With Colleagues and Families, if you go to the effort of evaluating a patient when on call or if you spend time communicating with the attending physician or the family, document this in a note! It takes only a moment to document, "Asked to evaluate [the patient's name] for [fever, chest pain, wheezing, etc.]. Vital signs stable. Cardiorespiratory exam normal. No signs of sepsis, shock, or meningitis. Tylenol ordered for fever control. No studies at this time. Supervisor notified [or will be notified in AM]. Discussed with family." Always make sure that the date and time are recorded in on-call documentation. Charting on-call encounters not only is for your protection but also serves a vital role in communicating with the team caring for the patient during the daytime. It is too important to neglect.

Each of these mistakes occurs when physicians are busy, but none of these actions is so time consuming that this is prohibitive. Each is a fundamental part of conscientious care and ultimately improves your efficiency. Improved efficiency will give you the time to call home, grab dinner, or even potentially catch a little sleep while on call.

CHAPTER 4

Remembering Your ABCs

Rainer G. Gedeit, MD

Nothing strikes fear in a house officer more than the "code page." When the "code team" is activated, there is a flurry of activity not seen at any other time or place in the hospital. The "code team" responds, as does everyone else within earshot of the page. A frenzied group of doctors, nurses, medical students, respiratory therapists, chaplains, pharmacists, phlebotomists, security guards, and anyone else who is curious enough to see what the commotion is all about show up. The team awaits orders from the "team leader." As you view the chaotic scene of a cardiac arrest in the hospital, many people are busy doing things but may not truly be helping. When you arrive at the scene, you must not be one of these people. You need to be caring for the patient, not getting in the way. The most important thing to remember comes from the novel *House of God* by Samuel Shem, MD. "AT A CARDIAC ARREST, THE FIRST PROCEDURE IS TO TAKE YOUR OWN PULSE!" Stop, take a breath, assess the situation, determine what you should be doing, and do it. Your role in the "code" will depend on the situation. You may be the first person on the scene, the first MD on the scene, the fifth MD on the scene, or the team leader. Think about what you need to do and do it. If you are not needed, move away.

THE ABCS

When you walk into a code situation, the things you learned in kindergarten will come in handy. Go back and think about the ABCs. You will probably not know the patient in front of you or why that patient is dying; that is not what is important. The thing to do is to try to reverse that process.

ELEVATOR THOUGHTS

Do I know the patient? If so, why would he or she be in trouble? Think about what you know and how this could help in the treatment of this patient.

What is my role in this situation? Am I a member of the code team? Is this my patient? If you are a member of the code team, remember your role and check in with the team leader to let him or her know you are there and ready to assist. If this is your patient, be ready to give a brief summary of the patient to the team leader.

BEDSIDE

When coming upon the scene, assess the situation. Are you the first physician there? If so, take the lead until others arrive. Otherwise, assume your role or take the role you are assigned by the team leader.

Quick-Look Test

Who is in the room, and what is being done for the patient? The activity in the room can usually tell you how critical the problem is. If you need to proceed with patient assessment and management, start your ABCs.

A = Airway

See whether the patient responds to stimulation. Call the child's name or gently shake the child; if there is no response, open the airway. A jaw thrust or chin lift along with placing the patient supine is the first thing to do. Make sure that suction equipment is available in case the child vomits or has excessive airway secretions. If it is not within reach, direct someone to get the equipment needed.

B = Breathing

Is the patient breathing? Look, listen, and feel. Is the chest rising, can you feel air moving in and out, are there breath sounds? If yes, maintain the airway and assess for cardiac output. If the patient is not breathing, begin assisted breathing. Most hospital rooms will have some type of resuscitation device (know where these are in your institution), or the "code cart" that should have been brought to the bedside will have a self-inflating bag and mask. Get the correct size mask and begin respirations. If this is not available, begin mouth-to-mouth or mouth-to-mask rescue breathing. Two people are often needed to accomplish effective bag-mask breathing: one to open the airway and hold the mask in place and the other to ventilate with the bag. Once intubation equipment arrives, an artificial airway should be placed. This is the best way to assist breathing and can be used as a portal to deliver drugs if intravenous (IV) access is absent. The size of endotracheal tube that should be used can be estimated by the formula (age in years/4) + 4. Make sure that all the equipment never works before attempting intubation. Nothing is worse than placing a laryngoscope and having a dead lightbulb. Use the personnel at the bedside to get the equipment; do not leave the patient.

C = Circulation

This is the most difficult part of the entire assessment. Feeling a weak pulse in an infant who is receiving artificial respirations is difficult, if not impossible. Your own adrenaline is rushing and your hand is shaking. Take time to feel multiple areas for a pulse (brachial, femoral, carotid). If there is no pulse, begin chest compressions. Use the appropriate rate and method for the patient's age and size.

Placement of an IV catheter is required for drug delivery. Using a large vein such as the antecubital should be attempted. If a catheter is already in place, flush it to ensure patency. Placing a second IV catheter is never wrong, in case the first one fails. Place the largest catheter possible. If an IV catheter cannot be placed within 15 to 30 seconds, place an intraosseous catheter. If available, place the patient on a cardiorespiratory monitor to evaluate the heart rate and rhythm. If needed, give a dose of epinephrine.

As the basics are started, it is important to get an idea of what might have precipitated this event. Someone familiar with the patient (nurse, medical student, resident) must be available to consult with the team leader, and the chart must be brought to the bedside. Always show up if a patient you know is in trouble.

If you are the team leader, you must take control of the situation at the bedside. Your job is to ask for information and request that medications be given, as well as control flow in the room. The most difficult part of running the "code" is keeping control. Keep control of your own emotions; a panicked leader makes a panicked team. Make sure that everyone in the room is supposed to be there. Excuse extraneous persons. If there are persistent "pests," give these people a job to do to keep them out of the way. The best team leader I ever saw was a senior resident who looked the extraneous personnel in the eye and gave them each a job to do, outside the room (get ice for labs, get the chart, check on the family, get equipment for a blood draw). This left only the needed team members in the room. Make sure that those performing ventilation and chest compressions are doing an adequate job, and replace them every few minutes as they fatigue (performing cardiopulmonary resuscitation [CPR] is physically and emotionally draining).

As a team member, know your role (perform CPR, get information, place an IV line, ventilate the patient, communicate with the family). Do that job until you are told otherwise, or tell the leader that you cannot perform the assigned duty or are becoming fatigued (while performing CPR).

In some institutions, rapid-response extracorporeal support is possible. Know your institution's policies and procedures so that this resource can be activated. Know what the response time will be and what needs to be done to prepare the patient.

If the child is successfully resuscitated, transfer to a higher level of care is required. The pediatric intensive care unit (PICU) should be notified of the patient's condition and needs (ventilator, pressors, etc.). The team leader should accompany the patient to inform the accepting team in the PICU of the situation.

The outcome of resuscitation becomes less favorable as time goes on. At some point the team leader must "call the code." This is the worst time for any physician, and how to do this is important. Verify how long the code has been ongoing, what medications were given, and that there has been no response to resuscitation. Make sure all agree that the code is to be stopped. Thank everyone for their hard work. Stay with the patient and help clean up. If the doctors help when it is over, it makes it easier for everyone, including yourself.

When a code is over, whether the patient survived or not, those involved are shaken. Take time to decompress. Get a drink of water, coffee, or soda. Talk with those involved. At times a formal debriefing may be needed, and most institutions can accommodate this. Ask about a debriefing if you think it is needed.

CHAPTER 5

Teaching (and Learning) While On Call

James J. Nocton, MD

Although the first priority for physicians on call is always to care for the patients, the hours spent on call are also of tremendous educational value. Every question, every call from a nurse, every discussion with a family, and every problem provide you with opportunities to learn something new and to share things you already know. The number of questions received from nurses and families, the number of patients who require evaluation, and the number of problems that you will need to manage will often be far greater while you are on call than at other times. Although you will probably be very busy responding to these situations, your on-call experience will be much more rewarding and useful to you if you remember to make an effort to teach, as well as remember to learn, while you are taking care of patients.

Teaching while on call may initially seem to be an impossible task. You may ask yourself, "How will I possibly find time to teach when I will be taking care of so many patients, getting so many pages, admitting so many new patients, and evaluating the other problems that will invariably arise?" The answer to this question involves understanding something about adult learning and using some very effective methods of efficient teaching. Most of us think of teaching as the active process of sharing information and learning as the passive process of receiving information from the teacher. This is how we recall most of our formal education, with heavy emphasis on "the lecture." Needless to say, it will generally be impossible for you to plan on giving lectures while you are on call, and as it turns out, this is not a very effective way for adults to learn anyway. Adults learn best when they are invested in the learning process and take an active role in their own education. Therefore the optimal way to teach is to allow your learners to be actively involved in everything you are doing. When evaluating a problem, evaluate it together with your student: inform the student of the problem as it was presented to you, and give the student an opportunity to think about it. Most importantly, give students an opportunity to commit to a specific plan of action, whether it be diagnostic testing, treatment, or both. Whenever possible, do this before informing the student of your own plan of action. It is the commitment on the part of students that gets them actively invested in the learning process and permits you to teach more effectively. After a student has thought the problem through independently, developed an assessment, and formulated a plan, you are then in a position to discuss that student's thought process and explain why or why not the assessment and plan are appropriate. You will be a better teacher, and your student will learn far more in this way than if you simply told the student what should be done.

Two specific types of teaching can be very effective when time is at a premium. The first is known as "priming." Priming involves setting a specific expectation for learners before engaging them actively in the learning process. For example, if you are called to see a child who has a sudden onset of abdominal pain, you might ask your student, "When we go in to examine this patient, how will we determine whether or not this may be appendicitis?" The student can then respond, hopefully with a reasonable answer, and you can comment on the answer and then proceed to examine the patient. This process should not take a great deal of time, it allows you to teach about a specific topic (the expected physical findings in someone with appendicitis), and it permits the learner to be invested in the learning process by making a commitment in responding to your question.

"Modeling" is an even more efficient method of teaching. Modeling is a more passive learning process than priming, but it can also be very effective; it involves preparing the student for a specific behavior or skill that you are about to demonstrate. For example, if you are called to a child's room by the nurse because the child has a high fever, you may say to the student, "I want you to watch how I discuss the significance of a fever with this child's parents." Modeling requires that you choose a specific teaching point and make sure that the student focuses on learning about this specific topic. In this case the teaching point is the significance of fever and how to explain it to families. You will be discussing many other issues when you go into the room to see the patient, but your student will understand what you would like him or her to learn from this individual patient interaction. You have been able to teach, while not spending any more time than you would have had the student not been present.

When teaching an adult learner, particularly when using priming or modeling as a teaching method, it is important to keep two additional things in mind. First, teaching needs to occur at a suitable level for the learner. It may be appropriate to ask an average third-year medical student about the expected physical findings in someone with abdominal pain and appendicitis. It may not be appropriate, even for the most advanced third-year student, to ask about the expected physical findings, genetics, and treatment of familial cold autoinflammatory syndrome. Of course, students will vary with regard to their knowledge and skill, and you will need to determine the individual level that is appropriate for each student. This can be accomplished by asking students questions and evaluating the appropriateness of their responses. Initially, the questions may be very basic or superficial ("What are the physical findings in appendicitis?"). If the student answers the initial questions easily, you can then determine the depth of the student's understanding by asking additional questions ("What are the expected laboratory and radiographic findings in appendicitis? Which patients should be taken to surgery? What is the prognosis and long-term outcome of appendicitis?"). In this way, you should be able to approximately determine the appropriate level at which to teach.

The second principle to keep in mind is that teaching should involve general rules that will be relevant to all learners. Physical examination of the abdomen is a skill that nearly every physician will need. Teaching about the genetics of familial cold autoinflammatory syndrome may be interesting, but it will not necessarily be relevant to most medical students. They will remember a general rule that they are able to apply repeatedly to the care of their future patients. They will forget the specific minutiae regarding a rare disease that they are unlikely to see very often.

As you are making efforts to teach while on call, you may not realize quite how much you have learned. When called regarding a problem that you have never been confronted with before, you may need to quickly review a textbook or an online database for information. You may need to discuss the problem with a consultant. It is to your educational benefit to take advantage of as many of these resources as you can, as time permits. Sharing what you are learning from these resources with your student will sharpen your understanding of the problem. Reviewing published information and discussing the problem with those who have more experience will also enable you to feel reassured regarding your evaluation and treatment of the patient.

Much of the learning that you will experience while on call will occur as you discuss problems with colleagues, either while you are on call or at a later time, such as during morning rounds. Presenting your patients at rounds and discussing how you evaluated and managed problems will give you an opportunity to ask how others might have proceeded in certain situations. This will permit you to reflect on your own decisions and allow you to ask the question to yourself, "What could I have done differently?" By doing so, you will increase your knowledge, improve your decision making, and improve the care you will provide to your patients the next time you are on call.

Teaching (and learning) can occur while you are on call. All that is required is some effort on the part of the teacher and willingness to invest in learning by the student. Hopefully, this chapter has explained how teaching can be very effective without taking a great deal of time away from patient care responsibilities. By making the effort to teach, the physician on call can make the on-call experience more educational, rewarding, and satisfying.

Patient-Related Problems

CHAPTER 6

Abdominal Pain

Rachel Weigert, MD

Abdominal pain in a hospitalized pediatric patient should always be evaluated promptly. Although it is an extremely common and often benign complaint in all children, abdominal pain should never be dismissed as insignificant until a thorough evaluation has excluded potentially serious causes. In addition, abdominal pain should not be empirically treated with analgesics until a thorough evaluation has determined that the patient does not have a surgical or other life-threatening condition. In some instances the cause of the abdominal pain may not be clear. After an initial evaluation, it may be necessary to adopt an expectant approach that involves performing serial examinations at regular intervals, prescribing analgesics when necessary for discomfort, and continuing to consider possible diagnoses until the cause becomes clear or the pain resolves.

PHONE CALL

Questions

1. How old is the patient?
2. Why is the patient in the hospital?
3. What are the patient's vital signs?
4. How does the patient rate the pain?
5. How long has it been present?
6. Is it localized?
7. Does the child have any nausea, vomiting, or diarrhea?
8. Is there blood in the emesis or stool?
9. Has the child complained of abdominal pain previously during this admission?

The patient's vital signs, the degree of severity, and the duration of pain allow a quick determination of the urgency of the situation. Stable vital signs with mild pain present for several hours are reassuring and not suggestive of an acute intra-abdominal process.

Understanding the location of the pain, the age of the child, the reason for hospitalization, and any associated symptoms will allow you to begin to consider a specific diagnosis. Previous complaints may signal that an evaluation has been performed before or that the cause of the pain is already known.

Orders

1. Nil per os (**NPO**). The patient should have NPO until further evaluated.
2. **Place IV**. If pain is severe and the vital signs indicate shock (tachycardia and hypotension), an intravenous (IV) line should be placed and a 20-mL/kg bolus of isotonic fluid (normal saline or lactated Ringer's solution) should be infused.

Inform Registered Nurse (RN)

If the pain is severe or the vital signs make you concerned about an intra-abdominal emergency or shock, alert the RN that the patient will be evaluated immediately. If the pain is mild and vital signs are normal, the nurse should be informed of when you expect to see the patient.

ELEVATOR THOUGHTS

On your way to evaluate the patient, you can contemplate the many causes of abdominal pain. You may consider the location of the organs within the abdomen, pelvis, and retroperitoneum and the potential pathologic processes that may affect each organ, the source of blood supply to each area, and whether the pain is related to that organ or referred. When abdominal pain is generalized or cannot be localized (e.g., in an infant or toddler), a wide differential should be considered. Abdominal pain may also result from systemic metabolic abnormalities (e.g., diabetic ketoacidosis, porphyria), as well as processes at distant anatomic sites (e.g., streptococcal pharyngitis, pneumonia):

Epigastric pain	Aortic dissection
	Carditis (pericarditis, myocarditis)
	Pancreatitis
	Peptic ulcer (perforation)
	Gastroesophageal reflux (heartburn)
	Gastritis
	Esophagitis
Left upper quadrant pain	Splenic rupture
	Splenic infarct
	Splenic abscess
	Subphrenic abscess
	Left lower lobe pneumonia

Right upper quadrant pain	Hepatitis
	Cholecystitis
	Biliary obstruction (gallstones)
	Liver abscess
	Subphrenic abscess
	Fitz-Hugh–Curtis syndrome (gonococcal perihepatitis)
	Right lower lobe pneumonia
Left lower quadrant pain	Ovarian torsion
	Mittelschmerz (ovulation)
	Ovarian cyst
	Psoas abscess
	Ectopic pregnancy
	Pelvic inflammatory disease
	Renal stone
	Colitis (infectious or inflammatory)
	Incarcerated hernia
	Testicular torsion
	Epididymitis
Right lower quadrant pain	Appendicitis
	Ruptured appendix/abscess
	Mesenteric adenitis
	Ovarian torsion
	Ovarian cyst
	Psoas abscess
	Ectopic pregnancy
	Pelvic inflammatory disease
	Renal stone
	Incarcerated hernia
	Testicular torsion
	Epididymitis
Hypogastric pain	Cystitis
	Bladder obstruction
	Ovarian torsion
	Pelvic inflammatory disease
	Testicular torsion
Generalized pain	Any of the preceding conditions
	Mesenteric adenitis
	Typhlitis
	Constipation
	Ileus
	Gastroenteritis
	Viral infection (e.g., mononucleosis)
	Inflammatory bowel disease
	Lactose intolerance

	Vasculitis (Henoch-Schönlein purpura, polyarteritis nodosa, systemic lupus erythematosus)
	Mesenteric thrombosis
	Trauma (including nonaccidental)
	Pharyngitis
	Diskitis
	Porphyria
	Bezoar
	Peritonitis
	Sterile peritonitis (systemic juvenile idiopathic arthritis, familial Mediterranean fever, lupus)
Generalized pain	Abdominal epilepsy
	Hereditary angioedema
	Abdominal migraine
	Tumor
	Adrenal insufficiency
	Bowel obstruction (volvulus, malrotation)
	Superior mesenteric artery syndrome
	Sickle cell crisis
	Pregnancy
	Meckel diverticulum (with secondary intussusception)
	Intussusception
	Psychologic (somatization)

MAJOR THREAT TO LIFE

- Obstruction leading to perforation
- Ischemic bowel (e.g., from volvulus, intussusception, or vasculitis)
- Infectious peritonitis (with or without a perforated viscus)
- Gastrointestinal (GI) bleed
- Ectopic pregnancy
- Splenic rupture
- Pericardial tamponade or myocarditis
- Aortic dissection

The biggest concern is shock. Exsanguination and infection are the most immediate sequelae of the possible causes just listed because hypovolemic or septic shock may occur quickly. Cardiogenic shock may also occur if severe pericarditis or myocarditis is the cause of the abdominal pain. In addition to the major threats to life, torsion of an ovary or testicle can threaten their viability and are considered emergencies requiring prompt intervention.

BEDSIDE

How Does the Patient Look?

Does the patient appear comfortable, uncomfortable, or severely ill?

An uncomfortable or severely ill patient should be examined immediately to look for signs of peritonitis. If peritonitis is suspected, empiric antibiotics, IV fluids, and immediate surgical evaluation are indicated. In general, patients with peritonitis appear uncomfortable and may prefer to lie motionless and avoid any movement of the peritoneum. A patient who has recently ruptured a viscus (e.g., a perforated appendix) may suddenly appear more comfortable because the obstruction has been relieved. The discomfort may also be intermittent, as in intussusception or renal colic, with episodic pain being punctuated by periods of relative comfort. An infant or a child who has been receiving narcotics or steroids may appear deceptively comfortable despite a significant intra-abdominal pathologic condition, so it is important to obtain a medication history.

Airway and Vital Signs

Hypotension and tachycardia are signs that shock may be present, although tachycardia alone may be present due to fever, pain, or anemia. Fever and abdominal pain should raise suspicion regarding infectious causes, which could be relatively mild (gastroenteritis) or life threatening (peritonitis). Tachypnea suggests pneumonia or an attempt to compensate for a metabolic acidosis associated with diabetic ketoacidosis, shock, or ischemic bowel. If a patient has abdominal pain and is tachypneic with shallow respirations, they may be splinting due to pain.

Selective History

When gathering information about pain in any location, including the abdomen, precise characterization of the pain is essential.

Duration: How long has the pain been present?

If the pain has been ongoing for several days, it is most likely not an intra-abdominal emergency. Acute onset or sudden worsening of chronic pain is concerning and warrants immediate evaluation.

Location: Where is the pain? Does it radiate? Has it changed location?

As noted earlier, the location of the pain may help to narrow the diagnostic possibilities. Pain moving from the umbilicus to the right lower quadrant is strongly suggestive of appendicitis. Pain radiating to the shoulder suggests pericarditis or irritation of the diaphragm, as with a subphrenic abscess, perforated ulcer, or hepatobiliary pathology including (Fitz-Hugh–Curtis syndrome or biliary colic). Pain radiating to the back may occur with aortic dissection or pancreatitis. Pain with radiation to the groin suggests ureteral irritation, as with renal stones. In young children, the response to "Where does it hurt?" invariably involves pointing directly to the umbilicus and therefore may be less reliable than in older patients.

Character: Is the pain aching, burning, crushing, or sharp? Is it constant or intermittent? Does it vary in intensity? What makes it feel better? Worse?

Esophagitis, gastritis, or peptic ulcers may often be described as burning. Aching pain generally indicates a more diffuse or distant cause (e.g., pneumonia, porphyria), whereas sharp pain tends to be indicative of a more localized process. Biliary or renal colic and intussusception may cause severe but intermittent pain. If walking or moving seems to provide relief, peritonitis is much less likely.

Associated symptoms: Does the child have any related symptoms?

If diarrhea is present, infectious causes need to be considered further. In children, vomiting may occur with any intra-abdominal process but should raise suspicion of infection or bowel obstruction. Hematemesis is strongly suggestive of gastritis, esophagitis, or an ulcer. Bilious or feculent emesis implies bowel obstruction. Melanotic stools are suggestive of bleeding in the upper GI tract. Hematochezia indicates bleeding in the lower GI tract, whereas streaks of blood on the stool may indicate constipation. Pharyngitis, coughing, rashes, headache, fever, and other systemic symptoms may likewise help with the differential diagnosis. If the child has been eating normally and appears well, the likelihood of a significant problem is very small.

Selective Physical Examination

Vital signs	Hypotension may ensue rapidly; therefore repeating blood pressure and other vital sign measurements is a good idea. Remember that in infants and young children, tachycardia alone may be indicative of shock. By increasing the heart rate, cardiac output can be enhanced enough to maintain "normal" blood pressure; hypotension may not occur until relatively late in the course of septic or hypovolemic shock.
HEENT*	Scleral icterus (suggestive of hyperbilirubinemia and possible liver disease), pharyngeal erythema or exudate (streptococcal infection, infectious mononucleosis), periorbital edema (angioedema).
Neck	Adenopathy (streptococcal pharyngitis, mononucleosis), jugular venous distention (cardiac tamponade).

HEENT, Head, Eyes, Ears, Nose, and Throat.

Chest	Rales, wheezes, decreased breath sounds (pneumonia, congestive heart failure [CHF] from myocarditis, pericarditis).
Heart	Muffled or distant heart sounds (pericardial effusion), friction rub (pericarditis).
Abdomen	1. Observe. Protuberance may be a sign of bowel obstruction, ascites, or an intra-abdominal mass (intussusception, hernia).
	2. Auscultate. The purpose of auscultation is twofold. You can begin to listen to the abdomen but also lightly palpate simultaneously. The absence of bowel sounds is consistent with ileus (which may occur with any condition). High-pitched bowel sounds are associated with obstruction, and hyperactive bowel sounds may be appreciated with gastrointestinal infection.
	3. Palpate. Rigidity, rebound tenderness, and guarding all suggest peritonitis. Localized tenderness may be present even if the pain is described as generalized. A fluid wave may be appreciated if ascites is present. Cautiously palpate the liver and spleen because an enlarged spleen may be more easily ruptured.
	4. Percuss. Evaluate the size of the liver. Shifting dullness is indicative of ascites.
Rectal	Tenderness (appendicitis, pelvic inflammatory disease), impacted stool (constipation), positive occult blood test result (gastritis, bleeding peptic ulcer, ischemic bowel, Meckel diverticulum, inflammatory bowel disease, intussusception, vasculitis). Note: A patient with abdominal pain has not been fully evaluated without a rectal examination!
Genitourinary	All adolescent girls should undergo a pelvic examination for any unexplained abdominal pain (pelvic inflammatory disease, ectopic pregnancy); prepubescent and pubescent boys should undergo testicular examination (torsion, edema associated with vasculitis).
Skin	Rashes (vasculitis, lupus, systemic juvenile idiopathic arthritis, scarlet fever), Cullen sign (purpuric discoloration of the skin of the abdomen seen in hemorrhagic pancreatitis), hyperpigmentation (adrenal insufficiency).

| Extremities | Peripheral edema (CHF, renal disease, vasculitis), pulses and capillary refill (assess for potential shock). |
| Neurologic | Altered mental status (shock, toxin, porphyria, diabetic ketoacidosis). |

Selective Chart Review

After the history and physical examination, the cause of the abdominal pain may still be unclear. Selectively reviewing the medical record may provide useful information.

What medications is the patient taking?

Some medications are notorious for causing abdominal symptoms, and abdominal pain is listed as a potential side effect of nearly all drugs. Attributing pain to a medication may be reasonable but should be considered a diagnosis of exclusion. Steroids and nonsteroidal antiinflammatory medications may potentially cause gastritis, esophagitis, and peptic ulcer. Narcotics and other medications may induce constipation and thereby result in abdominal pain. Pancreatitis and hepatitis are also side effects of multiple medications. Remember that *Clostridium difficile* infection, colitis, and subsequent abdominal pain may develop in any patient who has been receiving antibiotics. Conversely, both narcotics and steroids can mask abdominal pain.

If the child is an adolescent girl, when was the last menstrual period? Is she sexually active?

Missed menses is suggestive of pregnancy, ectopic or intrauterine. Known sexual activity confirms the possibility of pelvic inflammatory disease.

Has the child complained of this type of pain before?

If the same pain has prompted several previous calls, the problem is much less likely to be an acute one requiring extensive evaluation and emergency management in the middle of the night. However, acute changes in chronic pain need to be evaluated. The child may have a significant problem causing the pain (lactose intolerance, inflammatory bowel disease), but further evaluation may be able to be deferred after life-threatening possibilities are excluded.

Management

At this point, either a specific diagnosis is evident or you will be able to shorten the list of potential causes. If the specific cause of the abdominal pain remains questionable, you should at least be able to determine whether the patient (1) is critically ill and requires immediate intervention, (2) is in discomfort but has no evidence of an immediately life-threatening process, or (3) is only mildly uncomfortable and life-threatening processes can be excluded. If the patient is critically ill, you need to pursue management and additional diagnostic studies simultaneously. A patient who is stable but uncomfortable may require further diagnostic studies before appropriate management is begun. A mildly uncomfortable patient may not require any specific diagnostic tests or management at the moment and may often be managed expectantly.

Critically Ill Patients

A critically ill patient with abdominal pain usually has hypovolemic shock, septic shock, or a combination of both as a result of perforation, peritonitis, or exsanguination. Immediate management involves addressing the issues of shock and infection simultaneously and necessitates consultation with pediatric surgeons. Management should proceed as follows:

1. Volume

Immediate expansion of intravascular volume helps to improve tissue perfusion. Normal saline or lactated Ringer's solution can be given as a 20-mL/kg IV bolus as fast as possible. Evaluate the response of the heart rate, capillary refill, and blood pressure and repeat if indicated. If cardiogenic shock is a possibility, volume expansion should be performed cautiously, assessing for signs of fluid overload including hepatomegaly, rales, and jugular venous distention (JVD) after each bolus administration. If the patient is known to be bleeding, whole blood can also be used to expand intravascular volume. If time does not permit cross matching, O-negative blood should be used.

2. Oxygenation

Oxygen should be administered and an arterial blood gas measurement obtained to assess the adequacy of oxygenation and tissue perfusion.

3. Laboratory Studies

Additional laboratory tests include a complete blood count with differential, prothrombin time, partial thromboplastin time, blood culture, urinalysis, urine culture, human chorionic gonadotropin-β (HCG-β) if female, amylase, lipase, lactate dehydrogenase, blood gas, and electrolyte determinations, as well as blood for typing and cross matching. Additional labs are dictated by your differential diagnosis. If concerned about a renal etiology, add blood urea nitrogen (BUN) and creatinine. If the liver or biliary tract is concerning, aspartate transaminase (AST), alanine transaminase (ALT), γ-glutamyltransferase (GGT), and bilirubin would be appropriate.

4. Paracentesis

If sepsis is suspected and the patient has ascites, diagnostic para-centesis should be performed and the fluid cultured to evaluate for bacterial peritonitis.

5. Antibiotics

After cultures are obtained, broad-spectrum antibiotics should be started immediately to empirically treat gut anaerobes, as well as gram-positive and gram-negative pathogens (the combination of ampicillin, gentamicin, and metronidazole is one possible choice).

6. Radiography

Radiographic studies need to be performed with a portable machine at the patient's bedside and should include anteroposterior (AP) views of the abdomen, supine and erect if possible. If the patient is an infant, a cross-table lateral view allows the detection of free air in the peritoneum. A patient who cannot stand should have a lateral decubitus view. An AP view of the chest should also be obtained to evaluate the lung fields (the potential exists for acute respiratory distress syndrome, pneumonia) and heart size (to exclude pericardial effusion, myocarditis, CHF) and to look for free air under the diaphragm indicating perforation. Air-fluid levels suggest bowel obstruction or ileus. A "sentinel" loop suggests pancreatitis. Lead may be seen as radiopaque "chips" throughout the bowel. Constipation should be fairly obvious, as should an intra-abdominal mass. A fecalith in the right lower quadrant is suggestive of appendicitis.

7. Consultation

Surgical consultation is mandatory if a perforated viscus, splenic rupture, intra-abdominal abscess, aortic dissection, appendicitis, intussusception, volvulus, malrotation, psoas abscess, incarcerated hernia, ischemic bowel, Meckel diverticulum, tumor, or testicular torsion is suspected. Gynecologic consultation may be necessary if ovarian torsion, pelvic abscess, or ectopic pregnancy is suspected.

8. Vasopressors

If fluid resuscitation alone does not improve the signs of shock, vasopressors may be necessary (see Chapter 25, Hypotension and Shock).

9. Pain Control

Once the initial work-up is underway, pain control is paramount. IV opioid medications including morphine or hydromorphone should be given and patient or nurse-controlled analgesia should be considered if the cause of pain is determined to be ongoing, such as in the case of pancreatitis or renal or biliary colic. Consideration should be taken of the constipating nature of these medications.

Patients Who Are Uncomfortable but Do Not Have Cardiorespiratory Compromise

If the patient is not in shock, additional evaluation may proceed before any specific intervention is made. However, one should remain alert for the possibility that the patient may suddenly become critically ill (e.g., if ischemic bowel progresses to a perforated bowel or if intussusception progresses to ischemia and necrosis). Laboratory studies and radiographs as outlined for critically ill patients may be helpful diagnostically. If gastroenteritis is a consideration, stool may be tested for rotavirus, *Salmonella, Shigella, Yersinia,* and *Escherichia coli,* and if the patient has been taking antibiotics, *C. difficile* toxin. If laboratory testing and initial radiographs do not lead to a diagnosis, consideration may be given to performing abdominal or pelvic ultrasound studies (to exclude an abscess, tumor, ovarian or testicular torsion, ectopic pregnancy, urolithiasis, intussusception), computed tomography (CT) of the abdomen and pelvis (abscess, tumor, appendicitis), angiography (mesenteric thrombosis or vasculitis), or a Meckel scan. Whether these tests are performed immediately or not depends on clinical suspicion and the potential for morbidity if the diagnosis is delayed. If significant abdominal pain persists, the patient should remain NPO with IV hydration at a maintenance rate until the cause is found. Further management depends on the diagnosis.

Patients With Mild Discomfort

In some cases a patient with mild discomfort may need additional studies immediately to exclude the possibility of bacterial infection or a surgical abdomen. Laboratory studies and radiographs, as outlined earlier, may provide additional evidence of infection (dramatic increase in the white blood cell count with a left shift) or a surgical abdomen (free air), or they may help to exclude these possibilities. However, not every patient requires further study beyond a history and physical examination. If a potentially serious cause of the abdominal pain is unlikely, expectant management is reasonable, provided that the patient is observed and examined frequently. If the patient wants to eat, maintenance of NPO status is usually unnecessary. Acetaminophen, 10–15 mg/kg every 4 to 6 hours, or a hot pack may be used to alleviate pain. Tramadol may be considered if pain is not alleviated with initial measures.

CHAPTER 7

Altered Mental Status

Michael Girolami, MD

Altered mental status (AMS) may be defined as a change in consciousness. Almost any pathologic process involving the central nervous system (CNS) may cause AMS. Changes that may be caused by these processes include irritability, lethargy, syncope, seizures, and unresponsiveness. Immediately recognizing that there has been a change in mental status is initially more important than defining the exact type of alteration. The history of how the patient's mental status has changed and the physical examination will help narrow the list of diagnostic possibilities and guide the initial approach to management. This chapter discusses the evaluation and management of children in whom irritability, lethargy, syncope, delirium, or coma develop while in the hospital. Delirium is defined as an acute change in attention, awareness, and cognition and is usually manifested as inappropriate speech or bizarre behavior. Lethargy implies profound fatigue and lack of interest in any activity or conversation. If the lethargy is severe, the term *obtundation* is sometimes used. Typically a lethargic child can be awakened but then will return to a state of slumber. Stupor refers to a state characterized by lapses of consciousness. A stuporous child can only be awakened by repeated stimuli. Finally, coma is a state of profound unconsciousness. Irritability in an infant (see Chapter 12) and seizures (see Chapter 29) are discussed elsewhere.

PHONE CALL

Questions

1. How old is the patient?
2. What is the patient's reason for admission?
3. What are the patient's vital signs?
4. How is the child breathing? Is the airway compromised?
5. How is the child behaving? Was there a brief period of unresponsiveness suggesting seizure or syncope?

6. Has this occurred in the past? What is the child's baseline mental status?
7. Were any new medications started, or stopped recently? When was the last time any narcotics were given?

The patient's reason for admission is vitally important because it can help to acutely determine the etiology of the AMS. Assessment of vital sign trends, respiratory pattern, and current behavior help to determine whether the change in mental status is associated with a critical ongoing process, such as increased intracranial pressure (ICP), or a self-limited event, such as a seizure or syncope. If the airway is compromised, plans should be made to intubate the child immediately. The responses to these questions also help to differentiate between the various types of alterations in mental status. If this was only a brief episode and mental status is improving, an "event" may have occurred that does not require immediate treatment. However, if mental status remains altered, an ongoing process should be considered and management started immediately. For example, if the Cushing triad of systolic hypertension (widening pulse pressure), bradycardia, and irregular respirations is present, increased ICP should be suspected and management begun immediately. If the child has a history of similar events, this may help to direct your initial thoughts regarding the cause of the change in mental status. Defining the child's baseline mental status and history of previous alterations in mental status helps to clarify the significance of the current change. Review of the patient's medications can also be very helpful. New medications, missed doses, and pain medications may all cause acute changes in a patient's mental status.

Orders

1. Immediate blood glucose should be checked. If hypoglycemia is present (<40 mg/dL), give intravenous (IV) bolus of 2.5 mL/kg of 10% dextrose (D10) in infants or children up to 12 years of age; if older than 12 years, give 1 mL/kg of 25% dextrose (D25), or 0.5 mL/kg of 50% dextrose (D50). If there is no IV access, glucagon 0.03 mg/kg intramuscularly (IM) or subcutaneously (SQ; max 1 mg) may be administered. Keep in mind, hyperglycemia may also be associated with AMS, as in diabetic ketoacidosis.
2. Continuous pulse oximetry should be ordered if the patient has abnormal respirations or a cardiac or respiratory illness.
3. If vital signs changes indicate increased ICP or the airway appears to be compromised, preparation should be made for intubation.

4. If the history is suspicious for syncope, an electrocardiogram (ECG) should be performed at the bedside to evaluate for cardiac dysrhythmia. One should also consider continuous cardiac or telemetry monitoring.

5. An intravenous (IV) line should be placed in patients with delirium, obtundation, stupor, or coma. If an IV line is to be placed, you may ask the nurse to draw off some blood in anticipation of the need for laboratory studies. A complete blood count (CBC), basic metabolic panel (BMP), magnesium, and phosphate should be obtained, and, depending on the clinical history, other labs may need to be considered.

Inform RN

Acute AMS always requires immediate evaluation and may require immediate treatment. It is critical that the etiology be determined as soon as possible so that appropriate management can be initiated.

ELEVATOR THOUGHTS

As previously mentioned, AMS may have multiple etiologies. It may be due to systemic infection or disorder, metabolic disturbances, or a primary intracranial process. In young children, almost any illness can lead to irritability or lethargy. Therefore, in this population, it is important to also consider illnesses localized to organ systems other than the CNS. If consciousness is impaired, the process must be affecting both cerebral hemispheres or the brain stem. The mnemonic AEIOU TIPS (Table 7.1) covers most of the etiologies of AMS. A more detailed list of potential causes:

Intracranial Processes	Infection (meningitis, encephalitis, abscess)
	Hemorrhage (subarachnoid, subdural, epidural parenchymal) secondary to aneurysm, trauma (including shaken baby syndrome), coagulopathy, or arteriovenous malformation
	Tumor
	Concussion secondary to head trauma
	Cerebral edema secondary to trauma
	Cerebral thrombosis
	Cerebral vasculitis
	Cerebritis
	Psychosis
	Hydrocephalus
	Seizure disorder
	Acute confusional migraine ("Alice in Wonderland" syndrome)
	Acute disseminated encephalomyelitis
	Autoimmune encephalitis

Metabolic disturbances	Diabetic ketoacidosis
	Hyperammonemia (e.g., Reye syndrome, urea cycle disorders, liver disease)
	Hypoglycemia
	Hyponatremia, hypernatremia
	Hypocalcemia, hypercalcemia
	Hypokalemia
	Hypoxemia (e.g., carbon monoxide poisoning, cardiac failure, respiratory failure)
	Drugs and toxins (e.g., narcotics, lead, barbiturates, alcohol, salicylates, acetaminophen)
	Mitochondrial encephalomyopathies (e.g., Leigh disease, Zellweger syndrome)
Systemic illnesses	Hypothyroidism, hyperthyroidism
	Uremia (e.g., hemolytic-uremic syndrome)
	Addison disease
	Congestive heart failure
	Cardiac dysrhythmia
	Pulmonary failure
	Hypertension with encephalopathy
	Heat stroke
	Shock (distributive, obstructive, hypovolemic, cardiogenic, or combined)
	Fever
	Human immunodeficiency virus encephalopathy
	Systemic lupus erythematosus with cerebritis
	Malnutrition (with thiamine deficiency)
	Thrombotic thrombocytopenic purpura
	Burn encephalopathy
	"Hospital" or "intensive care unit" encephalopathy
	Posterior reversible encephalopathy syndrome (PRES)

In children and adolescents whose history is consistent with syncope, the following should also be considered:
Vasovagal episode
Cardiac conduction disturbance (heart block)
Dysrhythmia (e.g., supraventricular tachycardia, long QT syndrome)
Narcolepsy
Cough syncope
Severe anemia
Breath-holding
Hyperventilation
Cervical vertebral anomalies

TABLE 7.1	Differential of Altered Mental Status

A	Alcohol, Abuse
E	Epilepsy, Encephalopathy, Electrolytes, Endocrine
I	Ingestion, Insulin, Intussusception, Inadequate Fluid
O	Overdose, Occult Trauma, Obstructed ventriculoperitoneal (VP) shunt, Oxygen Deficiency
U	Uremia
T	Trauma, Temperature Abnormality, Tumor
I	Infection
P	Poisonings, Psychiatric, Postictal
S	Shock, Stroke, Space Occupying Lesion (Intracranial)

MAJOR THREAT TO LIFE

- CNS infection
- Intracranial hemorrhage
- Increased ICP
- Metabolic disturbance
- Shock
- Dysrhythmia
- Organ failure (e.g., heart, lung, liver, or kidney)
- Status epilepticus
- Aspiration resulting from an inability to protect the airway

The most worrisome etiologies in the acute phase include infection, hemorrhage, and mass lesions leading to increased ICP and possible herniation. Other etiologies with high morbidity and potential mortality include metabolic disturbances, shock, dysrhythmias, and organ failure. Status epilepticus may also have substantial deleterious effects on the CNS. Regardless of the underlying cause, a stuporous, obtunded, or comatose patient may not be able to protect their airway and is therefore at greater risk for aspiration.

BEDSIDE

Quick-Look Test

Is the patient currently alert, comfortable, and oriented (suggesting an episodic event, e.g., a self-limited seizure or syncope), or is the patient actively seizing, unconscious, lethargic, irritable, combative, or sleepy (suggesting an ongoing process)?

The latter patient needs an immediate focused exam with attention to signs that would suggest increased ICP, shock, infection, brain herniation, or a combination of these conditions. If the patient is actively seizing, management to control the seizure should begin simultaneously with further examination (see Chapter 29). Isolated irritability is present in many hospitalized children and, in the absence of other abnormal neurologic findings, is not necessarily an indicator of CNS pathology. However, keep in mind that mental status may change rapidly and a child who is irritable may progress to stupor, obtundation, or coma and should be closely monitored.

Airway and Vital Signs

Can the child protect his or her airway? (Are cough and gag reflexes present?)

If the answer is no, the child should be intubated as soon as possible.

A full set of vital signs should be evaluated, with particular attention paid to signs of infection or increased ICP—two of the major threats to life. Fever should raise the suspicion of CNS infection, certain toxins, or septic shock. Although the absence of fever makes infection less likely, patients with brain abscesses are not necessarily febrile. Cushing triad is an ominous finding that occurs as a **late** sign of significantly increased ICP and suggests impending herniation. Normal vital signs may be present in a patient in whom increased ICP is developing. Management should begin immediately if Cushing triad is present.

Hypertension may also be the cause (rather than the result) of an encephalopathy, usually associated with renal disease. Hypotension implies shock (distributive, obstructive, hypovolemic, cardiogenic, or combined) and also requires immediate management (see Chapter 25). Tachycardia may be present in several etiologies, including sepsis and hyperthyroidism, but may be an early finding in shock. Keep in mind, heart rates greater than 220 beats per minute (BPM) in infants and 180 BPM in older children are suggestive of supraventricular tachycardia. Tachypnea may reflect pulmonary disease, pain, intoxication/ingestion, or compensation for acidosis, as in diabetic ketoacidosis.

Focused Physical Examination I

After the quick-look test and a check of vital signs, an initial focused physical examination should be performed with the goal of determining the likelihood of increased ICP, impending brain herniation, or CNS infection (meningitis, encephalitis, or abscess) because immediate management is necessary if any of these conditions is suspected.

Head	Bruising over the mastoid (Battle sign), "raccoon eyes," or depressions or deformity of the skull (all indicators of significant head trauma); bulging or sunken fontanelle
Eyes	Pupil size and reactivity to light. A single dilated, unreactive pupil may indicate herniation of the ipsilateral temporal lobe. Bilateral dilatation is associated with a postictal state and certain drugs (e.g., atropine, cocaine, mydriatic agents). The pupillary reflex is typically intact in medical causes of AMS; however, if there is a structural CNS insult, one would expect the pupils to be unequal, sluggish, or unreactive.
	Fundi retinal hemorrhage is associated with trauma. Papilledema suggests increased ICP (Fig. 7.1)
	Extraocular movements. Third nerve palsy (dilated pupil, lateral and inferior displacement of the eye, ptosis) may be associated with temporal lobe herniation. Sixth nerve palsy (absence of lateral movement) may be associated with increased ICP and may be unilateral or bilateral
Ears	Hemotympanum or blood in the external canal (head trauma)
Nose	Cerebrospinal fluid rhinorrhea (trauma)
Neck	Nuchal rigidity (meningitis), Kernig and Brudzinski signs (meningitis)
Chest	Respiratory pattern (Table 7.2) (may indicate herniation)
Cardiac	Bradycardia (increased ICP), extreme tachycardia, or abnormal rhythm
Extremities	Posturing (see Table 7.2) (may indicate herniation)
Neurologic	Level of consciousness, orientation, focality, Glasgow Coma Scale score (asymmetry in muscle tone, strength, spontaneous movement, reflexes)

What is the Glasgow Coma Scale (GCS) (Table 7.3)? GCS is a 15-point neurologic scale used to record and describe the general level of consciousness in patients. A GCS score less than 8 is an indication that severe CNS abnormalities are present and the child is at risk for respiratory compromise. Intubation is indicated.

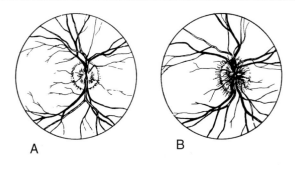

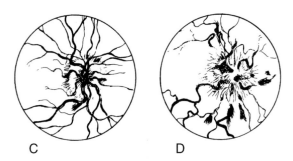

FIGURE 7.1 **Disk changes seen in papilledema. A,** Normal. **B,** Early papilledema. **C,** Moderate papilledema with early hemorrhage. **D,** Severe papilledema with extensive hemorrhage. (From Marshall SA, Ruedy J: On Call: Principles and protocols, ed 4, Philadelphia, 2004, Elsevier, p 123.)

Management I

Increased Intracranial Pressure

If elevated ICP is suspected, treatment must be initiated in an attempt to reduce the volume of the intracranial contents (i.e., brain, cerebrospinal fluid [CSF], and blood) and ensure adequate cerebral perfusion pressure (CPP). Mean arterial pressure (MAP) must be kept greater than ICP to maintain CPP (CPP = MAP − ICP). This is done by the following techniques:

1. Positioning. Elevate the head of the bed to 30 degrees. Maintain the head in the midline position. Do not elevate above 40 degrees because this can lead to decreased CPP.
2. Treat hypoxia, hypercarbia, and hypotension if present. Vasopressors may be necessary to maintain appropriate MAPs.

TABLE 7.2 Localization of Cerebral Dysfunction

Level of Hemispheres	Respiratory Pattern	Pupils	Vestibuloocular Reflex	Motor Response
Diencephalon	Regular or Cheyne-Stokes[a]	Small reactive	Present, normal	Localized noxious stimuli with nonparetic limb; later decorticate posturing
Midbrain-upper pons	Hyperventilation or Cheyne-Stokes	Mid position, fixed	Absent or abduction only	Decerebrate or no movement
Lower-pons to upper medulla	Ataxic	Mid position, fixed	Absent	Triple flexion response[b] or no movement
Medulla	Irregular or none	Mid position, fixed	Absent	Absent

[a]Cheyne-Stokes breathing refers to alternating hyperpnea and apnea.
[b]Triple flexion reflex is flexion of the thigh, leg, and dorsiflexion of the foot upon noxious stimulation of the foot.
Modified from Plum F, Posner JB: The Diagnosis of Stupor and Coma III, Philadelphia, FA Davis, 1995, p 103.

TABLE 7.3	Modified Glasgow Coma Scale

Score	Eyes Opening		
	>1 Year Old		<1 Year Old
4	Spontaneously		Spontaneously
3	To verbal command		To shout
2	To pain		To pain
1	No response		No response
Best Motor Response			
6	Obeys		Spontaneous
5	Localizes pain		Localizes pain
4	Flexion: withdrawal		Flexion: withdrawal
3	Flexion: abnormal (decorticate rigidity)		Flexion: abnormal (decorticate rigidity)
2	Extension (decerebrate rigidity)		Extension (decerebrate rigidity)
1	No response		No response
Best Verbal Response			
	>5 Years Old	2-5 Years Old	0-23 Months Old
5	Oriented	Appropriate words and phrases	Smiles, coos appropriately
4	Disoriented	Inappropriate words	Cries, consolable
3	Inappropriate words	Persistent cries	Persistent, inappropriate cries
2	Incomprehensible	Grunts	Grunts, agitated, or restless
1	No response	No response	No response

3. Osmotherapy. Increasing serum osmolarity to 300 to 320 mOsm/L may establish a gradient that allows brain water to be drawn into the circulation. Mannitol 0.25 to 1.0 g/kg can be given over 20 to 30 minutes; it can be given every 4 hours, and serum osmolality should be monitored with each dose. Typically a patient given mannitol should also have a urinary catheter because it will cause significant diuresis. Three percent saline, 5 mL/kg bolus, may also be given and may be repeated hourly until serum Na reaches 160 mEq/L. After this threshold is reached, there is typically minimal additional effect on ICP. Mannitol is usually preferred over 3% saline because mannitol lowers ICP more rapidly.

4. Hyperventilation. This method reduces blood flow to the brain and is the quickest way to decrease ICP; however, it also may reduce cerebral blood flow enough to cause cerebral ischemia

and therefore is reserved for acute situations. If the patient is intubated, they may be ventilated with the goal of keeping the arterial partial pressure of CO_2 between 30 and 35 mm Hg. One should ventilate only below 30 mm Hg if there are signs of acute herniation.

After these steps have been performed, computed tomography (CT) should be performed to help confirm the presence of a mass lesion, hemorrhage, or cerebral edema as a potential cause of the increased ICP. Neurosurgical consultation may be helpful because surgery and/or an ICP monitor may be necessary to further manage the increased ICP.

Infection

If meningitis, abscess, or encephalitis is suspected, further evaluation should be expedited and empiric treatment begun as quickly as possible. Ideally, blood and CSF cultures should be obtained before the administration of antibiotics. However, in a critically ill child, there should be no more than a 15-minute delay in the administration of antibiotics for suspected meningitis. If suspicion of increased ICP necessitates a CT scan before lumbar puncture, blood cultures should be drawn, the antibiotics should be administered immediately after, and the lumbar puncture performed after the CT scan. An opening pressure should be obtained during the lumbar puncture because high pressure is suggestive of bacterial meningitis. IV ceftriaxone (200 mg/kg/day, max 4 g/day divided every 12 hours) and IV vancomycin (60 mg/kg/day divided every 6 hours) are the empiric treatments of choice for suspected bacterial meningitis. The administration of dexamethasone (0.15 mg/kg) should be individualized. Studies have not shown that dexamethasone improves mortality or survival; however, there has been evidence that it decreases hearing loss in patients with *Haemophilus influenzae* meningitis. In geographic areas that are endemic for Rocky Mountain spotted fever, the addition of IV doxycycline may be considered. The presence of focal abnormalities on physical examination, hemorrhagic CSF, or associated focal seizures should raise suspicion of herpes encephalitis, and empiric treatment with acyclovir (30 to 45 mg/kg per day divided every 8 hours) is then indicated.

Selective Physical Examination II

If the patient has no signs of significant cardiorespiratory compromise, there is no evidence of increased ICP or CNS infection, and the patient is not actively seizing, a more detailed physical examination can be performed before further evaluation and management. The goal should be to identify findings that can help to narrow the list of diagnostic possibilities.

HEENT[*]	Intracranial bruits (arteriovenous malformations), periorbital edema (anaphylaxis), or mastoid edema and erythema (cellulitis); perioral cyanosis (hypoxemia), fruity breath (diabetic ketoacidosis)
Neck	Jugular venous pulsations (congestive heart failure), goiter (thyroid disease)
Chest	Rales, intercostal retractions, tachypnea (respiratory failure, pneumonitis)
Cardiac	Murmurs, friction rub, muffled heart sounds (endocarditis, pericarditis, pericardial effusion)
Abdomen	Hepatomegaly (liver disease, congestive heart failure), splenomegaly (portal hypertension)
Extremities	Paresis, paralysis, arthritis (systemic lupus erythematosus, vasculitis), edema (congestive heart failure)
Skin	Palpable purpura (vasculitis), petechiae, ecchymoses (hemolytic-uremic syndrome, thrombotic thrombocytopenic purpura, coagulopathy, abuse), jaundice (liver disease, hemolytic diseases)
Neurologic	Responsiveness (see Table 7.3, Modified Glasgow Coma Scale); cranial nerves; doll's eyes reflex; muscle bulk, tone, and strength; reflexes (to evaluate the extent of and potentially localize a nervous system lesion); if possible in an adolescent, assessment of mood, affect, and thought processes (psychosis)

*HEENT, Head, eyes, ears, nose, throat.

Selective History and Chart Review

After the airway and vital signs have been stabilized, treatment of increased ICP or infection has been initiated if necessary, and the patient has been examined, further information should be obtained from the patient, family members, and the chart.

Is there a known history of trauma?

Keep in mind that a traumatic event may have occurred before hospitalization. Symptoms due to a subdural hematoma may occur well after the injury.

Are there any concerns for shaken baby syndrome?

Recall that infants may not have any external signs of injury.

Has the child been complaining of headaches? Nausea or vomiting? Visual disturbances?

Symptoms of increased ICP that have been present for some time suggest a mass lesion such as tumor or abscess.

Has the child had any recent infections?

A recent infection raises the suspicion of encephalitis, meningitis, or abscess.

Does the child have any underlying illnesses that may affect the CNS? Have there been any symptoms to suggest a systemic illness that might be affecting the CNS?

Diabetes; chronic pulmonary, cardiac, renal, or liver disease; HIV infection; and lupus are examples of underlying conditions that may affect the CNS. Approximately 25% of diabetic children are diagnosed with diabetes upon presentation with ketoacidosis.

What medication is the child receiving? Do any of these medications have CNS effects? What medications are other family members taking (ask this to elicit what medications may be available to the child)? In an adolescent, is there a history of drug or alcohol use?

Accidental or intentional overdosing of numerous medications may alter mental status. In addition, secondary metabolic effects from medications, such as hypoglycemia or hypokalemia, may be contributing to the AMS.

Is there a family history of migraine or psychosis? Has the child been acting depressed or abnormal lately?

Acute confusional migraine or psychosis may begin suddenly but should be considered after the more life-threatening possibilities have been ruled out. In addition, keep in mind that a psychotic or depressed child is at increased risk for toxic ingestion.

If known, what was happening at the time of and prior to the event? Did the child feel anxious, flushed, nervous, or sweaty? Is there a family history of heart disease or premature death? Did the child feel palpitations?

Such symptoms suggest vasovagal syncope. A family history of early death raises the suspicion of long QT syndrome or cardiomyopathy. Palpitations also increase suspicion for a dysrhythmia.

Management II

Nearly all children and adolescents who have had an alteration in mental status require additional laboratory or radiographic evaluation. The exceptions to this generalization include young children who are irritable but consolable, have normal neurologic examination findings, and have been hospitalized for an illness that might be expected to cause some irritability. Such children may be observed as their illness is being treated, with the expectation that the irritability will resolve as they are feeling better. However, if there is suspicion of CNS pathology, additional evaluation is warranted.

The following tests should be performed in patients in whom syncope has been excluded and the cause of the AMS remains unclear:

1. CBC and differential (infection, anemia, thrombocytopenia)
2. Electrolytes, glucose, calcium, ammonia
3. Blood and urine toxicology screen
4. Head CT or magnetic resonance imaging (mass lesion). (CT is preferred in the acute phase.)
5. Lumbar puncture with an opening pressure. (Unless there are signs of increased ICP, focal neurologic findings, risk of cardio-respiratory compromise, or a skin/soft tissue infection overlying the site of the lumbar puncture.)

Additional blood and CSF should be collected and saved because further studies (e.g., autoantibodies) may be necessary if the diagnosis remains unclear.

The following tests may be helpful if some evidence suggests a specific illness:

1. Hepatic transaminases, blood urea nitrogen, creatinine, urinalysis (liver or renal disease)
2. Arterial blood gas (hypoxemia, hypercapnia)
3. Chest radiographs (cardiac or pulmonary failure)
4. Peripheral blood smear, prothrombin time, partial thromboplastin time (microangiopathy, coagulopathy)

If the alteration in mental status is thought to be consistent with syncope or if cardiac failure with decreased cerebral perfusion is suspected, an ECG should be obtained. In addition, a patient should be placed on telemetry monitoring because an ECG may not capture the inciting rhythm.

Additional diagnostic evaluation such as thyroid studies, cerebral angiograms, electroencephalograms, echocardiograms, antinuclear antibody studies, and other tests aimed at excluding specific diseases should be considered for individual patients. Similarly, further evaluation of a patient with syncope, such as electroencephalographic studies or tilt table testing, may need to be scheduled the next day. In most cases the cause of the AMS is apparent after the history, physical examination, and laboratory evaluation, as outlined earlier. At a minimum, the major threats to life are considered, and if necessary, the child is receiving treatment aimed at reducing increased ICP or resolving a possible CNS infection. Definitive treatment depends on the cause of the AMS.

Infection

As outlined previously, suspected bacterial meningitis is treated with antibiotics. IV ceftriaxone and vancomycin are a good choice of initial empiric therapy beyond the neonatal period because it is effective against the most common pathogens: *Streptococcus pneumoniae* (including penicillin- and cephalosporin-resistant strains) and *Neisseria meningitidis*. Brain abscess may be caused by a large group of aerobic and anaerobic bacteria, and therefore empiric treatment with appropriate broad-spectrum IV antibiotics is necessary. In addition, neurosurgical consultation is helpful because most children require excision or drainage of the abscess. Encephalitis should be treated empirically with acyclovir if herpes infection is suspected.

Mass Lesion

Intracerebral hemorrhage or tumor requires surgical evacuation or resection, and a neurosurgeon should be consulted promptly. Any alteration in mental status associated with trauma is also an indication for neurosurgical consultation.

Metabolic Disturbance

Diabetic ketoacidosis should be managed with insulin, hydration, and correction of associated electrolyte abnormalities. Likewise, other electrolyte disturbances should be corrected. Inborn errors of metabolism (particularly partial/incomplete forms) can occur at any age and require prompt evaluation and possible consultation with a geneticist to ascertain the cause and begin emergency therapy (i.e., reducing the serum ammonia level in patients with urea cycle defects).

Drugs and Toxins

If overdose is suspected, treatment should be directed at decontamination and supportive therapy. Treatment of ingestions includes activated charcoal, diuresis, and specific antidotes, depending on the substance ingested. Dialysis or exchange transfusion is reserved for the most severe cases.

Psychosis

A psychotic child should be managed in consultation with psychiatrists. Chlorpromazine, haloperidol, or diazepam may be considered in an extremely agitated or violent child.

Systemic illnesses such as liver or renal disease, thyroid disease, lupus, or vasculitis should be managed appropriately while keeping in mind that associated increased ICP may also need to be treated.

Analgesics and Antipyretics

Danielle DuMez, MD

Analgesics and antipyretics are two classes of medications that are among the most commonly prescribed in hospitalized pediatric patients. Although writing orders for these medications can become very routine, it is important to remember that like all medications, these drugs are to be prescribed with careful thought and attention to detail. When asked to write an order for analgesics and/or antipyretics, it is important that you (1) determine the need for the medication, (2) understand why the child needs these medications, and (3) realize the potential consequences of using these medications in the individual patient, including adverse effects, as well as the effect that limiting pain and/or fever will have on your ability to accurately evaluate a patient's status.

Analgesics

PHONE CALL

Questions

1. Why is an analgesic being requested?
2. Where is the pain?
3. How severe is the pain?
4. Is this pain new?
5. What interventions have been tried thus far?
6. What is the child's admitting diagnosis?
7. How old is the child?
8. How much does the child weigh?
9. Does the child have any allergies?
10. Are there other symptoms in addition to the pain?

The answers to these questions should allow you to consider potential causes of the pain and understand the child's need for an analgesic, as well as the urgency of the situation.

In children, it is sometimes difficult to know whether the problem is truly one of pain. Parents, nurses, and physicians may assume that pain is present because a young child is crying or screaming. Temper tantrums, night terrors, nightmares, and/or fear may be the problem rather than pain. Similarly, pain may be the result of behavioral issues, depression, anxiety, or other psychogenic and psychosocial factors, in which case analgesics may be ineffective. It is important to consider these possibilities before immediately ordering medication.

If the child's diagnosis is unclear or if masking the pain will make it difficult to evaluate the child's status or make an accurate diagnosis (e.g., abdominal pain that may require surgery or joint pain that may be associated with rheumatic fever), you must carefully consider these factors before immediately prescribing an analgesic.

Orders

Table 8.1 lists selected analgesics and antipyretics. In most situations, acetaminophen is the best initial choice because it is well tolerated, it does not usually mask significant pain, and there are no concerns regarding dependency. Ibuprofen or another nonsteroidal antiinflammatory drug (NSAID) is generally the next best choice if acetaminophen is insufficient. However, in children with abdominal pain, liver disease, or renal disease, one needs to be aware of the potential for gastritis or, less commonly, hepatotoxicity or nephrotoxicity with these drugs. Because of their antiinflammatory effect, NSAIDs also have greater potential to mask symptoms and signs associated with disease.

Narcotics should not be ordered unless the cause of the pain is clearly understood and not until either (1) the child has already failed a trial of acetaminophen and NSAIDs or (2) acetaminophen and NSAIDs are contraindicated or felt to place the child at significant risk. Narcotics have greater potential for serious adverse events such as respiratory depression. They may alter mental status; their potency results in significant masking of signs and symptoms; and they may result in dependency.

Inform RN

"Will arrive at the bedside in …minutes to assess the patient."

Any child with a new need for analgesics should be evaluated. The urgency of this evaluation will depend on the severity of the pain and the potential for life-threatening causes of pain.

ELEVATOR THOUGHTS

If there is any doubt regarding the origin or cause of the pain, if the pain is a new complaint, if the character of the pain has changed, or

TABLE 8.1 Commonly Used Analgesics and Antipyretics

Generic Name	Brand Name	Dose	Max Dosing	Use of Drug
Acetaminophen	Tylenol	10-15 mg/kg PO q4-6 h	Max daily dose: 75 mg/kg/day or 4000 mg/day	Analgesic and antipyretic
Ibuprofen—Avoid in children less than 6 months old	Motrin or Advil	5-10 mg/kg PO q6-8 h	Max single dose: 400 mg Max daily dose: 40 mg/kg/day up to 1200 mg	Analgesic and antipyretic
Naproxen	Aleve	Analgesia: 5-7 mg/kg q8-12 h Antipyretic: 10-15 mg/kg/day PO divided twice a day	Max daily dose: 1000 mg/day	Mostly used for analgesia and antiinflammatory but also has antipyretic effects
Codeine[a]	—	0.5-1 mg/kg PO q4-6 h; Requires dose adjustment in renal impairment	Max single dose: 60 mg	Analgesic can be used in combination with acetaminophen: Tylenol No. 2 = 15 mg codeine + 300 mg acetaminophen; Tylenol No. 3 = 30 mg codeine + 300 mg acetaminophen; Tylenol No. 4 = 60 mg codeine + 300 mg acetaminophen
Oxycodone[a]	Oxycontin[a]	Less than 6 months old: 0.025-0.05 mg/kg PO q4-6 h Greater than 6 months old: 0.1-0.2 mg/kg PO q4-6 h	Max single dose: 10 mg if <50 kg & 20 mg if >50 kg	Analgesic can be used in combination with acetaminophen (Brand: Percocet)
Morphine[a]	—	Less than 6 months old: 0.08-0.1 mg/kg/dose PO q3-4 h or 0.025-0.03 mg/kg/dose IV or SQ q2-4 h Greater than 6 months old: 0.2-0.5 mg/kg PO q3-4 h 0.1-0.2 mg/kg IV, IM, or SQ q2-4 h	Max single PO dose: 15-20 mg; Max single IV/IM/SQ dose for infants greater than 6 months old: 2 mg dose; IV/IM/SQ dose for infants greater than 1 year old: 5-10 mg	Analgesic 10 mg of morphine = 100 mg meperidine Antidote = naloxone
Meperidine[a]—Use with caution in renal and liver failure patients	Demerol[a]	Infants less than 6 months: 0.5-0.75 mg/kg PO q3-4 h and 0.2-0.25 mg/kg and IM/IV/SQ q2-3 h; infants greater than 6 months: 2-3 mg/kg PO q3-4 h and 0.8-1 mg/kg IM/IV/SQ q2-3 h	Max single PO dose for infants less than 6 months old: refer to dose section; max single dose for infants greater than 6 months: 150 mg PO and 75 mg IM/IV/SQ	Analgesic Antidote = naloxone

[a]Narcotics are addictive and may cause respiratory distress; therefore, they should be used only for severe pain and when the cause of pain is understood.

if the pain is severe, you must evaluate the child at the bedside before ordering an analgesic.

Remember

1. It is easy to both overestimate and underestimate the severity of pain in pediatric patients. You need to make sure that you understand the cause of the pain as clearly as possible while making the patient as comfortable as possible. Overprescribing narcotics and other analgesics and withholding medication from a child in pain should both be avoided. The severity of pain can be assessed and monitored over time with a simple 0 to 10 scale for older children or with the Bieri faces scale (see Fig. 21.1) for younger children.

2. Escalating the potency of the analgesic you order without ree-valuating the patient should also be avoided. After ordering acetaminophen or an NSAID for a patient, if the nurse calls you several hours later to tell you the child is still in pain, you must see that patient before simply ordering a more potent analgesic, such as a narcotic.

3. When the cause of pain is poorly understood, you should not order analgesics as "PRN pain." You must instead be notified if the patient remains in pain and how severe it is. In this situation, ask the nurse to call you back in several hours if the child remains in pain.

4. When the cause of pain is clearly understood and there is an anticipated need for multiple doses of intravenous (IV) narcotic medication, patient-controlled analgesia (PCA) should be considered. PCA should be ordered after consultation with an anesthesiologist or other pain specialist.

5. Narcotic overdosage can be reversed with naloxone, 0.01 to 0.1 mg/kg per dose intramuscularly (IM), IV, or subcutaneously (SQ; maximum, 2 mg per dose). This dose can be repeated every 2 to 3 minutes as needed. Reversal may induce nausea and vomiting. Therefore, be prepared to protect the airway because the child is at risk for aspiration.

Antipyretics

PHONE CALL

Questions

1. How old is the child?
2. How high is the fever?
3. What is the child's admitting diagnosis?
4. How much does the child weigh?

5. Is the fever a new finding?
6. Any other associated symptoms?
7. When did the patient receive the last dose of an antipyretic?

Orders

See Table 8.1 for dosing of antipyretics.

Inform RN

"Will arrive at the bedside in … minutes to assess the patient."

Any child with a new fever must be evaluated (see Chapter 18) before ordering antipyretics.

Remember

1. Although you are ordering these medications for fever, they also have an analgesic effect, and therefore you need to consider this potential effect on your ability to evaluate the patient as described earlier under "Analgesics."
2. There is no longer any need to use aspirin as an antipyretic. Aspirin has been associated with Reye syndrome and therefore should be avoided. Acetaminophen and ibuprofen are alternatives that in general are better tolerated and entail less risk.
3. There are fewer concerns with the use of antipyretics in a patient in whom the diagnosis remains unclear. Decreasing the fever rarely results in difficulty arriving at a diagnosis, and it allows the child to be much more comfortable.
4. When fever is persistently high and unresponsive to acetaminophen alone, acetaminophen and ibuprofen may be ordered together (acetaminophen every 4 to 6 hours and ibuprofen every 6 hours). You may alternate acetaminophen and ibuprofen every 3 hours (therefore each is administered every 6 hours) to maximize benefit if needed.

CHAPTER 9

Bleeding

Laura Adams, MD

Bleeding may potentially occur at any anatomic location in a hospitalized child. When evaluating a patient who has bled or is bleeding, the goals are simple: (1) stop the active bleeding, and (2) prevent further bleeding. How one achieves these goals depends on the answer to a basic question: "Is the bleeding secondary to an anatomically localized problem (e.g., trauma), or is it secondary to a generalized bleeding disorder (coagulopathy)?" Coagulopathies are further discussed in detail in Chapter 33. Epistaxis, hemoptysis, hematemesis, melena, hematochezia, rectal bleeding, hemarthrosis, and hematuria are terms used to describe bleeding from various locations. In addition, bleeding into the skin and soft tissues may produce ecchymoses, petechiae, or purpura. This chapter discusses bleeding that does not involve the gastrointestinal or urinary tract. These subjects are addressed in detail in Chapter 19 and Chapter 23.

PHONE CALL

Questions

1. What are the child's vital signs?
2. Where is the bleeding?
3. What is the child's underlying illness and reason for hospitalization?
4. What medications is the child receiving?

The vital signs allow you to quickly determine whether the blood loss has been severe enough to result in depletion of intravascular volume. Tachycardia and/or hypotension might indicate such a state. If the child is febrile and has petechiae or purpura, one must immediately consider the possibility of sepsis with associated coagulopathy. The location of the bleeding allows you to develop a more specific differential diagnosis. In addition, the patient's underlying illness may give you clues regarding potential causes of the bleeding. Discovering that the patient is receiving a medication that might affect platelets or clotting factors is obviously of significance.

Orders

If the vital signs suggest shock, an intravenous (IV) bolus of either normal saline or lactated Ringer's solution should be given (10 to 20 mL/kg), and blood should be sent to the blood bank for typing and cross matching. If bleeding is massive, type O-negative whole blood (as well as plasma and platelets if a coagulopathy is suspected) should be ordered immediately. A complete blood count, prothrombin time (PT), and partial thromboplastin time (PTT) should also be ordered to determine the degree of anemia and the potential need to correct deficiencies in platelets or clotting factors.

If active bleeding is apparent from an accessible site (e.g., skin, external nares, or oral cavity), firm pressure should be applied and held.

If the child is receiving anticoagulating medications, his or her use should be suspended.

Inform RN

Active bleeding, abnormal vital signs, and fever with purpura and petechiae all require immediate attention. In the absence of these concerns, you should inform the RN when you will be at the bedside.

ELEVATOR THOUGHTS

Potential causes of bleeding depend on the site of the blood loss. The basic question of whether the bleeding reflects a localized problem or a systemic one should be kept in mind. Local trauma to a blood vessel or vessels is in general far more common than a coagulopathy, particularly with epistaxis and hemoptysis. Generalized petechiae or ecchymoses should make you consider a systemic coagulopathy more carefully. Potential causes are listed by anatomic site:

Epistaxis	Blunt trauma
	Self-inflicted trauma (picking)
	Nasal congestion, crusting
	Excessive sneezing
	Foreign body
	Hypertension
	Polyp
	Tumor (e.g., angiofibroma)
	Nasal hemangioma
	Congenital syphilis ("snuffles")
	Granulomatosis with polyangiitis

Hemoptysis	Aspiration of blood from the mouth and upper airway
	Foreign body
	Infection
	Tuberculosis
	Pneumonia
	Pneumonitis
	Lung abscess
	Bacterial tracheitis
	Cystic fibrosis
	Chest trauma
	Pulmonary vasculitis (systemic lupus erythematosis, granulomatosis with polyangiitis, eosinophilic granulomatosis with polyangiitis, Goodpasture syndrome)
	Pulmonary embolus
	Pulmonary hypertension
	Severe congestive heart failure
	Idiopathic pulmonary hemosiderosis
	Heiner syndrome
	Arteriovenous malformations
Petechiae, purpura, ecchymoses	Trauma (e.g., blood pressure cuff)
	Sepsis
	Septic emboli (endocarditis)
	Vasculitis (e.g., Henoch-Schönlein purpura)
	Viral infections
	Drugs (salicylates, steroids, nonsteroidal agents)
	Scurvy
Any site	Thrombocytopenia
	Decreased platelet production (e.g., marrow failure, leukemia)
	Increased platelet destruction (disseminated intravascular coagulopathy [DIC], idiopathic thrombocytopenic purpura [ITP], hemolytic-uremic syndrome [HUS], thrombotic thrombocytopenic purpura [TTP], splenic trapping)
	Abnormal platelet function (inherited defect, drugs, uremia)
	Clotting factor abnormality
	Hemophilia (factor VIII or IX deficiency)

Other factor deficiency (inherited or from liver disease)

Consumptive coagulopathy (DIC, cavernous hemangioma)

Von Willebrand disease

Vitamin K deficiency

MAJOR THREAT TO LIFE

- Exsanguination
- Hypoxia from pulmonary hemorrhage or embolism
- Sepsis
- Intracranial hemorrhage secondary to a clotting abnormality
- Severe systemic necrotizing vasculitis

Exsanguination is possible as long as bleeding remains active. Similarly, persistent or recurrent hemoptysis indicates active pulmonary bleeding and is dangerous. A febrile child with petechiae and/or purpura needs immediate evaluation and empiric treatment of presumed sepsis. Severe clotting defects should be corrected as quickly as possible because they may lead to secondary bleeding in other locations, including intracranially. Vasculitides are rare but must be considered and treated promptly because they may quickly lead to multiorgan failure.

BEDSIDE

Quick-Look Test

Is the patient comfortable, alert, and in no distress, without any evidence of active bleeding?

If so, your evaluation may proceed in a more relaxed manner without the need for immediate intervention. However, if the child is actively bleeding, has persistent hemoptysis (particularly if the vital signs are abnormal), or is febrile with petechiae or purpura, immediate intervention is necessary.

Airway and Vital Signs

A child with epistaxis or hemoptysis may rarely have such excessive bleeding that the airway becomes compromised. Labored respirations, cyanosis, tachypnea, grunting, and retractions of accessory muscles may all be signs that the airway is compromised. In many instances, simple suctioning and turning the child to the side to clear the airway of blood alleviate the problem. However, if the airway cannot be maintained in this manner, the child needs to be intubated. Tachycardia and/or hypotension is indicative of shock secondary to either hypovolemia or sepsis and requires immediate management (see Chapter 25). Hypertension may result in rupture of small intranasal blood vessels and can thus lead to epistaxis. Fever may be associated with infection or vasculitis. Fever with petechiae or purpura should be treated as sepsis (e.g., meningococcemia) until proven otherwise.

Selective Physical Examination I

After a quick look and check of the airway and vital signs, the child should be examined briefly to determine the likelihood of a major threat to life, in which case immediate intervention is necessary before obtaining more historical information and reviewing the chart. The goal of this initial selective examination is to search for signs that (1) bleeding remains active (usually obvious), (2) pulmonary bleeding or emboli are causing significant hypoxia and/or respiratory distress, (3) sepsis is a possibility, or (4) the child is also bleeding intra-abdominally or intracranially.

HEENT	Pupil size and reactivity, papilledema (intracranial bleeding with increased intracranial pressure [ICP]), persistent epistaxis, meningeal signs (sepsis with meningitis)
Chest	Grunting, retracting, breath sounds (respiratory distress); chest wall trauma
Abdomen	Distention, tenderness, bruising, rebound tenderness, rigidity
Skin	Petechiae, purpura (meningococcemia, vasculitis)
Neurologic	Alterations in consciousness, focality (intracranial bleeding)

HEENT, Head, Eyes, Ears, Nose, Throat.

Management I

After the quick look, check of the airway and vital signs, and brief examination, the next step is intervention. You may need to intervene quickly if the patient is actively bleeding or if you suspect pulmonary embolism, pulmonary hemorrhage, sepsis, or intracranial bleeding.

Active Bleeding

Bleeding from the nose, oral cavity, or mucocutaneous sites usually abates with the application of pressure. Pressure should be applied firmly for 5 minutes or longer while trying to avoid the temptation to frequently visualize the site of bleeding. With epistaxis, the child should be positioned on the side, gauze should be placed or packed within the nares, and pressure should be held over the bridge of the nose. Epistaxis most often occurs as a result of ruptured vessels in Kiesselbach plexus, an area of anastomosed arterioles just within the nares on the septum. If the bleeding remains active or is profuse, blood should be sent for a stat complete blood count, platelet count, prothrombin time (PT), partial prothrombin time (PTT), and typing and cross matching. While these tests are performed, pressure should continue to be applied.

If bleeding is massive and/or the child is in shock, type O-negative blood should be requested from the blood bank and transfused as soon as possible. A consultation to general surgery or otolaryngology (depending on the site of bleeding) should be made immediately to assess for the need for operative management.

Coagulopathies detected by laboratory testing should be corrected with appropriate blood products (platelets, fresh frozen plasma, or cryoprecipitate; see Chapter 33). If bleeding persists after correction of clotting abnormalities, surgical consultation should be considered.

Pulmonary Embolus

Pulmonary embolism is a rare childhood event that should be suspected in a child with hemoptysis who is tachypneic and hypoxic, although these signs are not invariably present. Pulse oximetry analysis or arterial blood gas determinations help to establish the degree of hypoxia. If the child has a known deep venous thrombosis or hypercoagulable state, suspicion should be high and anticoagulation with heparin considered while further evaluation is proceeding. Once the child's airway and vital signs are stabilized, a helical computed tomographic (CT) scan of the chest should be performed as soon as possible to determine the probability of an embolus. If the diagnosis remains uncertain, pulmonary angiography should be considered to definitively diagnose or exclude an embolus. After pulmonary embolism is diagnosed, anticoagulation is the treatment of choice. Large emboli may require surgical intervention.

Pulmonary Hemorrhage

Cystic fibrosis and vasculitides are conditions that may lead to acute pulmonary hemorrhage. With cystic fibrosis, persistent inflammation of the lung parenchyma may eventually lead to erosion into a major vessel and the sudden onset of massive pulmonary hemorrhage and hemoptysis. Emergency bronchoscopy, pulmonary angiography, and percutaneous catheter embolization of bronchial arteries may be necessary to localize and treat the involved vessels. If the patient has a history of systemic vasculitis or systemic lupus erythematosus or if such a diagnosis is being considered because of associated symptoms and physical findings, aggressive treatment of the underlying illness with corticosteroids and cytotoxic agents may be effective.

Sepsis

A child with fever and petechiae or purpura should be considered to have sepsis, and further evaluation and empiric treatment of sepsis should begin immediately. Blood, urine, and cerebrospinal fluid (if signs suggestive of meningitis are present) should be obtained and antibiotics administered as quickly as possible. If the child is critically ill, antibiotics should not be delayed while awaiting the performance of a lumbar puncture. Ceftriaxone, 50 mg/kg per dose every 12 hours empirically, covers pneumococcus, meningococcus, and *Haemophilus influenzae*. Vancomycin should be added if there are concerns regarding resistant organisms. In a child younger than 2 months, the combination of ampicillin and cefotaxime should be used to provide additional coverage of the potential neonatal pathogens *Listeria monocytogenes*, group B streptococcus, and *Escherichia coli*.

Intracranial Bleeding

If intracranial bleeding is suspected because of focal neurologic findings or altered mental status, immediate CT scanning and neurosurgical consultation are required. If signs of increased ICP are present, management should proceed as outlined in Chapter 7. Immediate measurement of the platelet count, PT, and PTT is necessary with appropriate correction of deficiencies (see Chapter 33, for guidelines regarding the administration of blood products).

Selective Physical Examination II

If the child is not actively bleeding and your suspicion of pulmonary hemorrhage, pulmonary embolism, sepsis, or intracranial bleeding is not high, you should proceed with a more detailed physical examination:

HEENT	Fundi (retinal hemorrhage), hemotympanum, nasal deformity ("saddle nose" of granulomatosis with polyangiitis), palatal petechiae, dental trauma
Neck	Adenopathy (infection, malignancy), Kernig and Brudzinski signs
Chest	Breath sounds, rales, external trauma, friction rub
Heart	Murmurs (endocarditis), friction rub
Abdomen	Bowel sounds, tenderness (vasculitis), hepatosplenomegaly (malignancy, DIC, ITP, liver disease, secondary coagulopathy), rectal examination for occult blood
Musculoskeletal	Swollen joints (hemarthrosis, vasculitis), bone pain (malignancy), absent radii (thrombocytopenia–absent radii syndrome)

Genitourinary	Testicular swelling, tenderness (vasculitis)
Skin	Rashes, splinter hemorrhages (vasculitis, infectious), hemangiomas (Kasabach-Merritt syndrome), Grey Turner sign (pancreatic hemorrhage or retroperitoneal hemorrhage)
Neurologic	Abnormal sensation, motor deficits (peripheral neuropathy or weakness with vasculitis)

DIC, Disseminated intravascular coagulopathy; *ITP*, idiopathic thrombocytopenic purpura.

Selective History and Chart Review

Has the child bled excessively before?

A history of previous episodes should raise suspicion of an inherited coagulopathy or chronic thrombocytopenia. Recurrent epistaxis may be self-inflicted and is also suggestive of a potential anatomic lesion (e.g., polyp or hemangioma).

Has the patient had a recent infection?

If the patient has been hospitalized with a bacterial infection, sepsis with associated disseminated intravascular coagulopathy (DIC) is a possibility. A recent viral infection might suggest idiopathic thrombocytopenic purpura or Henoch-Schönlein purpura. Recent diarrhea, particularly if bloody, might indicate hemolytic-uremic syndrome (HUS).

What drugs has the patient received?

Multiple drugs may be associated with thrombocytopenia or decreased platelet function, including salicylates, nonsteroidal anti-inflammatory drugs, and antibiotics. Oral contraceptives may increase the risk for pulmonary embolism.

Is there a family history of coagulopathies? Has there been bleeding after childbirth or circumcision, menorrhagia, or epistaxis in family members?

If yes, this is a clue to a potential inherited coagulopathy.

Is there any reason to suspect liver or renal failure, either secondary to the child's underlying illness or as a consequence of treatment?

The answers to these questions may be diagnostically helpful.

If hemoptysis is present, has the child been exposed to tuberculosis? Have there been numerous upper and/or lower airway infections? Has the child undergone recent dental treatment? Is there any history of heart disease?

Numerous infections should raise suspicion of cystic fibrosis. Recent dental procedures might suggest lung abscess. A history of heart disease might increase the risk for endocarditis.

Has the child been hospitalized with severe traumatic injuries?

Chest trauma may result in hemoptysis. Crush injuries, burns, or severe head trauma may lead to DIC.

If the child is a newborn, is there a history of maternal thrombocytopenia or lupus? Has the mother been treated with any drugs that may cause vitamin K deficiency (e.g., anticonvulsants) or suppress platelet production? Has the neonate received vitamin K?

Neonatal immune thrombocytopenia may be the result of transplacental passage of maternal immunoglobulin G (IgG) antiplatelet antibodies, such as those seen in lupus or ITP. Vitamin K deficiency typically results in bleeding on the second or third day of life.

Management II

After the selective history and physical examination, further laboratory testing may be necessary to determine the cause of the bleeding or to exclude possible diagnoses. In many instances the bleeding is minimal, self-limited, and not life threatening. If epistaxis has occurred and resolved, additional testing may be unnecessary. It may be presumed that the bleeding was secondary to local trauma, and a simple "wait and see" approach may suffice. Similarly, self-limited bleeding localized to one area of the skin may often be presumed to be secondary to trauma and frequently does not require further evaluation. Excessive bleeding, hemoptysis, hemarthrosis, and generalized petechiae and purpura should be further evaluated with laboratory testing. Likewise, recurrent episodes of bleeding should be additionally evaluated. The following tests should be performed to assess the degree of anemia, possible thrombocytopenia, possible microangiopathy, or possible clotting factor abnormality:

1. Complete blood count
2. Platelet count
3. Peripheral blood smear
4. PT
5. PTT

Although not usually necessary immediately, a bleeding time may also be useful to determine whether abnormalities in platelet function are present.

For those with hemoptysis, a chest radiograph should be performed. Additional testing may be done selectively, depending on the clinical situation. If DIC is suspected, fibrinogen and D-dimer determination would be helpful. Hepatic enzymes, blood urea nitrogen, creatinine, and urinalysis are indicated if liver or renal disease is a consideration. Helical CT scanning should be performed if pulmonary embolism is suspected. Specific clotting factor assays should be performed if unexplained PT and/or PTT abnormalities are present.

Definitive management of bleeding depends on the cause. Management of life-threatening conditions has been outlined earlier. Less acute disorders should be managed as follows.

Infections

Chest radiographic studies should be performed in all patients with suspected lung infection. If possible, sputum should be sent to the laboratory for culture (including mycobacterial), Gram staining, and acid-fast staining. A purified protein derivative skin test should be performed if tuberculosis is suspected. Empiric treatment of suspected pneumonia can be initiated with ceftriaxone. The decision to empirically treat for *Mycoplasma pneumoniae* with erythromycin or azithromycin should be individualized. Cold agglutinins, often present in patients with *M. pneumoniae* infection, can be detected at the bedside by placing a small amount (2 to 3 mL) of blood in a purple-top tube and placing it on ice for several minutes. In the presence of cold agglutinins, clumping of cells can be seen along the glass walls of the tube as it is rolled in the hand. Lung abscesses should be treated with antibiotics effective against *Staphylococcus aureus* and anaerobes, such as clindamycin.

Vasculitis

Granulomatosis with polyangiitis, eosinophilic granulomatosis with polyangiitis, lupus, Goodpasture syndrome, and less commonly, polyarteritis nodosa and Henoch-Schönlein purpura may result in pulmonary hemorrhage. Prompt treatment with corticosteroids may be life saving. Consideration should also be given to the use of cytotoxic therapy. Consultation with a rheumatologist is recommended.

Coagulopathies

Disorders of coagulation may be divided into thrombocytopenias, abnormalities in platelet function, and clotting factor deficiencies. Depending on the cause (or presumptive cause), the treatment of these conditions varies (see Chapter 33).

Chest Pain

Stephen E. Wilkinson, MD

Acute chest pain is a nonspecific complaint with etiologies stemming from many organ systems. Although children generally have noncardiac causes of chest pain, each case must be evaluated for possible life-threatening pathology (see later). As with other types of pain described by children, the imprecision of the term may include any abnormal sensation, such as palpitations or dysphagia. A systematic approach to determining the etiology of the pain is generally done either by mentally reviewing all thoracic organ systems or by "thinking through the chest" in an anteroposterior manner. When evaluating patients for chest pain, consider if transfer to a higher level of care is needed. If more resources are needed during bedside evaluation and treatment, consider calling a rapid response team (RRT) or code team to assist.

PHONE CALL

Questions

1. What are the vital signs, including temperature?
2. How severe is the pain? How uncomfortable is the child? When did the pain start?
3. What is the child's underlying illness and reason for hospitalization?
4. Has the child complained of chest pain before?

The vital signs and degree of pain severity help to triage the urgency of the complaint. If vitals are severely abnormal, immediately calling for an RRT or code team to assist you is likely warranted; having such support often expedites medication availability, lab draws, imaging, electrocardiographic (ECG) studies, and, if needed, transfer to a critical care unit. Tachycardia may be present regardless of the cause of the pain. Extreme tachycardia (>200 beats per minute) suggests a tachyarrhythmia, often a supraventricular tachycardia (SVT). Bradycardia in a patient with chest pain is an ominous sign that often denotes impending cardiac arrest. This is symptomatic bradycardia, and Pediatric Advanced Life Support protocols should be initiated immediately. Tachypnea may likewise be secondary to the pain or to associated anxiety about the pain. However, organic causes of tachypnea are often concurrent and should be suspect, particularly cardiopulmonary pathology. Respiratory rate trends may help you to determine whether a pulmonary process was "brewing" before the chest pain became apparent. Bradypnea may connote impending respiratory failure. Hypertension may reflect anxiety, although organic, particularly cardiovascular and systemic causes should be ruled out. As with bradycardia, hypotension is an ominous sign and should be treated as an indicator of shock until this is ruled out. A fever should raise suspicion of an infectious cause for the chest pain, such as pneumonia, pleuritis, myocarditis, pericarditis, or osteomyelitis. The child's underlying illness and reason for hospitalization may offer clues to the cause of the pain. Sickle cell disease with acute chest syndrome (ACS), systemic juvenile rheumatoid arthritis (JRA) with pericarditis, and cystic fibrosis with pneumothorax are examples of illnesses associated with specific causes of chest pain.

Orders

If the vital signs reveal bradycardia or hypotension, have the RN call for an RRT or code team to assist. The patient should be placed on a cardiopulmonary monitor. An intravenous (IV) line should be placed, if not yet present, and a 10 mL/kg bolus of normal saline or lactated Ringer's solution should be prepared. You should evaluate the patient for congestive heart failure before administering fluids, given of the risk of exacerbating this condition if it is present. Signs to look for include pulmonary crackles, jugular venous distension, and hepatomegaly. Further fluid boluses (normally dosed at 20 mL/kg each, if no congestive heart failure or other fluid overload syndrome is present) may be needed to maintain blood pressure if the patient is septic or in noncardiogenic shock. When the IV line is placed, labs should be drawn, including a stat complete blood count (CBC), basic metabolic panel (BMP), troponin, and fractionated creatine phosphokinase (CK or CPK along with CK-MB); some labs run the troponin and the fractionated CK/CK-MB together as a "cardiac panel." If a hematocrit can be determined on the ward, this should be done because a decreasing hematocrit raises suspicion of hemorrhage, such as from a ruptured vascular aneurysm or a perforated gastrointestinal (GI) viscus. Keep in mind that slow bleeds may have compensated, and that normal hematocrits and such pathology should not be ruled out on the basis of this lab alone. Continuous pulse oximetry should be going with the cardiopulmonary monitoring; if the patient is in extremis, an arterial blood gas analysis should be obtained and oxygen administered, initially 100% by mask. Often, bedside ECG and chest radiographic studies may need to be performed soon after your evaluation. A portable supine anteroposterior chest x-ray should be obtained if the child is hemodynamically or otherwise clinically unstable. If the child is hemodynamically stable but tachypneic without a suspicion of impending respiratory failure, consider ordering posteroanterior and lateral chest views. These films may reveal pulmonary infiltrates and consolidations (including findings suggestive of pneumonia, ACS, and acute respiratory distress syndrome), pleural effusions, an enlarged cardiac silhouette, pneumothorax, pneumomediastinum, or rib fractures (additional views may be needed for rib evaluation).

Inform RN

A patient with abnormal vital signs or severe discomfort requires immediate evaluation. Otherwise, let the nurse know when you plan to arrive. If the patient's condition is severe, nursing staff should stay with the patient until you have arrived.

ELEVATOR THOUGHTS

Potential causes of acute chest pain in children are most easily categorized according to organ system or anatomic location. During inspiration, the superior liver edge goes as high as the nipple line, so upper abdominal and diaphragmatic pathology should also be considered.

Cardiac	Pericarditis (viral, inflammatory, metabolic [uremia, thyrotoxicosis], bacterial, fungal)
	Myocarditis (viral, inflammatory conditions including juvenile rheumatoid arthritis [JRA], systemic lupus erythematosus [SLE], and rheumatic fever)
	Dysrhythmias (consider metabolic and electrolyte causes)
	Bradycardia
	Supraventricular tachycardia
	Ventricular tachycardia
	Myocardial ischemia or infarction secondary to:
	Sickle cell disease
	Kawasaki disease with coronary artery aneurysms
	SLE (with or without a lupus anticoagulant)
	Antiphospholipid antibodies

	Oral contraceptives
	Cocaine or amphetamines
	Exertion/physiologic stress with a coronary artery anomaly/aberrancy
	Severe aortic stenosis, pulmonary stenosis, mitral valve prolapse
	Cardiomyopathy (including hypertrophic obstructive cardiomyopathy)
	Aortic dissection or rupture (Marfan syndrome or Takayasu arteritis)
Pulmonary	Pneumonia
	Pneumothorax (including tension pneumothorax)
	Pleuritis (infectious, JRA, SLE, familial Mediterranean fever, medication induced)
	Pulmonary embolism
	Pulmonary infarction (acute chest syndrome)
	Asthma exacerbation
	Foreign body aspiration
Gastrointestinal	Esophagitis (gastroesophageal reflux, pill esophagitis, eosinophilic esophagitis)
	Esophageal rupture (known as Boerhaave syndrome)
	Gastritis
	Peptic ulcer (including hemorrhages and perforations)
	Biliary colic
Musculoskeletal	Costochondritis
	Rib fracture
	Pectoral insertion pain or muscle strain
	Clavicular fracture
	Osteomyelitis
	Precordial catch syndrome ("Texidor's Twinge")
	Mastalgia
	Trauma (both accidental and nonaccidental)
Neurologic	Thoracic radiculopathy
	Neurotoxins from black widow (*Lactrodectus*) spider bites
Psychogenic	Anxiety
	Somatization
	Other regional considerations:
	Mediastinum
	Mediastinitis (infectious, caustic ingestion with ruptured esophagus, trauma including recent thoracic surgery)

Pneumomediastinum
Thymus cancers
Thymitis
Diaphragmatic (irritation can come from
    above or below the diaphragm)
Diaphragmatic hernia
Subdiaphragmatic abscess
Splenic infarction or abscess
Pancreatitis

MAJOR THREAT TO LIFE

- Pericarditis with tamponade
- Pneumothorax, pneumomediastinum, or pneumopericardium
- Aortic dissection or rupture
- Myocardial ischemia or infarction
- Unstable dysrhythmias
- Pulmonary embolism (PE)
- Pulmonary infarction/ACS
- Perforated or hemorrhaging GI viscus

All of these conditions are rare in children, but each must be considered for every patient complaining of chest pain given the high rates of morbidity and mortality if missed. Often, these pathologies occur in children with predisposing risk factors (e.g., aortic dissection with Marfan syndrome, pneumothorax with cystic fibrosis).

BEDSIDE

Quick-Look Test

Does the child appear well and comfortable, with no signs of distress?

If so, suspicion of major threat to life pathology is low. An ill-appearing child requires prompt attention. Providers should stay at the bedside until clinical stability is ensured. Body position may offer clues to the source of the chest pain because pericarditis and pericardial effusions may make it difficult for the child to lay supine; patients with these pathologies often prefer to sit and lean forward, sometimes in a tripod position.

Airway and Vital Signs

Labored respirations, tachypnea, central (oral) and peripheral cyanosis, nasal flaring, retracting, grunting, and hypoxemia (suggested by pulse oximetry or definitive by lab study) are signs of respiratory compromise. If there is *any* concern regarding the current or future ability to protect the airway, intubation must be considered; call a code for critical care support. As noted earlier, fever suggests infectious causes of pain. Blood cultures, chest imaging, and an ECG should be included in the work-up. Tachycardia and tachypnea are nonspecific and may occur as a result of the pain or may be indicative of cardiac or pulmonary processes. Cardiopulmonary monitoring should be used. Extreme tachycardia suggests SVT, and an ECG study should be obtained immediately (see Chapter 22). Hypotension should be considered a result of shock until proven otherwise. Critical care support is warranted. Key in treating this will be determining the underlying type of shock (often categorized as distributive [including septic and neurogenic], cardiogenic, hypovolemic, and obstructive). Fluids should be given serially to help maintain adequate perfusion pressure except in cases of cardiogenic shock; vasopressor or inotropic therapy may be needed. Critical care staff should help in the management of these patients. Adrenal insufficiency should be considered in hypotensive patients. Narrow pulse pressure suggests pericardial tamponade or tension pneumothorax. *Pulsus* paradoxus, an exaggerated decrease in systolic arterial pressure during inspiration (>10 mm Hg), is also suggestive of these conditions. During inspiration, there is normally a slight decrease in the filling of the left ventricle. This decrease becomes exacerbated by the presence of a large amount of pericardial fluid or by a tension pneumothorax. Normally, when manual blood pressure readings are obtained, if the pressure is decreased slowly, a systolic Korotkoff sound will initially be heard only as the patient is exhaling. Continuing to decrease the pressure slowly (2 to 3 mm Hg per heartbeat), the provider will hear the systolic Korotkoff sound with both inspiration and expiration. The degree of difference between these two points will indicate if *pulsus paradoxus* is present (Fig. 25.2).

Selective Physical Examination

General	Distressed breathing or cyanosis (initiate critical care efforts)
	Distressed posture (particularly tripod/anterior lean position)
	Confusion (uremia, other electrolyte and metabolic abnormalities, drugs)
	Marfanoid body habitus: tall, thin, long arms and fingers (marfan.org for physical exam calculator once stabilized)
HEENT	Pupillary dilatation (cocaine, amphetamine)
	Conjunctivitis (Kawasaki disease is classically bulbar and nonexudative; infectious can lead to systemic disease)

HEENT, Head, Eyes, Ears, Nose, Throat.

	Uveitis (primary inflammatory conditions: juvenile rheumatoid arthritis, systemic lupus erythematosus)

Uveitis (primary inflammatory conditions: juvenile rheumatoid arthritis, systemic lupus erythematosus)

Dislocated lenses (Marfan syndrome)

Blood in oropharynx (esophagitis, gastritis, gastrointestinal viscus perforation, pulmonary embolism [PE], acute chest syndrome, pneumonia)

Neck   Distended neck veins with or without prominent venous pulsation (pericardial effusion)

Deviation of the trachea (tension pneumothorax)

Goiter (thyrotoxicosis)

Lymphadenopathy (Kawasaki disease, lymphoma, leukemia)

Subcutaneous emphysema (pneumomediastinum with tracking)

Chest   Reproducible chest wall tenderness (costochondritis, wall trauma, radiculopathy)

Localized point tenderness (rib or clavicular fracture, osteomyelitis)

Suprasternal subcutaneous emphysema (pneumomediastinum)

Pectoral stress maneuvers (Fig. 10.1; pectoral muscle strain)

Erythema (cellulitis, myositis, mastitis)

Ecchymoses (trauma)

Heart   Arrhythmias (intrinsic electrical, ischemia, myocarditis)

Muffled or distant heart sounds (pericardial effusion, pneumopericardium)

Murmur (numerous causes)

Rub (pericarditis)

Gallop (cardiomyopathy)

Crunching or grating sound (Hamman sign for pneumomediastinum or pneumopericardium)

Lungs   Grunting, nasal flaring, muscle retractions (respiratory distress)

Absent breath sounds (pneumothorax until proven otherwise, pleural effusion)

Rales (pneumonia, congestive heart failure, acute chest syndrome, pulmonary embolus)

Wheezing (asthma, foreign body aspiration, acute chest syndrome)

Pleural rub (pleuritis: infectious and primary inflammatory)

Intrathoracic borborygmus (diaphragmatic hernia)

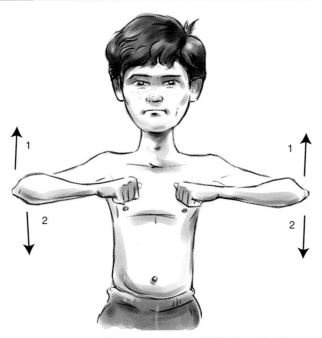

FIGURE 10.1 **Pectoral stress maneuvers.** With the patient's arms extended and elbows bent, ask the patient to move against resistance, first upward and then downward.

Abdomen	Rigid with guarding and rebound tenderness (surgical abdomen with peritonitis)
	Abdominal tenderness (gastrointestinal ulcer, viscus perforation, biliary pathology, intra-abdominal infection or infarction, empyema)
Extremities	Swollen or tender extremity (deep venous thromboses and PE)
Pulses	Unequal right upper extremity to other pulses (coarctation, dissection)
	Absent femoral pulses (aortic dissection)
Skin	Rash (Kawaski disease, infectious pericarditis or myocarditis)
	Livedo reticularis (antiphospholipid syndrome)

Selective History

What does the pain feel like? Where is it?

No descriptor of chest pain is pathognomonic, although many are suggestive of certain etiologies. Acute dyspnea may often be called chest pain by children. This complaint should raise suspicion for pneumothorax, PE or infarction, ACS, and pneumonia. Pericardial pain is usually sharp or stabbing; it is frequently referred to the shoulder. Ischemic or infarction cardiac pain is often described as crushing or squeezing and may be described with a clenched hand (Levine sign). Tearing pain radiating to the back, classically intrascapular, or neck suggests aortic dissection, although this should be highly suspected with any tearing chest pain. Pleuritic pain is sharp and intermittent with position and respiratory cycle dependency. Biliary pain is colicky and may have a postprandial temporal relationship. As mentioned previously, "pain" may also imply dyspnea, palpitations, dysphagia, or anxiety. Pain from chest wall pathology often feels superficial and may be localized. Attempting to elicit the specific characteristics of what the child is feeling may require careful questioning. Care should be taken not to use leading questions.

What exacerbates the pain?

Pain from the major threat to life pathology identified previously is usually progressive, often with no known exacerbating factors. Pericarditis is worse in the supine position and is relieved by leaning forward. Pain with inspiration suggests pleuritis or a musculoskeletal cause. Pain with palpation of the chest is consistent with musculoskeletal causes. Dysphagia suggests esophagitis. Pain after eating may be secondary to esophageal reflux, biliary pathology, or pancreatitis.

Has the child complained of chest pain previously?

A history of previous complaints and the results of previous evaluations, if any, may provide clues to the cause of the current complaints.

Selective Chart Review

What medications has the child received?

Amphetamines may cause tachyarrhythmias. Oral contraceptives predispose to thrombosis and may lead to cardiac or pulmonary infarction. Corticosteroids and nonsteroidal antiinflammatory agents may cause esophagitis, gastritis, and peptic ulceration.

If not already done, a urine drug screen should be obtained if there is any suspicion of recent amphetamine or cocaine use.

Review stat labs listed in Orders earlier. Correct electrolyte abnormalities as needed to prevent arrhythmias. Be mindful of kidney function when considering imaging studies with contrast. See Chapter 32 regarding ABG interpretation.

Management

Pericarditis With or Without Tamponade

If your work-up suggests pericarditis, a pericardial effusion may be present. Chest radiography may reveal an enlarged cardiac silhouette or a "water bottle"–shaped heart. Pericardial effusions are confirmed by echocardiography. Various ECG abnormalities may be present, notably decreased voltage, particularly in the QRS complexes, and generalized, nonregional ST-segment changes. Therapeutic management of pericarditis depends on the presence or absence of an effusion and the suspected cause. Tamponade physiology (which clinically shows a narrow pulse pressure, hypotension, *pulsus paradoxus*, and distended neck veins, as well as distinct echo findings) is an emergency, and a therapeutic and diagnostic pericardiocentesis should be done by a cardiologist or an interventional radiologist. A drain is often left in place. If needed, a pericardial window may be placed by a surgeon. Pericardiocentisis may be done on smaller, nontamponade effusions for diagnostic work-up, if needed. This is particularly the case with concerns for infectious pericarditis if it is presumed to be nonviral and a source eludes other detection. Studies on the fluid should at least include Gram staining, culture, and cell counts. Polymerase chain reaction (PCR) studies and cytology may also be performed. Antibiotics may need to be empirically started and later geared to findings. Pericarditis secondary to viral infections or primary systemic inflammatory diseases, such as JRA, may respond to IV nonsteroidal antiinflammatory drugs (NSAIDs; ketorolac or indomethacin are generally used). Similarly, oral prednisone may be sufficient for pericarditis secondary to systemic lupus erythematosus, although if the pericarditis is severe, IV methylprednisolone may be needed. Pericardial effusions secondary to thyroid disease or uremia should respond to treatment of the underlying condition.

Pneumothorax

Absent lung sounds in one hemithorax in a patient with respiratory or cardiac distress, or a patient with acute chest pain, should be treated emergently and empirically (before imaging confirmation) at bedside for a presumed tension pneumothroax. This is done by needle decompression. To accomplish emergency pneumothorax evacuation:

1. Either the second intercostal space along the midclavicular line or the third or fourth intercostal space along the midaxillary line (this spot may be easier in infants) should be chosen and cleaned in rapid but sterile fashion.
2. A 20- or 22-gauge angiocatheter should be used. Some new models of angiocatheters have a mechanism that allows blood to flash followed by a damming of the line to prevent blood loss; these should be strictly avoided because this will prevent decompression. The needle and catheter should be inserted directly perpendicular to the skin along the upper surface of

the inferior rib (i.e., at the bottom of the intercostal space). This protects the nerves and vessels that run adjacent to the inferior margin of the ribs. Once the pleural space is entered, a "pop" may be felt, and a rush of air may be heard through the angiocatheter. The risk of causing a pneumothorax, should one hit lung parenchyma, is low when using these gauges; that worry should not prohibit nor delay this emergency procedure.

3. The needle should then be withdrawn while keeping the catheter in place. The catheter should be secured against the chest tightly. Do not stopcock the line, because tension would accumulate.

4. Chest radiography should be done to evaluate the pneumothroax and catheter placement. The patient should be transferred to a critical care unit for monitoring and possible chest tube placement.

If breath sounds are reassuring but a pneumothorax is seen on imaging, treatment depends on its size. Giving 100% oxygen by mask (or by hood in an infant) may result in quicker resolution of the pneumothorax. Small pneumothoraces may resolve spontaneously. Large pneumothoraces require closed thoracostomy with chest tube placement as prophylaxis against tension pneumothorax and to aid in healing.

Pneumomediastinum and Pneumopericardium

Pneumomediastinum may be secondary to a pneumothorax; in these cases, it should be treated as an extension of the pneumothorax and may resolve with hemithorax decompression. Spontaneous pneumomediastinum lacks an associated pneumothorax and is often related to underlying pulmonary disease, particularly asthma and lower respiratory tract infections. This develops when a small parenchymal leak allows for air to track up along bronchovascular bundles into the mediastinum without developing a pneumothroax. Tracking often continues into neck and upper extremity soft tissues, causing palpable crepitus. Tracking may also continue into the pericardial sac, causing a pneumopericardium. Pneumomediastinum may also occur with esophageal perforation (often caused by medication overuse, alkali or other caustic ingestion, or as a complication to intraesophageal studies) and mechanical ventilation. It may be iatrogenic from intrathoracic procedures or surgery or may be idiopathic. Complications from tension accumulation are rare, particularly in non-neonates. Chest radiographs reveal a sharper cardiac border and may also disclose subcutaneous air. ECG studies may have low voltages and nonspecific segment and interval changes. Echocardiography may be helpful in determining if pneumopericardium is present, particularly if tamponade physiology is suspected. Treatment is directed at the underlying cause. Unless there is cardiovascular compromise, the air in the mediastinal and soft tissue space need not be evacuated and resolves spontaneously. Pneumomediastinum after esophageal perforation requires emergent surgical repair with empiric aerobic and anaerobic antibiotics for presumed concurrent mediastinitis. Blood cultures should be obtained in these cases.

Aortic Dissection or Rupture

These conditions have notably high mortality and morbidity rates. Life is preserved with early high indices of suspicion. Any patient with a suspected dissection or rupture requires critical care management. Imaging is required to make the diagnosis. Computed tomography (CT) angiography is generally the fastest modality for making a radiographic diagnosis. Magnetic resonance angiogram has a role. For patients who are hemodynamically unstable or unable to tolerate IV contrast, bedside echocardiography may be used. A widened mediastinum on a chest film raises suspicion but is not diagnostic, and this should not be used as a screening test. Any dissection should have a stat cardiothoracic surgery consult. Blood for a CBC, BMP, prothrombin time (PT), partial thromboplastin time (PTT), and blood typing and cross matching should be sent to the laboratory immediately. Large-bore IV access in at least two sites should be ensured. Propagation of the dissection may be limited with decreasing shear stress through beta-blockade or other medical suppression of cardiac output. Pain control should be ensured because this will help to decrease adrenergic drive. The surgery team will help to decide if emergent surgical intervention is indicated or if medical management will suffice.

Myocardial Ischemia and Infarction

These pathologies are generally due to sickle cell vasoocclusion, vasculitides, cocaine or methamphetamine use, or compression of an aberrant coronary artery. When myocardial ischemia or infarction is suspected, an ECG should be obtained to look for patterns consistent with these diagnoses (Table 10.1). Serum troponin and fractionated CPK (CK or CPK and CK-MB) levels should also be determined; as previously stated, many hospitals bundle these studies as a "cardiac panel." These levels should be trended over time (generally with three studies at 4- to 6-hour intervals) because enzymatic leak takes time to occur after myocardial insult. A CBC, BMP, PT, PTT, and a sample for blood typing and cross matching should be sent to the lab. A stat cardiology consult should be placed if ECG or lab studies are in any way concerning or if clinical judgment leads to a high suspicion of ischemia. The patient should be immediately transferred for critical care and cardiology management. Nitroglycerin may relieve the chest pain. Morphine should

TABLE 10.1	Myocardial Infarction Patterns

Patterns of Changes (Q Waves, ST Elevation, or Type of Infarct Inversion)[a]	Depression, T Wave
Inferior	Q in II, III, AVF
Inferoposterior	Q in II, III, AVF, and V6 R > S and positive T in V1
Anteroseptal	V1 to V4
Anterolateral to posterolateral	V1 to V5; Q in I, AVL, and V6
Posterior	R > S in V1, positive T, and Q in V6

[a]A significant Q wave is greater than 40 msec wide or greater than a third of the QRS height. ST-segment or T wave changes in the absence of significant Q waves may represent a non–Q wave infarct.

From Marshall SA, Ruedy J: On Call: Principles and Practices, 2nd ed. Philadelphia, WB Saunders, 1993.

generally be avoided given the risk for respiratory depression but may be used in small doses if necessary. Aspirin should be given empirically. Oxygen should be administered to all patients, initially at 100%; this will help with potential sickling and will decrease myocardial demand. Patients with sickle cell disease may require an exchange transfusion and those with hypercoagulable states may require heparinization.

Stable and Unstable Dysrhythmias
See Chapter 22.

Pulmonary Embolism
The diagnosis of PE is often delayed due to low clinical suspicion. Suspicion should be raised for patients who are immobile (including those with recent surgery), those with central venous lines, and those with hypercoaguable states (including those using oral contraception). Approximately half of patients also have deep venous thromboses (DVTs). Signs and symptoms do not have high sensitivity or specificity but may include acute chest pain, hypoxemia, tachypnea or other signs of respiratory distress, and extremity evidence of DVT. Chest x-rays have no role in the work-up. Likewise, a negative D-dimer has been shown to not rule out PE in children and is not specific for PE if positive. No diagnostic probability scoring systems (such as the Wells score) have been validated in children to this point. CT angiography of the chest or ventilation-perfusion scan should be used for diagnosis. Oxygen should be given to all patients with suspected PE. Rapid response or critical care support may be needed if the child is unstable.

Systemic thrombolysis with tissue plasminogen activator may be needed in unstable patients; the critical care team will help guide the decision to use this. Initial therapy is usually a heparin drip or therapeutic Lovenox subcutaneous injections. Long-term anticoagulation will be needed.

Pulmonary Infarction/Acute Chest Syndrome

Pulmonary infarction may be caused by thrombi but is most commonly caused in children by vasoocclusion secondary to sickle cell disease exacerbation, which leads to a condition called the ACS. This is a common cause for hospitalization and death in children with sickle cell disease. Infections, asthma exacerbations, nonpulmonic vasoocclusion events, and anything leading to atelectasis may trigger the intrapulmonary sickling. Patients with ACS often have fevers, hypoxemia, and respiratory distress. Chest radiography is key in diagnosing this condition with consolidations being seen in many cases, sometimes in a diffuse pattern. A stat hematology consult should be placed for any patient suspected to have ACS. Continuous pulse oximetry should be monitored and any hypoxemia treated with supplemental oxygen. Respiratory distress should prompt a call for rapid response assistance with an ABG draw for evaluation. Although dehydration can lead to sickling and should be corrected, care should be taken not to overcorrect because pulmonary edema will worsen the patient's respiratory status. Bronchodilators should be given, particularly if asthma is triggering the event. Empiric antibiotics (a third generation and a macrolide) should be given. A CBC, CMP, and a sample for blood typing and cross matching should be obtained. Hematology should help guide decisions about transfusions. The patient will require critical care.

Perforated or Hemorrhaging Gastrointestinal Viscus

The presentation of these pathologies is usually obvious with severe pain and possible hematemesis and hemodynamic instability. These conditions very rarely happen without an overt underlying cause including caustic ingestion, medication (particularly NSAID) overuse, recent surgery or intralumenal endoscopic studies, connective tissue disorders, or severe retching (Boerhaave syndrome). Initial management should be focused on maintaining the airway and hemodynamic stability; rapid response assistance is appropriate if any help is needed. Stat surgery and GI consults should be placed. Blood work should include a CBC, BMP, PT, PTT, and blood typing and cross matching. Plain films of the chest and abdomen in the left lateral decubitus or the cross-table positions may be helpful in evaluating for free air. Empiric antibiotics should be started as soon as possible and should cover aerobic and anaerobic organisms; blood cultures may be useful but should not delay treatment.

The following diagnoses should be considered and treated *only* after the above diagnoses have been clinically ruled out.

Myocarditis

This diagnosis is often seen with concurrent pericarditis. When isolated, it is generally due to a viral infection, although it may be seen with primary inflammatory conditions or bacterial infections. Help with diagnosis and management should be sought through a cardiology consult. Because myocarditis may lead to arrhythmias, children suspected to have this diagnosis should be monitored on telemetry. ECG findings often suggest myocardial injury with ST segment changes and T wave changes. Cardiac enzymes (troponin, CK, and CK-MB) are generally elevated. Chest radiography is nondiagnostic. Echocardiography and cardiac magnetic resonance imaging (MRI) may provide strong evidence of myocarditis. Endomyocardial biopsy via a cardiac catheterization is the gold standard for diagnosis. Patients with fulminant myocarditis have heart failure, and diuretic, afterload reducing (angiotensin-converting enzyme [ACE]-I), and inotropic therapies may be needed.

Severe Valvular Disease and HOCM

A careful, thorough cardiac examination will at least suggest these etiologies and may allow for clinical diagnosis. Echocardiography will delineate the pathology and the degree of its severity. Medical manipulation of preloads or afterloads will likely be indicated in children with chest pain. In severe cases, interventional cardiology or surgical management may be needed. The patient should be monitored on telemetry and have frequent vital checks. A cardiology consult should be used to help with management.

Pneumonia

Focal adventitial lung sounds, hypoxemia, consolidation(s) on chest radiography, fevers, respiratory distress, and hemodynamic instability may be seen in patients with pneumonia. A CBC with differential and blood cultures, as well as sputum Gram stain and culture, if possible, should be obtained. If bacterial pneumonia is suspected from the clinical and chest radiography findings, antibiotics are required. Antibiotic choice should be determined based on whether the infection is considered community acquired, hospital acquired, or due to aspiration. Review of any past infections and *Pseudomonas* infection risk factors will also help to guide therapy. Continuous pulse oximetry with supplementation as needed is indicated. See Respiratory Distress, Chapter 28, for further management guidance.

Pleural Effusion

If the effusion is leading to hypoxemia, supplemental oxygen should be given. Incentive spirometry is indicated for all patients with effusions. Effusions in patients with any signs of infection, especially respiratory infections, should be considered empyemas until proven otherwise. Thoracentesis should be strongly considered for diagnostic purposes in all patients with new effusions and is indicated if any concerns exist about it being an empyema. If the effusion is large, thoracentesis may be therapeutic as well. This procedure is usually done under imaging, often by interventional radiology. Critical care support may help to perform this as a bedside procedure if the patient is unstable. Studies on the fluid should include Gram stain, culture, cell count, lactic acid dehydrogenase (LDH), and total protein determination. Concurrent serum LDH and total protein should be measured for evaluation using Light's criteria. If the tap is bloody, obtain a hematocrit on the sample. If it is turbid, obtain a triglyceride level on the sample. If there are concerns for malignancy, obtain cytology and fluid pH. If pancreatitis is suspected, a fluid amylase level may be helpful.

Pleuritis

This usually responds well to conservative, symptomatic treatment (e.g., NSAIDs).

Asthma Exacerbation

See Chapter 28.

Foreign Body Aspiration

See Chapter 28.

Esophagitis, Gastritis, or Peptic Ulcer

A "GI cocktail" of viscous lidocaine, liquid diphenhydramine, and an antacid may be therapeutic, with an improvement in symptoms suggesting these pathologies. Maintenance antacid, H_2-receptor antagonist, or proton pump inhibitor therapy may be used. Consultation with a gastroenterologist and endoscopic examination may be required to evaluate the underlying cause of pathology. A day-to-day trend of the hemoglobin/hematocrit (Hgb/Hct) may help to identify bleeding; a markedly elevated blood urea nitrogen (BUN), especially without a reflective rise in the creatinine, is suggestive of an upper GI bleed. If bleeding is suspected, more frequent Hgb/Hct checks may be appropriate.

Diaphragmatic and Peridiaphragmatic Pathology

Irritation of the diaphragm from either side may present as chest pain. Pleural effusions are discussed previously. Diaphragmatic hernias may be identified by intrathoracic borborygmus and chest radiography showing stomach or bowel contours above the diaphragm. Subdiaphragmatic abscess is usually diagnosed only if there is a high suspicion; CT imaging of the chest and abdomen with contrast may identify such pathology. Splenic infarction or abscesses are rare. Infarction may take place during sickle crises or with hypercoaguable states, including myeloproliferative cancers. Abscesses usually develop secondary to a bacteremia or endocarditis. Blood counts with differential, a peripheral smear, and blood cultures should be obtained if splenic pathology is considered. CT studies are often needed. Pancreatitis generally leads to abdominal pain, although chest pain may be concurrent. Serum lipase and amylase levels along with abdominal imaging (ultrasonography or CT) help make the diagnosis. Biliary colic has a distinct intermittent nature. Liver panel chemistries and right upper quadrant ultrasonography are helpful in making the diagnosis. See Chapter 23.

Chest Wall Musculoskeletal and Neurologic Pain

These conditions may lead to guarded or weak inspiratory effort, tachypnea with possible hyperventilation, and anxiety. The pain is often reproducible with palpation and positional changes. Pain control is key; NSAIDs and topical therapies are often helpful. Many of the underlying conditions spontaneously resolve. Consideration should be given to possible infections.

Psychogenic

Reassurance and efforts aimed at relaxing the patient are the best approach. As with abdominal pain, headaches, and extremity pain, idiopathic chest pain is common in children, particularly during the preadolescent years. Concern for family members who have heart disease may contribute to the child's fears and subsequent pain. Reassurance that they have a "normal heart," once clinically determined, may be all that is required to result in the resolution of the pain.

REMEMBER

Rapid response and critical care assistance should be sought quickly when needed. All life-threatening causes of chest pain should be considered and ruled in or out for every patient complaining of chest pain. Thinking through all of the organ systems in the thorax or mentally going "through the chest" in an anterior to posterior manner helps to make sure differential diagnoses are not overlooked.

chapter 11

Constipation

Maja Z. Katusic, MD

Constipation is a common problem in both outpatient and inpatient pediatrics. An estimated 3% to 5% of all pediatrician visits are due to constipation. Calls about hard stools or no stools are frequent in the hospital. Constipation is most often functional due to stool retention. However, additional rare etiologies must always be considered, especially in the hospital setting.

PHONE CALL

Questions

1. Is the stool hard with painful defecation or has there been no stool at all? When was the last time the child had a stool?
2. How old is the child?
3. Why is the child hospitalized?
4. Are there any associated gastrointestinal symptoms or signs, such as abdominal pain, poor oral intake, nausea, vomiting (especially bilious), or abdominal distention?
5. Does the child have a history of constipation?
6. What medications is the child taking?

Characterizing the "constipation" is the most important step. It may be normal for a formula fed infant to go up to 2 to 3 days without a stool. Breastfed infants generally have stools more often. Infants on average go 3 to 4 times per day. Toddlers have approximately 2 to 3 stools per day. By age 4 or older, stool patterns are about the same as adults. Constipation tends to happen in times of transition. For infants, this can occur when they go from breastfed to formula fed. In toddlers, difficulty with stools may develop when going through toilet training. Finally, school-age children may become more constipated when entering school and they have to use unfamiliar bathrooms.

In general, the nature of the stool is much more indicative of constipation than the frequency is. Straining in infants is a common concern for parents. Infant dyschezia occurs in healthy infants younger than 6 months who strain excessively due to difficulty coordinating increasing intra-abdominal pressure with relaxing the pelvic floor to allow passage of stool. Straining alone usually requires no further evaluation or intervention.

Once it is clear that the child does in fact appear to be constipated, the age of the child allows you to consider the likelihood of possible causes for the constipation. In addition, the reason for hospitalization and other clinical signs may suggest specific etiologies, including potential serious causes of constipation, such as bowel obstruction. A previous history of constipation suggests a chronic process, and medication side effects (i.e., secondary to opioids) are a relatively frequent cause of constipation.

Orders

Most calls regarding infrequent or absent stools do not require urgent action. If the problem is brought to your attention in the middle of the night and the child is stable with no associated symptoms, it may often be appropriate to defer further evaluation if you are busy with more urgent matters. In this situation, symptomatic treatment may be reasonable if it appears that it will be a while until you are able to evaluate the child further. The management section below discusses treatment options, including laxatives, stool softeners, and enemas. It should be emphasized that these orders should not simply be reflexively given. A child who has associated symptoms such as abdominal pain, vomiting, or abdominal distention needs to be evaluated promptly because a significant intra-abdominal process is then more likely.

ELEVATOR THOUGHTS

Potential causes of constipation differ depending on the age of the child and can be divided into general subgroups:

Infant

1. Anatomic
   - Imperforate anus or anal atresia
   - Malrotation of gut
   - Hirschsprung disease
   - Spinal cord lesions (meningomyelocele)
2. Dietary
   - Insufficient fluid intake
   - Insufficient fiber intake
3. Endocrine/electrolyte imbalance
   - Hypothyroidism
   - Hypokalemia
   - Hypercalcemia

4. Syndromes
   - Prune belly syndrome
   - Trisomy 21
   - Meconium ileus (cystic fibrosis)
5. Other
   - Infant botulism
   - Pseudo-obstruction

Older Child

1. Functional (i.e., withholding)
2. Dietary
   - Insufficient fluid intake
   - Insufficient fiber intake
3. Anatomic
   - Bowel obstruction
   - Painful defecation due to anal fissure
   - Hirschsprung disease
   - Spinal cord lesion (e.g., tumor)
   - Abdominal or pelvic mass
4. Endocrine/electrolyte abnormalities
   - Hypothyroidism
   - Hypokalemia
   - Hypercalcemia
5. Neurologic
   - Guillain-Barré syndrome
   - Food-borne botulism
6. Other
   - Drugs or toxins (e.g., opioids, anticholinergics, iron supplements, antacids, antidepressants, lead poisoning)
   - Ileus (postoperative, postviral)
   - Dysmotility

MAJOR THREAT TO LIFE

Constipation as the sole complaint is not suggestive of a life-threatening illness. The major threats to life are associated with other signs and symptoms, which should suggest a specific diagnosis.
- Bowel obstruction (abdominal pain, bilious vomiting)
- Botulism (weakness, hypotonia)
- Guillain-Barré syndrome (weakness, decreased deep tendon reflexes)
- Exposure to drugs or toxins (altered mental status)
- Hypokalemia (e.g., in patients admitted with eating disorder and at risk for refeeding syndrome)

BEDSIDE

Quick-Look Test

In nearly all cases the infant or child will likely be comfortable if constipation is an isolated symptom. If an infant is irritable or an older child appears distressed, one of the aforementioned major threats to life should be considered.

Airway and Vital Signs

A child with isolated constipation is expected to have normal vital signs and a stable airway. If this is not the case, a prompt search for signs to suggest one of the threats to life listed previously should be undertaken. Fever, tachycardia, and hypotension suggest bowel obstruction with perforation and consequent peritonitis. Labored respirations may be a sign of respiratory muscle weakness secondary to botulism or Guillain-Barré syndrome. Arrhythmias or altered heart rate may be seen with hypokalemia or a number of toxic syndromes (opioids, anticholinergics).

Selective History and Chart Review

Does the child have abdominal pain, nausea, vomiting, or abdominal distention?

Relatively mild pain or rarely severe pain may occur as a result of constipation. Other gastrointestinal symptoms such as distention or bilious vomiting should raise concern about bowel obstruction.

In a neonate, has there been a normal stool yet? Is there a history of a meconium plug?

Meconium plug at birth suggests Hirschsprung disease or cystic fibrosis. These disorders, as well as anatomic anomalies of the gastrointestinal tract, are possibilities if the neonate has not yet had their first stool.

What is the patient's diet? Has the infant (<12 months old) had honey?

Breastfed infants should have several relatively loose, light yellow or green stools every day, often after each feeding. Therefore constipation in an exclusively breastfed infant is rare and suggests either inadequate intake of breast milk or an explanation other than diet. Insufficient volume of intake because of either diet or intercurrent illness may cause defecation difficulties. In both infants and older children, low fecal bulk may result in an inadequate stimulus to peristalsis and subsequent constipation. A high-starch, high-protein diet or the continued use of puréed foods beyond infancy may not provide adequate fiber to promote defecation. Honey is a notorious source of *Clostridium botulinum* spores, the cause of infant botulism.

Has there been a history of constipation or fecal soiling?

Chronic constipation may lead to encopresis, characterized by retention of stool with leakage of fluid stool involuntarily around a large fecal mass. This may occur as a result of withholding secondary to a traumatic toilet training experience, painful defecation due to anal fissures, or another psychologic disturbance. Occasionally, Hirschsprung disease is diagnosed later in childhood after years of constipation. A history of never having a normal stool pattern may suggest such an underlying anatomic defect.

What medications has the child received?

Constipation may be secondary to a long list of possible medications. This includes opioids, iron supplements, or anticholinergics.

Selective Physical Examination

HEENT	Mydriasis (anticholinergic, botulism); miosis (opioids)
Cardiovascular	bradycardia (opioids, hypothyroid); tachycardia (anticholinergic); hypertension (anticholinergic, Guillain-Barré); hypotension (opioids, Guillain-Barré)
Lungs	Tachypnea (abdominal distention due to bowel obstruction); respiratory insufficiency (Guillain-Barré, botulism, bowel obstruction)
Abdomen	Hyperactive or hypoactive bowel sounds; rebound; rigidity; distention (bowel obstruction)
Rectal	Nonpatent rectum (imperforate anus); impacted stool in the vault or anal fissure (functional constipation)
Neurologic	Absent or delayed reflexes (Guillain Barré, spinal cord lesion); hypotonia (spinal cord lesion, Guillain-Barré, botulism)

HEENT, Head, Eyes, Ears, Nose, Throat.

Management

When you are on call, most patients with constipation can be treated symptomatically with plans to address a potential systemic cause at a later point. The exceptions would be if the patient appears to have signs or symptoms suggestive of a bowel obstruction, Guillain-Barré syndrome, a spinal cord lesion, an electrolyte disturbance, or botulism. If there are any concerns about bowel obstruction, the patient should be nil per os and a surgeon should be consulted as soon as possible. If Guillain-Barré syndrome or botulism is a concern, close monitoring, especially of respiratory status, and potential treatment with intravenous immunoglobulin (IVIG) or botulism antitoxin therapy, respectively, would be appropriate. If there is concern for a spinal cord lesion, imaging studies such as spinal magnetic resonance imaging (MRI) should be performed and a neurosurgeon should be consulted. Electrolyte disturbances should be identified with laboratory testing if the patient is at risk for these and corrected appropriately (see Chapter 34).

Imaging of a constipated child may be necessary if it is unclear whether constipation is present or to further evaluate a potential bowel obstruction. An abdominal radiograph may confirm a large amount of stool in the bowel. If bowel obstruction is suspected, an abdominal radiograph may reveal free air due to bowel perforation. Further imaging in such a case should be discussed with a surgeon. Additional imaging studies, such as computed tomography or MRI of the spine, abdomen, or pelvis, may be pursued if there is concern for spinal, abdominal, or pelvic masses leading to constipation.

Laboratory tests rarely need to be ordered urgently in the setting of constipation. If Guillain-Barré is suspected, lumbar puncture should be done to look for elevated protein in the cerebrospinal fluid prior to starting IVIG. If botulism is a possibility, *C. botulism* toxin in the stool can be ordered, but in most laboratories this result will likely not be available for several days. Therefore electromyography (EMG) may be performed when the diagnosis is suspected, and if the EMG reveals characteristic findings, treatment of botulism may be initiated while awaiting the results of the stool testing. Consultation with a neurologist in this situation will likely be necessary to perform and interpret the EMG. Rectal biopsy will confirm Hirschsprung disease. Serum thyroid-stimulating hormone and free thyroxine (T4) can be tested if hypothyroidism is suspected. A serum metabolic panel may be obtained to assess for electrolyte imbalances if there is concern that such abnormalities may be contributing to constipation.

Symptomatic treatment of constipation includes laxatives (osmotic or stimulant), stool softeners, and rectal enemas. Osmotic laxatives include polyethylene glycol (PEG) (Miralax), lactulose, or milk of magnesia. Mineral oil is an excellent stool softener. Some evidence suggests that PEG is more effective for functional constipation compared with lactulose, milk of magnesia, mineral oil, or placebo. Stimulant laxatives include bisacodyl (Dulcolax) and senna (Senokot). Enema options are sodium phosphate (also known as Fleet enema) or normal saline. For infants, a glycerin suppository or normal saline enema can be used. If these measures are unsuccessful, manual disimpaction may be necessary. Lubiprostone (Amitiza) is a recently developed oral chloride channel protein activator that has been well tolerated in the pediatric population; however, experience thus far with this treatment remains limited.

An inadequate diet is often a significant contributor to constipation. Several options are available to increase bulk or soften stool. Increasing the volume of fluid intake, as well as dietary supplements such as prune juice, olive oil, or mineral oil, may be helpful. Vegetables, fruits, bran, and whole grains add bulk. An easy way to remember the recommended grams of daily fiber in a child's diet is that it is equal to the child's age plus five.

Most of the time while on call, constipation can be treated symptomatically. However, it is always important to evaluate the patient for potential warning signs that might indicate the need for further evaluation. If there are no concerning symptoms or signs, initial treatment with laxatives and enemas as needed may be most appropriate, with further evaluation of potential systemic causes performed at a later time if necessary.

Bibliography

Biggs WS, Dery WH: Evaluation and treatment of constipation in infants and children, *Am Fam Physician* 73(3):469–477, 2006.

Colombo JM, Wassom MC, Rosen JM: Constipation and encopresis in childhood, *Pediatr Rev* 36(9):392–402, 2015.

Hyman PE, Di Lorenza C, Prestige LL, et al: Lubiprostone for the treatment of functional constipation in children, *J Pediatr Gastroenterol Nutr* 58(3):283–291, 2014.

Tabbers MM, et al: Evaluation and treatment of functional constipation in infants and children: evidence-based recommendations from ESPGHAN and NASPGHAN, *J Pediatr Gastroenterol Nutr* 58(2):258–274, 2014.

chapter 12

Crying and the Irritable Infant

Julia Richards, MD

Crying and irritability may be considered expected findings in hospitalized infants because these signs are frequently associated with any condition causing pain or discomfort. Usually it will be clear that the infant is irritable because of a known underlying illness. However, in some hospitalized infants the irritability or crying may be difficult to explain. There may not be a readily apparent cause for the irritability, or the character or degree of the irritability may differ from that present on admission. Evaluation of an irritable infant must be particularly thorough to search for clues that suggest a source of the irritability. Sepsis and other infections should always be at the top of the list of considerations, even in the absence of fever, but this should not keep you from thinking of other possible explanations. The age of the patient (whether they are younger or older than 2 months old) is also an important factor when considering infection as a potential cause because at a very young age, there may be few or no additional signs and symptoms. Crying in an infant in the absence of illness, such as that seen in infants with colic, should always be a diagnosis of exclusion.

PHONE CALL

Questions

1. What are the vital signs and trends?
2. Has the infant's degree of irritability changed since admission? Is this a new sign or simply a persistent one?
3. Why is the infant hospitalized?

The development of a new fever with irritability is strongly suggestive of infection and requires immediate action. Some tachycardia is expected in an infant who is irritable, but extreme tachycardia or progressive abnormalities in the vital signs should also raise your level of concern. Because at least some degree of irritability is likely to be present in most hospitalized infants, it is important to determine whether the current status of the infant is different. For example, an infant admitted with bacterial meningitis who has received only a few doses of antibiotics may continue to be irritable for several days until the infection and meningeal inflammation begin to resolve. In contrast, in an infant who has been gradually responding to treatment and then becomes increasingly irritable, a new condition may have developed to explain the change in status. It may be serious, such as a subdural effusion, or simple, such as an infiltrated intravenous (IV) site.

Orders

No orders should be given until the infant is further evaluated.

Inform RN

An infant with a change in the degree of irritability or new onset of irritability needs to be evaluated immediately.

ELEVATOR THOUGHTS

What might cause irritability in the infant? As mentioned earlier, almost any condition may be associated with irritability, and infection is a very common cause. The following list contains some of the more common possibilities, as well as some that may often be overlooked. Remember to prioritize this list based on the age of the infant:

Infection

Sepsis
Meningitis
Encephalitis
Brain abscess
Lymphadenitis
Pneumonia
Gastroenteritis
Myocarditis
Pericarditis
Viral syndrome
Cellulitis
Mastitis
Otitis media
Urinary tract infection
Pyomyositis
Osteomyelitis
Septic arthritis

Gastrointestinal and intra-abdominal conditions	Gastritis
	Gastroesophageal reflux and esophagitis
	Intussusception
	Volvulus
	Bowel obstruction
	Appendicitis
	Peptic ulcer disease
	Constipation
	Anal fissure
	Inguinal hernia
Inflammatory disorders	Kawasaki disease
	Systemic juvenile idiopathic arthritis
Metabolic and endocrine disorders	Hypocalcemia or hypercalcemia
	Hyponatremia or hypernatremia
	Hypokalemia
	Hypoglycemia
	Urea cycle disorders (early)
	Reye syndrome (early)
	Zinc deficiency
	Protein malnutrition
	Scurvy
	Hyperthyroidism
Cardiac processes	Supraventricular tachycardia
	Congestive heart failure
	Pericarditis
	Anomalous left coronary—artery from the pulmonary artery
Intracranial processes	Increased intracranial pressure
	Subdural hematoma
	Subdural effusion with meningitis
	Brain tumor
	Seizures
Toxic processes	Lead ingestion
	Vitamin A poisoning
	Narcotic withdrawal
	Fetal alcohol syndrome
Other disorders	Trauma, including nonaccidental
	Respiratory failure
	Foreign body ingestion
	Teething
	Colic
	Hunger

Mechanical problems	Infiltrated intravenous (IV) site
	Entanglement in monitor wires or IV tubing
	Skin irritation from monitor lines
	Blood pressure cuff
	Too small a diaper
	Lying on a foreign body in the bed
	"Hair tourniquet" of a digit

MAJOR THREAT TO LIFE

- Infections (sepsis, meningitis)
- Intra-abdominal conditions (bowel obstruction, appendicitis)
- Metabolic disturbances
- Increased intracranial pressure (ICP)
- Seizures
- Cardiac disorders (dysrhythmia, pericarditis, myocarditis)
- Respiratory failure

Immediate evaluation of an irritable infant should focus on searching for signs suggestive of one of the aforementioned threats and/or recognizing that the infant is at risk for one or more of these conditions because of an underlying illness or its treatment.

BEDSIDE

Quick-Look Test

Irritability can be intermittent, persistent, or progressive. If the infant is quiet by the time of your arrival, this is not necessarily reassuring. Intussusception, anal fissure, seizures, supraventricular tachycardia, gastroesophageal reflux, systemic juvenile idiopathic arthritis, teething, and colic should be greater considerations if the irritability is intermittent. As mentioned before, your differential should also be considered in the context of the child's age.

Airway and Vital Signs

Fever can be associated with irritability in an infant. Fever and irritability, especially in very young infants (younger than 2 months), is sepsis until proven otherwise. This warrants further evaluation, including blood, urine, and cerebrospinal fluid culture and the administration of IV antibiotics (see management section later).

In a critically ill infant, the risks of delaying antibiotic treatment need to be weighed against the benefit of obtaining as many of the cultures mentioned as possible.

Hypothermia: In an infant, hypothermia can also be a sign of infection.

Tachycardia: Tachycardia can be associated with fever. Extreme tachycardia can be suggestive of a cardiac etiology, such as supraventricular tachycardia (see Chapter 22), as well as myocarditis.

Tachypnea: Tachypnea may be secondary to respiratory distress or respiratory failure, infection, such as bronchiolitis or pneumonia, congestive heart failure, or metabolic acidosis.

Hypotension: Hypotension may be related to sepsis or may be related to hemorrhage.

Keep in mind that tachycardia and tachypnea can be secondary to crying and irritability.

Comprehensive Physical Examination

When evaluating an irritable hospitalized infant, the physical exam should be the initial step in your evaluation rather than the usual approach of history taking followed by physical examination. It is critical that the physical examination be especially thorough rather than selective. Particular attention needs to be paid to potential sources of infection (e.g., ears), the abdominal examination, and a careful examination of the extremities. It is very easy to overlook the fact that an infant is not moving an extremity normally because of pain. This may be seen with septic arthritis, osteomyelitis, "hair tourniquets," and trauma (including occult fractures). Carefully inspect any IV sites by removing tape and other coverings so that you can clearly visualize the skin. An infiltrated or infected IV site can easily be overlooked. Remember, the fontanelle exam is as important as the vital signs in an irritable infant. Meningeal signs are not reliable indicators of meningitis in an infant.

HEENT	Fontanelle (flat or bulging?), pupils, conjunctivitis (infections, Kawasaki disease), periorbital soft tissue (cellulitis), tympanic membrane (otitis), auditory canal (foreign body, trauma), nose (rhinorrhea), mouth, pharynx (stomatitis, trauma)
Neck	Adenopathy (Kawasaki disease); erythema, warmth (adenitis)
Chest	Breath sounds (pneumonia, foreign body aspiration, congestive heart failure); breast swelling, warmth (mastitis); erythema, tenderness (rib fracture)

HEENT, Head, Eyes, Ears, Nose, Throat.

Cardiovascular	Heart sounds (myocarditis, pericarditis, supraventricular tachycardia); thrills, heaves (congestive heart failure)
Abdomen	Bowel sounds, distention, masses (bowel obstruction)
Genitalia	Masses (inguinal hernia), testicular swelling or tenderness
Rectal	Masses, stool, bleeding
Extremities	Swelling, warmth (infections); bruising (trauma); cyanosis (respiratory failure), "hair tourniquet"; limited use, limited range of motion, tenderness (trauma, infection)
Neurologic	Focal signs (brain abscess, tumor), seizures (metabolic disturbance)
Skin	Rash, petechiae, purpura (systemic juvenile-idiopathic arthritis, meningococcemia); wounds (trauma)

Selective History and Chart Review

What has the infant's previous behavior been like? How is the infant described in previous notes?

An attempt should be made to determine whether the infant's status has changed. If so, this suggests that either a new problem has developed or the underlying illness being treated during this hospitalization is progressing.

Does the infant have a known infection that is currently being treated?

If so, you need to consider the possibilities of inadequate treatment and/or a complication of the initial infection (e.g., mastoiditis following otitis, meningitis, osteomyelitis, or septic arthritis following bacteremia). Look carefully at the fever pattern during the hospitalization. A recurrence following initial defervescence suggests "seeding" of a distant site after bacteremia.

What has the infant's oral intake been? Has there been any vomiting, constipation, or diarrhea?

The answers may suggest a gastrointestinal cause of the irritability. A change in oral intake may also suggest worsening of an underlying illness.

Has the infant received IV fluids?

Review the type and amount of fluids, as well as any recent electrolyte measurements, to determine the likelihood of a metabolic abnormality to explain the irritability.

What medications has the infant received?

Aspirin, as well as other drugs, may lead to Reye syndrome. Numerous other medications may result in seizures or metabolic disturbances. Recent narcotic or benzodiazepine use raises the possibility of withdrawal symptoms.

Management

Further evaluation and management of an irritable infant depends on the differential diagnosis that you develop after the quick look, physical examination, and history and chart review. It may be apparent at this point that the infant's irritability is not a significant change in status or can easily be attributed to the underlying reason for admission. If this is the case, continuing the present management with observation of the infant may be the most appropriate next step. However, it needs to be emphasized that continued and frequent observation is the key element of this approach and that further evaluation may become necessary if the irritability either changes in character or persists.

If the irritability of the infant is believed to be either "new" or different in character, further evaluation is necessary and depends on the suspected diagnoses. As mentioned earlier, if new or worsening fever is present, especially in infants less than 2 months of age, a complete evaluation for sepsis should be initiated. This includes obtaining a blood culture, urine culture, and cerebrospinal fluid (CSF) culture, followed by immediate administration of empiric antibiotics. The choice of antibiotics depends on the infant's age, as well as special considerations, such as the presence of a venticuloperitoneal shunt, recent surgery, or immunodeficiency (see Chapter 18 for further discussion). If an intra-abdominal process is suspected, the infant should be given nothing orally, and radiographs and surgical consultation may be necessary (see Chapter 6). If metabolic disturbances remain a possibility, serum electrolyte, calcium, glucose, and ammonia measurements are helpful, followed by appropriate correction of the disturbance if present. Neurologic signs suggesting seizures or increased ICP should be managed appropriately (see Chapter 7).

In some cases, no other identifiable clues may be present to help guide further evaluation. In these circumstances, it may be best to pursue additional studies and management, with the goal being to exclude and empirically treat the major threats to life. Ask yourself "What could be happening *at the moment* that is potentially life threatening?" Remembering that sepsis is always a possibility, blood, CSF, and urine cultures should be obtained and antibiotics begun empirically in a young infant (<2 months) and in an older infant who appears particularly ill. In an older infant, this decision requires clinical judgment and potentially a discussion with supervisors or consultants. Serum electrolyte, calcium, and glucose levels should be determined if a recent result is unavailable. As emphasized previously, repeated evaluations of the infant are necessary in this situation to ensure that the abdominal, cardiac, respiratory, or neurologic status is not changing. Additional studies depend on your findings as the process evolves.

Evaluation of an irritable infant requires a careful, thorough approach and is therefore often a time-consuming and potentially frustrating process. Remember that your goals while on call are to (1) identify a cause and treat it when possible and (2) exclude or empirically treat life-threatening illness. This should help you prioritize and prevent you from becoming as "irritable" as the patient.

CHAPTER 13

Cyanosis

Rachel T. Sullivan, MD

Cyanosis is blue to purple discoloration of the skin and is typically a clinical diagnosis made by visualization of the skin. Cyanosis is a result of decreased arterial oxygen saturation of hemoglobin or increased oxygen utilization in tissues. As with many problems in pediatrics, appropriate evaluation of a patient with cyanosis depends on the age of the child. The diagnoses you consider when confronted with cyanosis in a neonate differ from those you consider when evaluating an older child or adolescent. Regardless of age, the key distinction should be made between peripheral cyanosis and central, or generalized, cyanosis.

Peripheral cyanosis is, by definition, present in the extremities, with sparing of the central regions of the body. It is usually the result of localized vascular changes that lead to poor perfusion and/or venous stasis. Peripheral cyanosis may be secondary to vascular phenomena (e.g., "physiologic" acrocyanosis of the newborn, Raynaud phenomenon, sepsis), obstructive processes (superior vena cava syndrome, deep venous thrombosis, tourniquets), or blood disorders such as hypercoagulability (with subsequent thrombosis) and hyperviscosity (e.g., polycythemia). Typically, the presence of peripheral cyanosis without generalization suggests that primary lung or heart disease is not present.

In contrast, generalized cyanosis is more commonly associated with primary heart disease or respiratory insufficiency but may also occur if some of the processes that cause peripheral cyanosis are severe enough (e.g., sepsis). Generalized cyanosis indicates that a large amount of hemoglobin is in its reduced state (>5 g/dL) or that oxygen saturation is less than approximately 85%. This chapter focuses on generalized cyanosis because it is more common, more likely to be life threatening, and more likely to require extensive evaluation when on call.

The many causes of central cyanosis can be broadly divided into two groups: (1) decreased oxygenation of hemoglobin (often as a consequence of either respiratory insufficiency or cardiac disease) and (2) abnormalities of hemoglobin (methemoglobinemia or hemoglobin with reduced affinity for oxygen). The vast majority of cases encountered in infants and children are a result of decreased oxygenation because of lung or heart disease, but hemoglobin abnormalities should always be considered. In a full-term newborn, cardiac and pulmonary disease should be considered equally, whereas in an older child, congenital heart disease is a less likely consideration. This chapter is divided into two sections, with evaluation of a newborn discussed separately from evaluation of an older child.

Cyanosis in a Newborn

PHONE CALL

Questions

1. What are the vital signs?
2. Is the cyanosis central or peripheral?
3. Are there signs of respiratory distress (tachypnea, grunting, nasal flaring, retracting)?
4. Are there signs of poor perfusion (delayed capillary refill, cold extremities, weak pulses)?
5. How old is the child?
6. Is the infant alert and active and able to feed or lethargic and refusing to feed?

The vital signs and differentiation between central or peripheral cyanosis allow you to determine the urgency of the situation and may also provide clues to the potential cause of the cyanosis. Tachycardia, tachypnea, signs of respiratory distress, poor perfusion, and/or hypotension may indicate sepsis, cardiogenic shock associated with congenital heart disease, or severe respiratory insufficiency. Fever or hypothermia may raise suspicion of septic shock. The age of the infant may provide a clue to the cause. Peripheral cyanosis in the early newborn period may be "physiologic" and of little concern in an otherwise well-appearing neonate. Because the ductus arteriosus normally closes functionally by the third day of life, the onset or worsening of cyanosis at this age may indicate the presence of a congenital heart lesion that depends on ductal flow to perfuse the lungs (i.e., obstructions to pulmonary blood flow, such as with tricuspid atresia or pulmonary atresia) or to provide oxygenated blood to the systemic circulation (e.g., transposition of the great arteries with an intact ventricular septum). Congenital heart lesions with complete mixing of venous and arterial blood may present with cyanosis and hypoxia in the early newborn period without any significant associated respiratory distress.

Exacerbation of the signs of distress with feeding may suggest congestive heart failure. This occurs with congenital heart lesions that result in an increase in pulmonary blood flow (e.g., transposition of the great arteries, truncus arteriosus, and total anomalous pulmonary venous return) or with lesions associated with obstructed left heart outflow (as seen with coarctation of the aorta, valvular aortic stenosis, and hypoplastic left heart syndrome). Lethargy is expected if central nervous system (CNS) depression and secondary respiratory insufficiency are occurring.

Orders

1. If possible, an arterial blood gas sample should be obtained from a site distal to the ductus arteriosus (i.e., the left arm or either leg) while the infant is breathing room air. The infant should then be placed on 100% oxygen, and after at least 10 minutes, a second arterial blood gas sample should be obtained. This test, the hyperoxia test, may help to distinguish primary cardiac disease from lung disease and other potential disorders. In cyanotic congenital heart disease, the partial pressure of O_2 (PaO_2) is not expected to rise to a value greater than 150 mm Hg for mixing lesions or 100 mm Hg in the case of severely restricted pulmonary blood flow (Table 13.1). Pulse oximetry (oxygen saturation analysis) cannot be a substitute for measurement of PaO_2 because saturation reaches the maximum of 100% at approximately 90 mm Hg (see Appendix D, The Oxyhemoglobin Dissociation Curve of Normal Blood). Caution should be used in interpreting the hyperoxia test too strictly. Exceptions to the generalization may occur, and therefore the results should always be interpreted in conjunction with other clinical information.

2. A serum glucose (or Dextrostix) measurement, chest radiograph, and 12-lead electrocardiogram (ECG) should be ordered stat. Additional laboratory measurements that should be

TABLE 13.1	Hyperoxia Test Interpretation	
PaO_2 in Room Air[a]	**PaO_2 in 100% FiO_2**	**(mm Hg)**[a]
Healthy	70	>200
Lung disease	50	>150
Cyanotic Heart Disease		
Decreased pulmonary blood flow	<50	<100
Increased pulmonary blood flow	50	<150
Methemoglobinemia	70	>200

[a]Values are approximations.

obtained include a complete blood count and serum electrolyte determinations.

3. The infant should be placed on a cardiorespiratory monitor with continuous pulse oximetry.

4. An intravenous (IV) line should be placed, and the infant should be maintained without oral intake pending results of the work-up outlined previously.

Inform RN

"I will be there as soon as possible."

A newborn with cyanosis needs to be evaluated immediately.

ELEVATOR THOUGHTS

What is the differential diagnosis of cyanosis in a newborn?

Central cyanosis	See Table 13.2
Peripheral cyanosis	Physiologic acrocyanosis
	Arterial thrombosis
	Vasomotor instability

MAJOR THREAT TO LIFE

Cyanosis in a newborn is nearly always a threat to life, and all of the conditions just listed and in Table 13.2 (with the exception of methemoglobinemia and physiologic acrocyanosis) are potentially fatal. In particular, cardiac conditions that depend on a patent ductus arteriosus for pulmonary or systemic circulation may be fatal within the first few days of life if appropriate interventions are not undertaken in a timely manner.

BEDSIDE

Quick-Look Test

Is the infant alert, active, and breathing comfortably?

If so, you may proceed with slightly less urgency. An infant in obvious distress may need urgent intervention, such as intubation, blood pressure support, and/or initiation of a prostaglandin infusion (see later).

Airway and Vital Signs

Severe compromise of the airway by congenital masses (e.g., goiter, cavernous hemangioma, tumor) is an unusual cause of cyanosis and is obvious on physical examination. Hypotension is the most significant sign and suggests cardiogenic or septic shock (or rarely, salt-wasting congenital adrenal hyperplasia). If hypotension is

TABLE 13.2	Differential Diagnosis of Neonatal Cyanosis

Disease	Mechanism
Pulmonary	
Respiratory distress syndrome	Surfactant deficiency
Sepsis, pneumonia	Inflammation, pulmonary hypertension, shunting R → L
Meconium aspiration pneumonia	Mechanical obstruction, inflammation, pulmonary hypertension, shunting R → L
Persistent fetal circulation	Pulmonary hypertension, shunting R → L
Diaphragmatic hernia	Pulmonary hypoplasia, pulmonary hypertension
Transient tachypnea	Retained lung fluid
Cardiovascular	
Cyanotic heart disease with decreased pulmonary blood flow	R → L shunt as in pulmonary atresia, tetralogy of Fallot
Cyanotic heart disease with increased pulmonary blood flow	R → L shunt as in *d*-transposition, truncus arteriosus
Cyanotic heart disease with congestive heart failure	R → L shunt with pulmonary edema and poor cardiac output, as in hypoplastic left heart syndrome and coarctation of the aorta
Heart failure alone	Pulmonary edema and poor cardiac contractility, as in sepsis, myocarditis, supraventricular tachycardia, or complete heart block; high-output failure, as in patent ductus arteriosus, vein of Galen, or other arteriovenous malformation
Central Nervous System	
Maternal sedative drugs	Hypoventilation, apnea
Asphyxia	CNS depression
Intracranial hemorrhage	CNS depression, seizure
Neuromuscular disease	Phrenic nerve palsy, hypotonia, hypoventilation, pulmonary hypoplasia
Hematologic	
Acute blood loss	Shock
Chronic blood loss	Congestive heart failure
Polycythemia	Pulmonary hypertension
Methemoglobinemia	Low-affinity hemoglobin or red blood cell enzyme defect
Metabolic	
Hypoglycemia	CNS depression, congestive heart failure
Adrenogenital syndrome	Shock (salt losing)

CNS, Central nervous system; *R → L*, right-to-left intracardiac (foramen ovale), extracardiac (ductus arteriosus), or intrapulmonary shunting.

From Behrman RE: Nelson Textbook of Pediatrics, 14th ed. Philadelphia, WB Saunders, 1992, p 464.

present, support of blood pressure should proceed while you are pursuing your evaluation (see Chapter 25). In addition to standard support with maintenance of intravascular volume and vasopressors if necessary, consideration may need to be given to the use of prostaglandin E_1 infusion if any ductal-dependent lesion (e.g., hypoplastic left heart syndrome or critical coarctation of the aorta) is a possibility (see "Management," later). As noted earlier, tachypnea and/or tachycardia can be expected in many cardiac and pulmonary disorders. Weak respiratory effort may suggest CNS depression from maternal drugs, birth asphyxia, or neuromuscular disorders.

Selective Physical Examination

When evaluating a cyanotic newborn, you should ask three questions to help guide your further evaluation and treatment:

Are there signs of respiratory distress?

If none are present, primary lung disease is unlikely.

Are there signs of congestive heart failure and/or hypotension and poor perfusion?

Congestive heart failure suggests congenital heart disease associated with increased pulmonary blood flow; the additional findings of poor perfusion and/or hypotension suggest obstruction to left heart outflow. Sepsis, myocarditis, supraventricular tachycardia, adrenal insufficiency, or complete heart block may also produce these signs, but the degree of cyanosis is not usually as great in these conditions.

Are there signs of CNS depression?

The infant's mental status should be assessed immediately, with simultaneous questioning regarding irritability, lethargy, and general responsiveness. Any sign of a depressed level of consciousness is concerning.

General	Evaluation of a cyanotic newborn requires a fairly quick but complete physical examination.
	The presence of any dysmorphic features or extracardiac congenital malformations, especially midline defects (e.g., cleft lip or palate), increases the likelihood of congenital heart disease.
HEENT	Pupillary constriction (maternal narcotics); cyanosis of the oral and mucous membranes, usually the most easily recognized sites, implies generalized cyanosis; nasal flaring (respiratory distress); midline defects such as cleft lip or palate
Neck	Masses (airway compromise), deviation of the trachea (congenital heart disease, tension pneumothorax)
Chest	Grunting, retractions (respiratory distress); abnormal breath sounds (pneumonia, congestive heart failure)

HEENT, Head, Eyes, Ear, Nose, Throat.

Cardiac	Hyperdynamic precordium, thrills, heaves (ventricular hypertrophy, volume overload from left-to-right shunting); point of maximum impulse (situs inversus, cardiomegaly); silent precordium (pericardial effusion, cardiomyopathy); murmurs (congenital heart disease)
Lungs	Breath sounds (pneumonia, respiratory distress syndrome, meconium aspiration), absent breath sounds (pulmonary hypoplasia, diaphragmatic hernia, pneumothorax)
Abdomen	Scaphoid (diaphragmatic hernia); location of the liver, spleen (situs inversus)
Pulses	Weak (coarctation, hypoplastic left heart, aortic stenosis, sepsis), femoral and brachial pulses unequal (coarctation)
Genitalia	Ambiguous (congenital adrenal hyperplasia)
Neurologic	Lethargy, hypotonia, lack of response to stimuli (central nervous system depression from maternal drugs, birth asphyxia)
Skin	Cyanosis, petechiae, purpura (sepsis)

Selective History and Chart Review

Review the maternal history. Did the neonate's mother have any illnesses during pregnancy? What is the gestational age of the infant? Did the mother receive antibiotics or narcotics during labor and delivery? If so, why?

A maternal infection perinatally is a risk factor for neonatal sepsis. Maternal narcotics may be passed transplacentally and affect the infant postnatally, especially if administered close to the time of delivery. Maternal systemic lupus erythematosus is a risk factor for congenital heart block in a neonate. The gestational age can give you insight into how well developed the newborn's lungs are. When infants are born prematurely, they have a higher chance of incomplete lung development and subsequently higher risk of respiratory distress as a result. Whether antenatal steroids were given can be helpful as well because administration of steroids to a pregnant mother who is expecting a preterm delivery can help to promote lung development.

Was the delivery complicated? Was meconium present, and if so, was it visualized below the vocal cords of the infant at the time of delivery? What were the Apgar scores? What interventions were required as part of the neonatal resuscitation?

Meconium aspiration, which may lead to pneumonia and/or persistent fetal circulation, should be specifically investigated.

The Apgar scores may suggest birth asphyxia and subsequent CNS impairment.

Is there a family history of congenital heart disease?

A previous family history increases the risk for disease in the child being evaluated.

Management

By the time you have completed the quick-look test, check of the airway and vital signs, and selective physical examination and history, it may remain unclear whether the newborn has a primary respiratory problem, cardiac disease, or one of the other potential causes of cyanosis. An algorithm for the further evaluation of a cyanotic newborn is presented in Fig. 13.1. An abnormal hyperoxia test result (failure to detect an appropriate rise in PaO_2) effectively excludes causes other than lung or heart disease, makes congenital heart disease most likely, and allows you to concentrate on further differentiating heart from lung disease. The chest radiographic findings and ECG results can be extremely valuable tools to help differentiate congenital heart disease from lung disease and also to allow preliminary discrimination of the various forms of cyanotic heart disease. The presence of a specific congenital heart lesion can then be confirmed with echocardiography.

Abnormal Hyperoxia Test Result

Chest Radiograph

When interpreting the chest radiograph, several questions should be asked.

Is a primary lung process responsible for the cyanosis?

Infiltrates and/or consolidation, suggesting pneumonia or meconium aspiration, may be present. A diaphragmatic hernia may not be obvious by physical examination and should be ruled out by chest radiograph. If meconium aspiration, pneumonia, or a diaphragmatic hernia is present, persistent fetal circulation (persistent pulmonary hypertension) should be strongly suspected. This condition can be detected by obtaining arterial blood gas samples from both a preductal (right arm) and a postductal (left arm or legs) vessel. A decrease in PaO_2 in the postductal sample relative to the preductal sample suggests right-to-left shunting across the ductus as a result of pulmonary hypertension. If both determinations are extremely low (<40 mm Hg) and the other clinical findings suggest persistent fetal circulation, there may be significant intracardiac right-to-left shunting across the foramen ovale as a result of the same process.

If the lung fields do not reveal signs of inflammation, consolidation, or diaphragmatic hernia, heart disease is more likely (if the

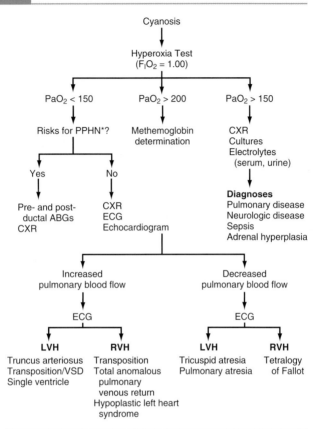

FIGURE 13.1 Approach to cyanosis in a newborn.

*PPHN, persistent pulmonary hypertension (also known as persistent fetal circulation)
ABG, arterial blood gases
CXR, chest radiograph
ECG, electrocardiography
LVH, left ventricular hypertrophy
RVH, right ventricular hypertrophy
VSD, ventricular septal defect

hyperoxia test result is abnormal), and one should then ask the next question.

Are there increased pulmonary markings, suggesting increased pulmonary blood flow, or is there a paucity of markings, suggesting diminished pulmonary blood flow?

As shown in Fig. 13.1, increased pulmonary blood flow is associated with a different set of congenital heart lesions than decreased pulmonary blood flow is.

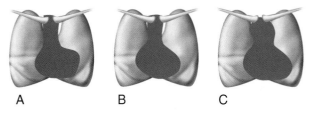

A   B   C

FIGURE 13.2 **Abnormal cardiac silhouette. (A)** "Boot-shaped" heart seen in a cyanotic child with the tetralogy of Fallot or tricuspid atresia. **(B)** "Egg-shaped" heart seen in transposition of the great arteries. **(C)** "Snowman" sign seen in total anomalous pulmonary venous return (supracardiac type). (From Park MK: Pediatric Cardiology for Practitioners, 2nd ed. Chicago, Year Book, 1988, p 54.)

What is the shape of the heart?

A few lesions may result in a characteristic cardiac silhouette (Fig. 13.2).

Shape	Defect
Boot	Tetralogy of Fallot
	Tricuspid atresia
Egg on a string	Transposition of the great arteries
Snowman	Total anomalous pulmonary venous return

Where is the aortic arch?

A right-sided aortic arch is associated with intracardiac defects 40% of the time.

Electrocardiogram

The most distinguishing features of the ECG in the various forms of congenital heart disease are the presence and pattern of ventricular hypertrophy (see Fig. 13.1).

Echocardiogram

Once congenital heart disease is suspected, you should consult with a pediatric cardiologist and arrange for an echocardiogram to confirm the diagnosis.

Normal Hyperoxia Test Result

If the hyperoxia test result is normal and the infant has no signs that suggest heart or lung disease, other potential causes need to be considered further. In this case, sepsis remains a possibility and appropriate cultures should be obtained before starting broad-spectrum antibiotic coverage for the most common neonatal pathogens (see Chapter 18). CNS disease should be easily excluded if there are no signs of CNS depression in the infant and the maternal and delivery history is unremarkable. Hypoglycemia should have been detected by Dextrostix testing and corrected appropriately. The salt-wasting variant of congenital adrenal hyperplasia in a female infant is suggested by the presence of abnormal genitalia. Because a male infant with this disorder may have normal genitalia, the diagnosis depends on laboratory measurement of serum and urine electrolytes. Methemoglobinemia should be suspected if the cyanotic infant appears well, the infant has an otherwise normal examination, and the infant's blood appears "chocolate brown" when exposed to room air.

Treatment

Further management depends on the diagnosis made after the evaluation just presented.

Cyanotic Heart Disease

If the clinical findings, arterial blood gas results, chest radiogram, and ECG findings are consistent with congenital heart disease, immediate consultation with a pediatric cardiologist is necessary. Admission to an intensive care unit, where appropriate monitoring can occur, is also necessary. If the infant has a suspected lesion that is dependent on flow through the ductus arteriosus, consideration should be given to initiation of a prostaglandin E_1 infusion. Prostaglandin E_1 vasodilates the ductus arteriosus and improves pulmonary or systemic blood flow, depending on the specific cardiac lesion that is present. The infusion can be initiated at 0.05 to 0.1 µg/kg/min and increased to 0.4 µg/kg/min if necessary to achieve therapeutic response with increased oxygenation or increased systemic perfusion. Once therapeutic response is achieved, reduce the rate to the lowest dosage where clinical effectiveness is obtained. The rate of infusion should be titrated according to the response in PaO_2 or the improvement in peripheral perfusion. The infant should be monitored closely because apnea is a potential complication. The infusion often adequately stabilizes the infant's condition until a full cardiac evaluation can be completed. Oxygen should be administered and respiratory status and oxygen saturations monitored closely.

Pneumonia or Respiratory Distress

Ventilatory support, antibiotics, selective pulmonary vasodilators, and extracorporeal membrane oxygenation may all be required. Admission to an intensive care unit and neonatology consultation may be necessary depending on the level of respiratory support that is required (see Chapter 28). If a diaphragmatic hernia is present, intensive care monitoring and surgical consultation are also necessary. Antibiotics are required as are cultures of blood and urine.

Sepsis

As mentioned earlier, appropriate cultures and broad-spectrum antibiotic coverage are required.

Hypoglycemia

Hypoglycemia may be seen alone or in connection with one of the other disorders causing cyanosis and should be appropriately corrected (see Chapter 35).

Central Nervous System Disorders

Brain or spinal cord injury from birth trauma can be confirmed by computed tomography (CT) or magnetic resonance imaging (MRI). Hypoxic-ischemic injury (asphyxia) may also result in cerebral edema that can be detected by CT scanning. Care should be supportive. Neurologic injury places these infants at higher risk for seizures. If clinical concerns arise for the presence of seizures, the infant may require monitoring with an electroencephalogram (EEG).

Narcosis causing cyanosis, hypotonia, and slow, shallow respirations is a result of heavy doses of opioids, meperidine, or barbiturates taken by or given to the mother shortly before delivery. It can be treated with naloxone, 0.1 mg/kg, intravenously, intramuscularly, subcutaneously, or intratracheally. If the initial dose is unsuccessful, repeated doses may be given at 2- to 3-minute intervals.

Methemoglobinemia

Methemoglobin is the product of oxidation of hemoglobin to the ferric state. It is present in healthy people, but the erythrocytic reducing system maintains amounts at less than 2% of the total hemoglobin content. Methemoglobinemia may be hereditary (a deficiency of the reducing enzyme nicotinamide adenine dinucleotide (NADH)_ cytochrome b_5 reductase) or may occur secondary to exposure to a toxin (aniline dye, benzocaine, nitrites). Methylene blue, 1 mg/kg intravenously, can be used to treat both hereditary and toxin-related methemoglobinemia. To confirm the diagnosis, methemoglobin levels in the blood can be measured.

Congenital Adrenal Hyperplasia

The salt-losing form of 21-hydroxylase deficiency causes virilization, vomiting, dehydration, and potentially cyanosis in the newborn period. As noted earlier, male infants may have normal genitalia. Low serum sodium and chloride and high potassium levels may be present. Plasma renin levels are elevated, as are serum levels of 17-hydroxyprogesterone and urinary 17-ketosteroids. Contrast imaging of the urogenital tract in virilized females may be helpful when the genitalia are particularly ambiguous. Treatment is aimed at replacing glucocorticoid and mineralocorticoid, as well as sodium. A dehydrated infant needs volume and sodium replacement initially (see Chapter 15, Diarrhea and Dehydration) and then hydrocortisone (10–15 mg/m^2/day orally in three divided doses), fludrocortisone 0.05 to 0.3 mg daily in one or two divided doses, and sodium chloride (1–3 g/day) as maintenance therapy.

Cyanosis in an Older Child

PHONE CALL

Questions

1. What are the vital signs?
2. Are there signs of respiratory distress?
3. Are there signs of altered mental status?
4. Is the cyanosis generalized or localized?
5. Why is the child hospitalized? Is there a history of lung or heart disease?

Cyanosis in an older child is seen most often in the context of lung disease, such as pneumonia, reactive airway disease, or an exacerbation of cystic fibrosis. Changes in mental status may suggest a neurologic cause for hypoventilation and secondary cyanosis. Alternatively, mental status changes may be a result of hypoxia. Remember, cyanotic older children frequently become acidotic and symptomatic more quickly than newborns do because they lack the adaptations that allow newborns to tolerate lower levels of oxygen, such as fetal hemoglobin, higher hematocrit, and increased levels of 2,3-diphosphoglycerate (2,3-DPG).

Orders

1. An arterial blood gas determination should be done as soon as possible. Oxygen should be administered and the patient placed on continuous cardiorespiratory monitoring and pulse oximetry.
2. An IV line should be placed if not already present.
3. A complete blood count and serum glucose (or Dextrostix) measurement should be obtained and extra blood drawn into a red-top tube and saved (if toxicology screening studies or serum chemistry studies are thought to be necessary after your further evaluation).
4. A stat chest radiograph and ECG should be obtained.
5. If the child is febrile or there are significant infectious concerns, appropriate cultures should be obtained.

Inform RN

"I will be there right away"

Cyanotic patients should be evaluated immediately.

ELEVATOR THOUGHTS

What are the causes of cyanosis beyond the newborn period?

Pulmonary	Pneumonia
	Reactive airway disease
	Foreign body
	Cystic fibrosis
	Pneumothorax
	Pulmonary hemorrhage
	Bronchiectasis
	Pulmonary embolism
	Aspiration
	Primary pulmonary hypertension
Cardiac	Congenital heart disease
	Myocarditis
	Tetralogy of Fallot "spells"
	Dysrhythmia
	Cardiomyopathy
Neurologic	Encephalopathy
	Encephalitis
	Toxins
	Metabolic disease
	Neuromuscular disease
	Seizure
Hematologic	Polycythemia
	Hypercoagulable state
	Methemoglobinemia
Peripheral or localized	Arterial thrombosis
	Raynaud phenomenon
	Compartment syndrome (traumatic)
	Superior vena cava syndrome
	Septic shock with poor peripheral perfusion
Infectious	Sepsis

MAJOR THREAT TO LIFE

Cyanosis in an older child nearly always indicates a critical underlying process. With the exception of Raynaud phenomenon and methemoglobinemia, the other possibilities are all life threatening.

BEDSIDE

Quick-Look Test

A cyanotic older child commonly has other signs of respiratory distress or may also appear lethargic or obtunded if neurologic disease is present or the hypoxia is severe and prolonged. The paroxysmal hypercyanotic episodes experienced by young children with the tetralogy of Fallot ("tet spells") may result in syncope after a short period of respiratory distress.

Airway and Vital Signs

Because most older children with cyanosis have lung disease, particular attention should focus on the airway and the presence of tachypnea. If there is any compromise, intubation may be required. Bradycardia and hypotension are ominous signs in a cyanotic child. Shallow, slow respirations suggest neurologic dysfunction and hypoventilation.

Selective Physical Examination

HEENT	Edema, proptosis, localized cyanosis (superior vena cava syndrome); pupillary constriction or dilation (narcosis or other ingestion); ptosis (neuromuscular disease); nasal flaring (respiratory distress)
Neck	Distended neck veins (congestive heart failure, superior vena cava syndrome), deviation of the trachea (tension pneumothorax), use of accessory muscles
Lungs	Breath sounds, grunting, retracting (respiratory distress, congestive heart failure, pneumothorax, foreign body); stridor; wheezing; weak respiratory effort (neuromuscular disease, central nervous system disease)
Heart	Rate and rhythm (dysrhythmias), single loud S_2 sound (pulmonary hypertension), murmurs (a temporary decrease in the intensity of a systolic murmur is associated with hypercyanotic spells in the tetralogy of Fallot), S_3 or S_4 sound (heart failure)
Extremities	Weak pulses (myocarditis or cardiomyopathy and congestive heart failure, arterial thrombosis, compartment syndrome, sepsis), edema (congestive heart failure), local cyanosis (thrombosis, vasospasm, compartment syndrome), clubbing (chronic lung or cyanotic

Neurologic	heart disease), transient pallor of the digits changing to cyanosis and then hyperemia (Raynaud phenomenon), muscle tenderness (compartment syndrome)
Neurologic	Weakness, decreased reflexes (neuromuscular disease); altered mental status (encephalitis, toxin)

Selective History and Chart Review

Has the cyanosis been chronic or recurrent, or is this an acute episode? Is there a history of chronic heart or lung disease?

Mild cyanotic heart disease may go undetected for years; therefore a history of previous cyanosis may be helpful. The same is true of chronic lung disease, such as cystic fibrosis or primary pulmonary hypertension. Suspicion of a "tet spell" is obviously high in those with a known history. These spells are characterized by rapid and deep respiration pattern, irritability, cyanosis, and decreased intensity of cardiac murmur. Cyanotic heart disease may be associated with polycythemia. Pneumothorax may occur in those with known lung disease, such as reactive airway disease or cystic fibrosis.

In a patient with respiratory distress, is the history suggestive of foreign body or chemical aspiration?

This should be considered, especially in a toddler.

Does the patient have any other known chronic medical conditions, in particular chronic CNS disease (seizure disorder, cerebral palsy, severe developmental delays, etc.)? How is the patient fed, orally or via tube? Is there any association of the onset of symptoms with timing of an episode of emesis, a choking event, or an oral feed?

Patients with known CNS disorder and developmental delays are at higher risk for aspiration. History and chest radiograph findings can be used in combination to determine the likelihood of aspiration as the etiology of cyanosis.

Has the patient had fever, upper respiratory symptoms, or "flu" symptoms?

This raises suspicion of lung infection, sepsis, or myocarditis. In a child with neurologic findings, this would lead more toward a diagnosis of encephalitis or postinfectious Guillain-Barré syndrome and secondary respiratory insufficiency.

What medications has the patient received? Has there been exposure to dyes or chemicals?

One should specifically look for narcotics, barbiturates, or substances known to produce methemoglobinemia.

Is the patient predisposed to a hypercoagulable state?

This may cause pulmonary embolism or arterial thrombosis. Oral contraceptive use, antiphospholipid antibodies, and immobilization are risk factors for hypercoagulability.

If cyanosis is localized to the distal end of an extremity and is associated with pain, is the patient at risk for compartment syndrome?

Trauma (e.g., fractures) or excessive exercise and muscle swelling can precipitate compartment syndrome.

Management

In nearly all cases of cyanosis in an older child, a respiratory, cardiac, or neurologic cause is readily apparent, and management should proceed as indicated by the underlying disorder (see Chapters 7, 10, 22, and 28). Management of a few selected processes that are associated with hypercyanosis and are not discussed elsewhere is presented here.

Tetralogy of Fallot

Placement of the child in the knee-chest position compresses the femoral arteries and increases systemic vascular resistance, thereby decreasing right-to-left shunting across the ventricular septal defect and improving pulmonary blood flow. Oxygen should be administered and the child calmed as much as possible. Morphine, 0.05 mg/kg to a maximum of 0.2 mg/kg subcutaneously or intramuscularly, may aid in relaxing a young child. If these measures are unsuccessful or if the attack is particularly severe, administration of IV sodium bicarbonate should be considered to correct the metabolic acidosis that quickly develops as the PaO_2 is maintained below 40 mm Hg. IV propranolol (0.1–0.2 mg/kg) may also be considered to alleviate the tachycardia that often accompanies episodes and may impede adequate pulmonary blood flow. IV ketamine (1–2 mg/kg IV or 3–5 mg/kg IM) may help by increasing systemic vascular resistance and providing beneficial sedating effects to the infant.

Polycythemia

If polycythemia is severe enough (hematocrit of 65% to 70%) and associated with hyperviscosity, plethora, and/or cyanosis, consideration should be given to phlebotomy and replacement of whole blood with plasma, 5% albumin, or normal saline solution. The volume replaced can be calculated as follows:

$$\text{Volume (mL)} = \frac{\text{Estimated blood volume (mL)} \times \text{Desired hematocrit change}}{\text{Starting hematocrit}}$$

Arterial Thrombosis

If there is concern for thrombosis, ultrasound study should be obtained to aid in diagnosis. Heparinization may relieve the clot and prevent further thrombosis in those with a hypercoagulable state. An initial IV bolus of 50 U/kg should be followed by a maintenance infusion of 10 to 25 U/kg/h. The partial thromboplastin time should be maintained at 1.5 to 2.5 times normal.

Raynaud Phenomenon

An episodic, triphasic (white-blue-red) color change of the digits, usually bilateral and symmetrical, associated with cold exposure or anxiety should suggest vasospasm. Most cases can be managed by simple rewarming. Refractory cases can be treated with nifedipine, 10 mg 1 to 3 times a day.

Compartment Syndrome

Immediate surgical consultation is required because fasciotomy is necessary to relieve pressure and restore adequate blood flow.

Summary

Cyanosis is a challenging problem and usually represents a true emergency. A stepwise approach as outlined here that combines a selective physical examination and a few laboratory and radiographic studies usually allows you to determine a cause in an efficient manner and begin appropriate treatment. It should be clear that by thinking logically about the problem, you can take the actions necessary to ensure that neither you nor the patient is "blue."

CHAPTER 14

Delivery Room Problems

Kathryn M. Rubey, MD

A call requesting the presence of a pediatrician at the delivery of a newborn may be received for several reasons. The call may be "routine" (e.g., request for a pediatrician to be present for cesarean section or instrument-assisted delivery), for premature delivery, multiple births, or because fetal monitoring during labor reveals fetal distress. For any type of call, you should always be prepared to resuscitate the newborn and to manage several other potential problems discussed in this chapter.

PHONE CALL

Questions

1. What is the expected gestational age?
2. Is the amniotic fluid clear?
3. How many babies are expected?
4. Are there any additional risk factors (e.g., no prenatal care, maternal infection, maternal substance abuse)?

The younger the gestational age, the more likely the presence of immature lungs in the newborn and subsequent respiratory distress at birth. Fetal tachycardia (>160 beats per minute [bpm]) or bradycardia (<120 bpm) or a fetal scalp blood pH less than 7.25 suggests fetal distress. Tachycardia may be seen with fetal hypoxia, maternal fever, or anemia. Bradycardia may be seen with hypoxia, inadvertent administration of anesthetic to the fetus, or congenital heart block. Understanding the relationship of bradycardia to uterine contractions (decelerations) may be helpful (Fig. 14.1). Late decelerations reflect fetal hypoxia from lack of sufficient uteroplacental blood flow, whereas early and variable decelerations are less worrisome. Hypoxia results in acidosis and a fall in fetal scalp blood pH. A value less than 7.20 indicates significant

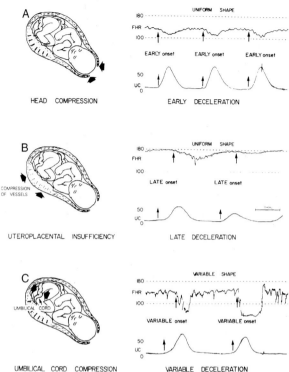

FIGURE 14.1 **Three types of decelerations. (A)** Early decelerations reflect head compression with contractions of the uterus. **(B)** Late decelerations occur when there is uteroplacental insufficiency as a result of compression of the blood supply to the placenta during uterine contraction. **(C)** Variable decelerations occur with umbilical cord compression during uterine contraction. *FHR*, Fetal heart rate; *UC*, uterine contraction.

distress and is generally a reason for immediate early delivery. Passage of meconium into amniotic fluid may be a sign of fetal distress and presents an added risk to the infant because this meconium may be aspirated into the lungs at delivery and result in obstruction of small airways and perhaps secondary complications (persistent fetal circulation, pneumonia).

Several maternal illnesses may potentially complicate delivery. Maternal infections may place the newborn at risk for sepsis, diabetes may result in macrosomia and a difficult delivery, and maternal systemic lupus erythematosus may give rise to congenital heart block.

Orders

You should ask the delivery room nurse to make sure that the infant warming table is prepared in the event that resuscitation is necessary. A laryngoscope, laryngoscope blades, several sizes of endotracheal tube (sizes 2.5 to 4.5), an umbilical catheterization tray, intravenous (IV) angiocatheters, butterfly needles, and syringes, in addition to oxygen and wall suction, should be present. Naloxone as well as epinephrine, atropine, sodium bicarbonate, surfactant, and dopamine should be readily available.

Inform RN

"I will be there right away."

You need to go directly to the delivery room. It is optimal to arrive well before the delivery so that you have time to briefly review the mother's chart.

ELEVATOR THOUGHTS

What possibilities do I need to anticipate?

Respiratory failure

Hyaline membrane disease (in a premature infant)
Secondary to birth asphyxia or CNS depression
Meconium aspiration
Sepsis
Choanal atresia
Diaphragmatic hernia
Mandibular hypoplasia
Pneumothorax
Cystic adenomatoid malformation
Phrenic nerve paralysis
Pulmonary hypoplasia

Severe anemia (and secondary hydrops fetalis)
Plethora (polycythemia)
Seizures
Congenital malformations (e.g., cleft lip or palate)
Birth injury
Shock

CNS, Central nervous system.

MAJOR THREAT TO LIFE

All of the aforementioned are major threats.

BEDSIDE

Quick-Look Test

You should look to see whether delivery is imminent. If not, you should find and review the maternal history.

Selective Maternal History

Does the mother have any medical illnesses?

Specifically, diabetes, hypertension, systemic lupus erythematosus, chronic renal disease, chronic lung or heart disease, and sickle cell anemia may affect the developing fetus and potentially predispose to problems at birth.

Does the mother use narcotics, alcohol, cocaine, tobacco, or other drugs? Has the mother received narcotics during labor?

All may affect the fetus and newborn infant. Narcotics administered within 1 hour of delivery may result in significant central nervous system (CNS) depression in the newborn.

Is there a history of previous high-risk pregnancies?

Such a history may increase the risk associated with the current pregnancy.

Has the mother had any infections during pregnancy? Does she have a current infection? Is she receiving or has she received antibiotics? Has a cervical culture for group B streptococci been performed, and if so, what are the results?

Rubella, human parvovirus B19, human immunodeficiency virus, cytomegalovirus, toxoplasmosis, herpes simplex, syphilis, tuberculosis, varicella, and hepatitis C may all be transmitted transplacentally and affect the newborn if present during pregnancy. Group B streptococci, *Escherichia coli*, hepatitis B, and herpes simplex may be acquired perinatally.

Have the maternal membranes ruptured, and for how long? What is the maternal white blood cell count?

The risk for neonatal infection secondary to ascension from the cervix and genital tract is greater if the membranes have been ruptured for 18 hours or more and/or maternal leukocytosis is present.

What is the mother's blood type and Rh status?

ABO or Rh incompatibility may result in hemolytic anemia in the newborn.

Has polyhydramnios or oligohydramnios been present?

Polyhydramnios is associated with anencephaly, hydrocephaly, bowel atresia, tracheoesophageal fistula, cleft lip or palate, cystic adenomatoid malformation, and diaphragmatic hernia. Oligohydramnios is associated with pulmonary hypoplasia, renal agenesis, growth retardation, twin-twin transfusion, and fetal anomalies.

Has amniocentesis been performed?

Chromosome abnormalities, neural tube defects (elevated α-fetoprotein level), and the degree of fetal lung maturity (a lecithin-sphingomyelin ratio >2:1 generally indicates maturity) may all be determined with amniocentesis.

Has a nonstress test, a contraction stress test, or a biophysical profile been performed?

Abnormal results of such testing may indicate fetal hypoxia. Interpretation of the nonstress test and contraction stress test may be difficult because of high false-positive rates with these tests.

Fetal Vital Signs

As noted earlier, tachycardia or bradycardia may indicate fetal distress. The pattern of decelerations and the beat-to-beat variability of the fetal heart rate should also be observed. Decreased beat-to-beat variability reflects fetal distress. Maternal fever may indicate infection, in which case the newborn is also at risk.

Management I

Three questions to determine if a newborn needs initial steps at the radiant warmer:
1. Is the newborn term?
2. Is the newborn breathing or crying?
3. Does the newborn have good muscle tone?

At the majority of deliveries, the newborn is crying and vigorous once removed from the perineum; and therefore does not require any immediate intervention other than drying and warming (skin-to-skin contact with mother is recommended), but they may need a period of observation (e.g., if there is prematurity, congenital malformation, or any question of meconium aspiration or sepsis). All infants whose delivery you attend should have an Apgar score assigned (see later) and should be examined thoroughly. If there are meconium-stained fluids, but the infant is vigorous, the child may stay with the mother and requires only bulb suctioning of the mouth and nose.

Newborns who are not breathing, are not vigorous, or are in distress need intervention. The key is to be an astute observer of the transition period to judge which infants need help and which do not.

Respiratory Failure

If the infant is received from the obstetrician and is not crying, is cyanotic, is limp, and has not initiated respirations, initial efforts should be directed toward suctioning the mouth then nose and vigorously stimulating the infant in an effort to provoke respiration. Of note, the seventh edition Neonatal Resuscitation Program (NRP) recommendations for nonvigorous newborns (depressed respirations or poor muscle tone) with meconium-stained fluids are to follow these initial steps of newborn care. Stimulation is best accomplished by rubbing the back of the torso while the infant is in a supine position. Throughout this time, another person should be monitoring the newborn's pulse by auscultating the left side of the chest. Although pulsations may be felt by holding the umbilical stump with the thumb and forefinger, this is less accurate and may underestimate the true heart rate. This person can help your evaluation by tapping out the heart rate on the surface of the warming table. Estimate the heart rate by counting the number of beats for 6 seconds and then multiplying by 10. If the child is not vigorous, a pulse oximetry sensor (placed on the right hand or wrist) and/or electronic cardiac (ECG) monitor leads should be connected to evaluate the heart rate. Continuous positive airway pressure (CPAP) may be used for infants who are breathing with a heart rate of at least 100 bpm but with labored respirations or oxygen saturation below target. If the infant does not respond with a spontaneous breath, improved color, and improved muscle tone within several seconds or if the heart rate is less than 100 bpm, positive pressure ventilation (PPV) with bag and mask should be started at a rate of 40 to 60 breaths/min with flowmeter set to 10 L and 21% oxygen (start between 21% and 30% for infants <35 weeks' gestation) should be administered while you continue to stimulate. Oxygen concentration should be titrated to goal oxygen saturation (see Fig. 14.2 for saturation goal by age in minutes). If you are alone, you should call for help when beginning PPV. Heart rate should be reassessed after 15 seconds. If heart rate is rising, continue PPV and recheck heart rate in 15 seconds. If heart rate is not increasing, assess ventilation. If chest rise is noted, continue PPV and recheck heart rate in 15 seconds. Address ventilation without chest movement with corrective steps (known as "MR. SOPA;" Table 14.1), and reassess after 30 seconds of ventilation with chest movement. If heart rate remains less than 60 bpm after 30 seconds of PPV that moves the chest, intubation with endotracheal ventilation is indicated. Providing 30 seconds of ventilation is strongly recommended; and then if heart rate remains less than 60 bpm, oxygen concentration should be increased to 100% and chest compressions begun. If the infant's mother received a narcotic during labor, they should be managed as above. There is insufficient evidence for the

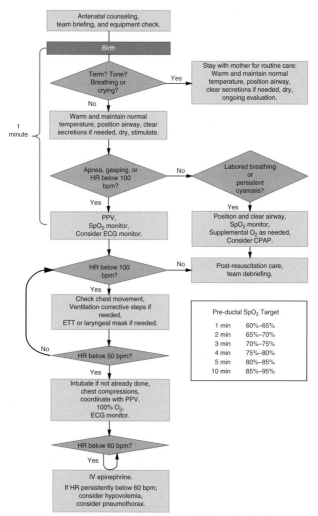

FIGURE 14.2 Seventh edition Neonatal Resuscitation Program flow diagram. *CPAP*, Continuous positive airway pressure; *ECG*, electrocardiogram; *ETT*, endotracheal tube; *HR*, heart rate; *IV*, intravenous; *PPV*, positive pressure ventilation.

TABLE 14.1	The Six Ventilation Corrective Steps: MR. SOPA

	Corrective Steps	Actions
M	Mask adjustment	Reapply the mask. Consider the two-hand technique.
R	Reposition airway	Place head neutral or slightly extended.
	Try PPV and reassess chest movement.	
S	Suction mouth and nose	Use a bulb syringe or suction catheter.
O	Open mouth	Open the mouth and lift the jaw forward.
	Try PPV and reassess chest movement.	
P	Pressure increase	Increase pressure in 5-10 cm H_2O increments, maximum 40 cm H_2O.
	Try PPV and reassess chest movement.	
A	Alternative airway	Place an endotracheal tube or laryngeal mask.
	Try PPV and assess chest movement and breath sounds.	

PPV, Positive pressure ventilation.

safety and efficacy of using naloxone, the narcotic antagonist, in the delivery room with the neonatal population. At this point, you need to call for more "hands" because an umbilical venous catheter or peripheral IV line should be placed and samples drawn for arterial blood gas measurement. Fluid volume, epinephrine, sodium bicarbonate, and vasopressors may all be necessary to resuscitate the infant. Remember, pulmonary hypoplasia, diaphragmatic hernia, or pneumothorax may interfere with adequate ventilation.

If the infant begins to breathe spontaneously and does not require immediate intubation, you should carefully observe the pattern of respiration and look for signs of respiratory distress. Labored breathing, intercostal and subcostal retractions, and tachypnea are worrisome signs and can quickly evolve in a new-born who is initially breathing comfortably. These signs may indicate any of the problems associated with respiratory failure in the newborn, and you should then proceed with a physical examination to determine the probable cause.

Shock

Internal hemorrhage from birth trauma, fetomaternal transfusion, placental abruption, hemolytic anemia, or umbilical cord trauma may result in shock in the newborn. Pallor, poor perfusion, cyanosis, respiratory distress, and cold extremities may all be present at birth. Resuscitation should begin immediately by maintaining the airway and respirations (see earlier) and supporting the circulation. Hypovolemia can be corrected with normal saline solution, plasma, or type O-negative blood after placement of a peripheral IV line or, ideally, umbilical catheters (both arterial and venous). Vasopressors may be necessary to support the blood pressure. Once the infant is stabilized, further evaluation, with a complete physical examination and laboratory studies, can proceed.

Physical Examination

HEENT	Swelling (caput succedaneum, cephalohematoma), indentations (skull fracture), subconjunctival hemorrhages (often considered a "normal" event with delivery), colobomas, ear anomalies, encephaloceles (may obstruct the nose or airway), cataracts, dysmorphic facies
Neck	Masses (goiter, cystic hygroma), tracheal position
Chest	Symmetry and adequacy of chest rise; equal breath sounds; rales; rhonchi; grunting, flaring, retracting (respiratory distress)
Heart	Location of heart sounds (right-sided sounds may indicate congenital heart disease or a shift secondary to diaphragmatic hernia, tension pneumothorax, or a lung mass), murmurs (congenital heart disease), bradycardia (congenital heart block, hypoxia)
Abdomen	Scaphoid, flat, distended (scaphoid suggests diaphragmatic hernia); liver and spleen position (situs inversus may be associated with cyanotic heart disease); umbilical cord inspection for two arteries and one vein (lack of a vessel may be associated with other congenital anomalies, including cardiac defects)
Genitalia	Testes palpable and descended in a male, external genitalia normal in a female
Extremities	Tone (generalized decrease associated with asphyxia or hypoxia, poor perfusion, or neuromuscular disorder), movement (nerve palsy secondary to birth injury), presence of all digits, color (cyanosis, plethora), perfusion
Neurologic	Alert, active, moving all extremities, responsive to stimuli

HEENT, Head, Eyes, Ears, Nose, Throat.

An Apgar score should be assigned at 1 and 5 minutes of life for all infants (Table 14.2). In those requiring resuscitation, 10-, 15-,

TABLE 14.2	Apgar Evaluation of a Newborn Infant		
Sign	**0**	**1**	**2**
Heart rate	Absent	Less than 100 bpm	Over 100 bpm
Respiratory effort	Absent	Slow, irregular	Good cry
Muscle tone	Limp	Some flexion	Active motion
Reflex irritability	No response	Grimace	Cry
Color	Pale	Body pink, extremities blue	All pink

Sixty seconds after complete birth of the infant (disregarding the cord and placenta), the five objective signs above are evaluated, and each is given a score of 0, 1, or 2. A total score of 10 indicates an infant in the best possible condition. An infant with a score of 0 to 3 requires immediate resuscitation.

Modified from Apgar V: A proposal for a new method of evaluation of the newborn infant. Curr Res Anesth Analg 32:260-267, 1953.

and 20-minute scores may also be necessary. The first Apgar score indicates the need for resuscitation, and later scores are more indicative of the potential for morbidity and mortality.

Management II

Severe Anemia

If the infant is born with pallor and shock and appears to be in distress, acute blood loss from a perinatal problem (abruption of the placenta, placenta previa, internal hemorrhage) is more likely than chronic intrauterine anemia. Chronic intrauterine anemia is more likely to produce fetal hydrops and signs of congestive heart failure at birth. In contrast to acute blood loss, laboratory measurements of hemoglobin, the reticulocyte count, and mean cell volume are often abnormal. A newborn infant who is symptomatic and anemic is likely to require a transfusion. Additional evaluation of a newborn with anemia is outlined in Fig. 14.3 and should include a complete blood count, reticulocyte count, Coombs test, peripheral smear review, and a determination of infant and maternal blood types.

Plethora (Polycythemia)

Delayed umbilical cord clamping, twin-twin transfusion, maternal diabetes, and chromosomal abnormalities are a few of the conditions that may result in polycythemia in the newborn, which is defined as a central hematocrit greater than 65%. Many newborns

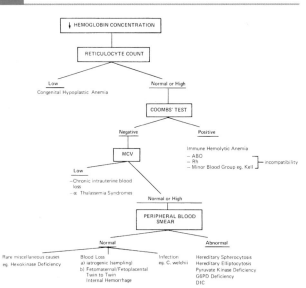

FIGURE 14.3 Algorithm for the evaluation of a newborn with anemia. *DIC*, Disseminated intravascular coagulation; *G6PD*, glucose-6-phosphate dehydrogenase; *MCV*, mean cell volume.

are asymptomatic, but respiratory distress, cyanosis, lethargy, and seizures may all occur. An infant who appears ruddy or reddish purple should be suspected of having polycythemia and should have a hematocrit determination immediately. If polycythemia is present, a partial exchange transfusion should be performed with the aim of reducing the hematocrit to 50%. The volume of the exchange is calculated as follows:

$$\text{Volume (mL)} = \frac{\text{Estimated blood volume (mL)} \times \text{Desired hematocrit change}}{\text{Starting hematocrit}}$$

Seizures

Seizures in the delivery room are most likely secondary to asphyxia and hypoxic or ischemic injury to the CNS. Other possibilities include a structural anomaly of the brain, intracranial bleeding, electrolyte disturbance, hypoglycemia, drug withdrawal, and meningitis or sepsis. A point of care blood glucose, hematocrit, arterial blood gas analysis, and serum electrolyte measurements should be obtained, oxygen administered, and the neonate treated with anti-convulsants (see Chapter 29). Blood cultures, a lumbar puncture, and administration of antibiotics to empirically treat potential causes of meningitis in the neonatal period are also necessary.

Congenital Malformations

Any malformations of the infant noted should be discussed immediately with one or, ideally, both of the parents. If you are unsure of the presence of an anomaly, you should state this to the parents and let them know that you will be discussing it with other physicians (senior residents, neonatologists, the infant's pediatrician) who will be available to examine the infant. If you are unsure of the significance of an anomaly, you should also say so to the parents and again let them know that other physicians will be available to them to fully discuss the particular anomaly and its implications. As the first physician to evaluate their child, the parents will be looking to you for an initial confirmation that all is "perfect" with their newborn. It is imperative that any potential problem be discussed with them immediately. If this is not done, their initial sense of reassurance will be crushed by bad news sometime in the next few days.

Many trips to the delivery room end with your handing over a healthy, swaddled infant to a mother or father, with little or no intervention required on your part. If there has been a problem, you should remember to phone and inform the infant's pediatrician-to-be (if one has been identified) of the problem.

chapter 15

Diarrhea and Dehydration

Karlo Kovacic, MD

Diarrhea is a common problem in the pediatric population. It is generally defined as multiple watery stools in a day. Although usually the result of a gastrointestinal infection, and usually mild and self-limited, it is important to recognize that diarrhea may have a number of potential causes and that the potential complications of diarrhea will vary according to the volume, frequency, and content of stool, as well as the duration of the symptoms and the presence of associated comorbidities.

When asked to evaluate a child with diarrhea, one needs to be aware of the potential for dehydration and anemia (if there is also blood in the stool). Significant anemia, hypovolemia, and electrolyte abnormalities can lead to increased morbidity or even mortality. When called regarding a child with bloody or nonbloody diarrhea, your priorities should be to (1) quickly assess the overall volume status of the child and the need for fluid resuscitation and/or a blood transfusion, (2) appropriately correct volume deficits, (3) appropriately correct electrolyte abnormalities, and (4) identify the most likely cause of the diarrhea. This chapter discusses diarrhea, as well as the general fluid management of hospitalized children. Specific electrolyte abnormalities are discussed in detail in Chapter 34 (Electrolyte Abnormalities).

PHONE CALL

Questions

1. Clarify whether diarrhea is present. Both increased frequency and increased water content define diarrhea.
2. Is there blood in the stool?
3. What are the child's vital signs?

4. How old is the child?
5. How long has the child had diarrhea?
6. Is there mucus or pus in the stool?
7. Why is the child in the hospital?

Hypotension implies significant hypovolemia and requires urgent attention and intervention (see Chapter 25). The infant may be able to maintain normal blood pressure in the face of significant hypovolemia; tachycardia may be the only finding initially. The duration of diarrhea may allow you to estimate the risk for dehydration. Blood or mucus in the stool and the reason for admission may provide clues to the cause of the diarrhea.

Orders

1. If hypovolemia is a concern, the patient should have an intravenous (IV) line placed.
   - If the patient is hypotensive, an immediate 10- to 20-mL/kg bolus of normal saline or lactated Ringer's solution should be ordered (see Chapter 25).
2. Labs: electrolytes, blood urea nitrogen (BUN), creatinine, venous pH, complete blood count with differential, and urinalysis.
   - The serum sodium concentration and hemoglobin are necessary for you to plan appropriate rehydration and/or blood transfusion if needed.
3. The patient should not receive any oral intake until your further evaluation.

Inform RN

"I will arrive at the bedside in … minutes." A child with abnormal vital signs or bloody diarrhea should be evaluated immediately.

ELEVATOR THOUGHTS

What causes diarrhea?

Mild diarrhea without dehydration is a nonspecific finding that may be present with nearly any illness in childhood. Diarrhea as a manifestation of a pathologic condition of the gastrointestinal tract is usually more severe and has greater potential to lead to dehydration.

Infections

Diarrhea in children may result from infection of the gastrointestinal tract itself (gastroenteritis, colitis) or from acute infections elsewhere, such as an upper respiratory infection, pneumonia, hepatitis, or a urinary tract infection.

Viral gastroenteritis	Rotavirus
	Norwalk virus
	Adenovirus
	Influenza
	Enteroviruses
Bacterial colitis	Salmonella, Shigella, Yersinia, or Campylobacter ("SSYC")
	Enteropathogenic *Escherichia coli*
	Staphylococcal food poisoning
	Clostridium difficile (pseudomembranous colitis)
	Vibrio cholerae
	Mycobacterium tuberculosis
Parasitic infection	Giardiasis
	Amebiasis
	Cryptosporidiosis
	Worms (strongyloidiasis, ascariasis, trichuriasis, hookworm, tapeworms)

Malabsorption

Secondary lactase deficiency (e.g., after gastroenteritis)
Eosinophilic gastroenterocolitis
Cystic fibrosis
Celiac disease
Primary immunodeficiencies (including human immunodeficiency virus)
Shwachman-Diamond syndrome
Abetalipoproteinemia

Diarrhea in the Neonate

Milk protein intolerance
Necrotizing enterocolitis
Overfeeding
Congenital diarrhea

Miscellaneous Causes

Medications
Illicit drugs
Laxative abuse
Starvation stools
Inflammatory bowel disease

Irritable bowel syndrome
Henoch-Schönlein purpura
Typhlitis
Appendicitis
Neuroendocrine tumors
Malignancy

MAJOR THREAT TO LIFE

- Dehydration
- Electrolyte abnormalities
- Severe blood loss (if diarrhea is bloody)
- Sepsis

BEDSIDE

Your initial goal should be to determine the degree and type of dehydration, if any. Dehydration can be classified as hyponatremic, isonatremic, or hypernatremic, depending on the serum sodium concentration. The appropriate management of each type of dehydration differs; therefore, it is critical to identify which type is present. Determining the degree of dehydration can usually be accomplished with a brief physical examination and the answers to a few selected questions. If dehydration is present, you should initiate therapy before returning to perform a more detailed physical examination, history, and chart review.

Quick-Look Test

Does the child look well (comfortable), sick (uncomfortable or distressed), or critical?

Infants are often irritable or lethargic if dehydration is present. Older children generally appear ill if the diarrhea is significant.

Airway and Vital Signs

Look carefully at the heart rate and blood pressure. These values provide you with a quick assessment of the degree of hypovolemia, if any. A child with a normal heart rate and blood pressure is unlikely to have severe hypovolemia or anemia. Orthostatic blood pressure should be determined in older children if tachycardia is present in the absence of hypotension. Fever suggests gastroenteritis or colitis.

Selective Physical Examination I

What is the child's volume status?

In addition to the vital signs, estimation of the hydration status of the child can be made by selectively examining the following:

1. Mucous membranes
   Are they moist or dry? How dry? Absence of tears suggests severe dehydration, as do very sunken eyes.
2. Skin turgor
   Normal or decreased? Is there "tenting"? Is the skin "doughy"? Skin turgor can be assessed by gently pinching and releasing the skin over the abdomen between the thumb and forefinger. Normally, in an adequately hydrated person, the skin retracts immediately and quickly. Slow retraction suggests moderate dehydration, and "tenting," or the lack of retraction, suggests severe dehydration. "Doughy" skin is suggestive of hypernatremic dehydration, a condition in which intracellular volume decreases as a means of attempting to maintain equal osmolality between the extracellular and intracellular spaces. In the case of hypernatremic dehydration, the child's appearance may be deceptive. Clinical signs of dehydration may not be as obvious as in the other two forms of dehydration, hyponatremic and isonatremic dehydration, which result in a decrease in extracellular volume and have an insignificant effect on intracellular volume.
3. Capillary refill and temperature of the extremities
   Normal or delayed (>2 seconds) refill? Warm or cool extremities? Delayed capillary refill and/or cool extremities imply inadequate distal perfusion secondary to hypovolemia.
4. Anterior fontanelle (in an infant)
   Flat or sunken?
5. Weight
   Determining the current weight of the child is necessary, and comparing it with a previous recent weight (if known) is also very useful. It is conventional to assign a "percent dehydration" to a dehydrated child (Table 15.1). Either a known amount of weight loss or the estimated percentage can then be used to determine the volume deficit.

Selective History and Chart Review I

Has a previous weight been recorded with which you can compare the current weight?

This allows you to most accurately estimate the volume deficit.
What has the child's urine output been?

TABLE 15.1	Estimation of Volume Deficit in a Dehydrated Child		
Infant	5%	10%	15%
Child	3%	6%	9%
Mucous membranes	Normal	Dry	Parched
Tears	Present	Decreased	Absent
Eyes	Normal	Slightly sunken	Severely sunken
Skin turgor	Normal	Slow retraction	Tenting
Skin temperature	Normal	Slightly cool	Cool, clammy
Capillary refill	<2 s	2-3 s	>3 s
Heart rate	Normal	Mild tachycardia	Severe tachycardia
Fontanelle	Flat	Slightly depressed	Sunken
Urine output	Normal	Decreased	Severe oliguria, anuria

Normal urine output (approximately 1–2 mL/kg/hr and similar to recent intake) suggests that the child is either euvolemic or only mildly dehydrated. Severe oliguria or anuria suggests a large volume deficit. In infants, you may need to base an estimate of urine output on the number of wet diapers per day that the child has had.

Has the child also been vomiting?

Vomiting and diarrhea often coincide, thereby potentially adding to the volume deficit.

Are there other factors that may contribute to volume loss, such as fever or recent surgery?

Management

Principles

Fluid therapy can be divided into three categories:
1. Maintenance therapy
2. Deficit replacement
3. Replacement of ongoing losses

Maintenance therapy is aimed at providing the body's normal daily requirements for fluid and electrolytes. In a healthy person, water is physiologically "lost" through urine, stool, and so-called insensible losses (pulmonary and cutaneous losses). Electrolytes (primarily sodium and potassium) are also lost in urine and stool. These water and electrolyte losses are usually replaced through eating and drinking; however, in those who are ill and hospitalized, oral intake is often greatly reduced or absent, and therefore IV replacement of maintenance fluids is necessary. Several methods are available for estimating a person's maintenance requirements. The simplest method is based on caloric requirements and assumes that 100 mL of water, 2 to 4 mEq of sodium, and 2 to 4 mEq of potassium are necessary for each 100 kilocalories (kcal) expended. The calories expended for a 24-hour period depend on body weight and are estimated by using the following rules for a hospitalized child:

100 kcal/kg for the first 10 kg
50 kcal/kg for the next 10 kg
20 kcal/kg for each kg above 20

Therefore a 30-kg child would expend approximately 1700 kcal/day and require 1700 mL of water and 34 to 68 mEq each of sodium and potassium. A solution of 5% dextrose and 0.2 normal saline with 20 mEq of potassium per liter at a rate of 70 mL/hour adequately approximates these requirements (0.2 normal saline solution contains 0.2×154 mEq/L $= 31$ mEq/L of sodium). This method can be used to calculate the maintenance requirements for a child of any weight, and by determining the appropriate volume (with the rules just presented), appropriate amounts of sodium and potassium can also be provided.

Deficit replacement is aimed at replacing the amount of water and electrolytes that have already been lost. A deficit is present when physiologic and pathologic losses are greater than oral or IV intake. As noted earlier, your initial goal when evaluating a potentially dehydrated child is to determine the severity and type of dehydration.

The severity of dehydration, or the percentage of body weight lost, is determined either by the known difference in weight or by the estimated "percent dehydration" based on clinical findings (see Table 15.1). In infants, total body water is a larger percentage of body weight than in children, and therefore clinical estimates of mild, moderate, or severe dehydration represent a slightly larger deficit.

The type of dehydration (hyponatremic, isonatremic, or hypernatremic) depends on the relative losses of water and sodium, as well as on attempts that have already been made to correct a deficit (e.g., replacement of losses with free water). Hyponatremic dehydration can be defined as a serum sodium concentration less than 130 mEq/L, isonatremic dehydration as a serum sodium concentration of 130 to 150 mEq/L, and hypernatremic dehydration as a serum sodium concentration greater than 150 mEq/L. Most infants and children with diarrhea and dehydration have the isonatremic form (approximately 70%), but certain clues may lead you to suspect either hyponatremia or hypernatremia. An infant who has been given large amounts of free water to replace diarrheal losses is probably hyponatremic. Conversely, an infant with fever and diarrhea who has ingested an inappropriately mixed, highly concentrated formula may have hypernatremia.

Replacement of ongoing losses is appropriate when there are reasons to believe that these losses are significant. For example, a patient with excessive vomiting may continue to lose large amounts of gastric fluid. A child with an ileostomy or excessive burns may also continue to have large fluid losses. These losses must be considered when determining appropriate fluid therapy, or the amount of water and electrolyte replacement may be significantly underestimated.

Treatment

For all but the most mildly dehydrated patients, management should begin with an initial IV fluid bolus of 10 to 20 mL/kg of normal saline solution. The goal is to rapidly expand the extracellular fluid volume, particularly intravascular volume. In severely affected children, the bolus may need to be repeated until signs of improved peripheral perfusion and stable hemodynamics are present. This initial approach is appropriate for hyponatremic, isonatremic, and hypernatremic dehydration and therefore should not be delayed while waiting for the serum sodium result. Hypotonic solutions and those containing potassium should not be used during this initial phase of therapy because the goal is to provide fluid that remains intravascular and potassium may be dangerous if renal function is abnormal or hyperkalemia is already present.

After the initial replenishment of intravascular volume, subsequent therapy is aimed at replacing the calculated deficits of water and electrolytes while also providing ongoing maintenance requirements and replacement of ongoing losses. When determining appropriate subsequent therapy, it is assumed that sodium is the only electrolyte to be replaced. Because calculations are based on the sodium deficit, the extracellular space is preferentially replenished (which is desirable).

The water deficit is determined by a known weight loss (1 kg = 1 L) or estimated by your clinical examination. For children with hyponatremic or isonatremic dehydration, the sodium deficit can be calculated by using the following formula, once the current serum sodium concentration is known:

$$\text{Deficit (mEq)} = (135 - \text{Na})(0.6)(\text{Normal Weight in kg}) +$$

$$(\text{Weight Loss in kg}) \text{Na}$$

where Na is the current measured serum sodium concentration (in mEq) and weight loss is either known or estimated from clinical findings.

Subsequent management depends on the type of dehydration present and is discussed in the following sections.

Isonatremic and Hyponatremic Dehydration

Isonatremic and hyponatremic dehydration are clinical states resulting primarily from loss of extracellular volume. They should be managed as follows:

1. Calculate or estimate the volume deficit (based on weight or clinical examination, respectively).
2. Calculate the sodium deficit with the formula presented earlier.
3. Estimate the daily maintenance requirements (based on normal weight) and add these to the deficit determination (step 1).
4. Subtract the amounts of fluid and sodium already given as boluses to determine the amount of fluid and sodium to be administered over the next 24 hours.
5. Replace half of these amounts in the first 8 hours and half in the remaining 16 hours with a concentration of saline that provides the appropriate amounts of water and sodium as determined by your calculations.
6. Add potassium to the fluids only after the child has voided and you have established that renal function is normal.
7. Replace ongoing losses at 8-hour intervals if they continue to be significant. Table 15.2 lists the estimated electrolyte composition of various body fluids that may be lost abnormally; such charts can be used to determine the concentration of replacement fluids.
8. Check the serum sodium and potassium concentration again in 4 to 6 hours. Also monitor the child's clinical findings and urine output and specific gravity closely as a guide to hydration status.

This plan assumes that symptomatic hyponatremia (altered mental status, seizures) is not present. If the child has symptoms secondary to severe hyponatremia, hypertonic saline infusion may be required initially (see Chapter 34). As noted earlier, the

TABLE 15.2	Estimated Electrolyte Composition of Body Fluids		
Fluid	Na (mEq/L)	K (mEq/L)	Cl (mEq/L)
Gastric	20-80	5-20	100-150
Pancreatic	120-140	5-15	40-80
Bile	120-140	5-15	80-120
Small bowel	100-140	5-15	90-130
Ileostomy	40-135	3-15	20-115
Diarrhea	10-90	10-80	10-110
Burns	140	5	110

amount of sodium administered should then be subtracted when calculating the deficit to be replaced.

Hypernatremic Dehydration

Hypernatremic dehydration results from an excessive loss of free water in the absence of a significant sodium deficit. In contrast to the other types of dehydration, replacement of the water deficit must occur slowly, over a period of 48 hours or more. Rapid decreases in the extracellular fluid sodium concentration may lead to cerebral edema secondary to a large intracellular shift of fluid. For this reason, the goal should be to reduce the serum sodium concentration by no more than 10 mEq/L/day. Management should proceed as follows:

1. Calculate the free water deficit. As noted previously, clinical findings in those with hypernatremic dehydration can be deceptive and may not reflect the severity of dehydration. Therefore, it is often reasonable to estimate a 10% loss of weight unless the weight loss is known. The free water deficit can also be calculated by using the following formula:

$$\text{Deficit}(L) = \text{Normal Total Body Water} - \text{Current Total Body Water}$$

where

$$\text{Normal Total Body Water} =$$

$$\frac{(\text{Current Total Body Water})(\text{Current Osmolality})}{\text{Normal Osmolality}}$$

$$\text{Osmolality} = 2(\text{Na}) + \frac{\text{BUN}}{2.8} + \frac{\text{Glucose}}{18}$$

Therefore

$$\text{Deficit}(L) = \frac{(\text{Current Weight in kg})(0.6)(\text{Current OsM})}{290}$$
$$- (\text{Current Weight in kg})(0.6)$$

2. Subtract the amount of water given as boluses. Add maintenance requirements for 48 hours.
3. Replace the remaining water deficit over a 48-hour period with a solution that is either a one-fourth or one-third normal saline solution initially and check the serum sodium level frequently (i.e., every 2–4 hours initially). It is usually necessary to make frequent adjustments in the concentration and/or rate to ensure an appropriate, slow steady fall in the serum sodium concentration.

4. Add potassium to the IV fluids only after the child has voided and you have established that renal function is normal.
5. Replace ongoing losses every 8 hours if they are significant.
6. After initiating therapy, you should return to perform a more detailed physical examination, history, and chart review to look for clues to the cause of the diarrhea.

Selective Physical Examination II

	Physical exam findings to look for	Conditions to consider
General	Wasted appearance	Starvation tools, laxative abuse, immunodeficiency, malignancy, celiac disease
Cardiac	Murmurs, rubs or gallops	Primary or secondary heart failure
Pulmonary	Rales, wheezes, cough, increased work of breathing	Cystic fibrosis, protein-losing enteropathy, tuberculosis
Abdomen	Bowel sounds, distention, tenderness, organomegaly, masses and protuberance	Gastroenteritis, colitis, appendicitis, celiac disease, inflammatory bowel disease, malignancy, Henoch-Schönlein purpura
Lymph nodes	Adenopathy	Immunodeficiency, malignancy, tuberculosis
Extremities	Edema, tenderness, limited range of motion	Protein-losing enteropathy, inflammatory bowel disease, Henoch-Schönlein purpura
Skin	Rashes	Viral and bacterial gastroenteritis, inflammatory bowel disease, Henoch-Schönlein purpura

Selective History and Chart Review II

Has the child been exposed to others with diarrhea?
If so, a common infection or perhaps staphylococcal food poisoning is suggested.
Is there blood, leukocytes, or eosinophils in the stool?
Blood and/or fecal leukocytes are more consistent with a bacterial cause than a viral one but may also be present with inflammatory bowel disease or some parasitic infections. The stool can be

examined easily for leukocytes by preparing a thin smear on a slide and adding a drop of methylene blue. A Wright stain allows you to identify eosinophils, which may lead to a diagnosis of milk protein allergy in an infant or a parasite in an older child.

In addition to these bedside tests, stool cultures should be considered if bacterial colitis is suspected. A stool sample for ova and parasite detection should also be considered if there is any possibility of this diagnosis.

Has the child received antibiotics? What other drugs has the child received?

Clostridium difficile infection should always be considered in a child older than 12 months in whom diarrhea develops while in the hospital or if the child has received antibiotics recently. There should be a low threshold for sending stool to the laboratory for toxin assays. Mild diarrhea is a common adverse effect of many drugs including antibiotics.

Is there a history of recent gastroenteritis?

Secondary lactase deficiency is a common sequela of gastroenteritis and may lead to persistent mild diarrhea.

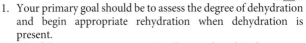

REMEMBER

1. Your primary goal should be to assess the degree of dehydration and begin appropriate rehydration when dehydration is present.
2. All of the management strategies discussed in this chapter are based on multiple estimations. The most critical aspect of managing a dehydrated infant or child is frequent monitoring and reassessment, with appropriate adjustments in therapy. This is especially true in cases of hypernatremic dehydration.
3. Initial management is aimed at rapidly replenishing intravascular volume. After this has been accomplished, you have time to plan your subsequent management.

chapter 16

Extremity Pain

Jennifer Lhost, MD

Extremity pain is a frequent complaint in children. The list of potential causes of extremity pain is extensive; however, very few of these causes are immediately life threatening. When called regarding a child with extremity pain, your primary goal while on call should be to determine the likelihood of an illness that is either life threatening or associated with significant morbidity if the diagnosis is delayed.

PHONE CALL

Questions

1. How old is the child?
2. What is the severity of the pain?
3. Is there pain in one site or in multiple sites?
4. Is there swelling, warmth, or erythema at the affected site?
5. Is the child febrile?
6. Why has the child been hospitalized?

The age of the child may help you narrow the list of possible causes. For example, benign nocturnal leg pains, commonly referred to as "growing pains," are more common in younger children. Similarly, the various malignancies that may produce extremity pain tend to affect children of different ages (e.g., neuroblastoma and leukemia in a younger child, osteogenic sarcoma in an adolescent). The severity of the pain helps you determine the need for an urgent evaluation, but it may not necessarily reflect the seriousness of the underlying problem, particularly in a young child. Multiple painful sites should raise suspicion of a systemic process, whereas a single site makes a localized process more likely. If the affected area appears erythematous and swollen, trauma or infection is suggested. Fever increases the likelihood of an infectious cause, and the child's reason for hospitalization or past history allows you to consider some specific causes (e.g., sickle cell crisis, deep venous thrombosis in a postoperative patient, hypertrophic osteoarthropathy in those with chronic lung disease).

Orders

If not recently administered, acetaminophen or ibuprofen may be given in an attempt to relieve the pain.

Inform RN

A child in severe pain, with fever, or with an extremity that appears abnormal should be seen immediately.

ELEVATOR THOUGHTS

What causes extremity pain? It may help to think anatomically and classify causes according to whether bone, muscle, joint, nerve, blood vessel, or skin and connective tissue are involved. Benign nocturnal pains (growing pains) and behavioral causes of pain are diagnoses of exclusion.

Bone	Osteomyelitis
	Fracture
	Infarction (e.g., in sickle cell crises)
	Malignancy (leukemia, neuroblastoma, primary bone tumor)
	Avascular necrosis
	Osteoid osteoma
	Hypertrophic osteoarthropathy
	Histiocytosis
Joint	Septic arthritis
	Transient synovitis (hip)
	Viral arthritis
	Benign hypermobility
	Slipped capital femoral epiphysis (hip) (9-16 years old)
	Legg-Calvé-Perthes disease (hip) (4-9 years old)
	Serum sickness
	Traumatic arthritis
	Hemarthrosis (e.g., hemophilia)
	Juvenile idiopathic arthritis
	Rheumatic fever
	Lyme disease
	Reactive arthritis
	Systemic lupus erythematosus

Muscle	Myositis
	Infectious
	Traumatic
	Inflammatory (dermatomyositis, polymyositis)
	Electrolyte disturbances
	Cramps
	Muscle strain
Nerve	Neuropathy
	Radiculopathy
	Complex regional pain syndrome
	Guillain-Barré syndrome
Vascular	Deep venous thrombosis
	Coarctation of the aorta
	Arterial thrombosis
	Vasculitis (which may also cause secondary neuropathy, arthritis, or myositis)
Connective tissue	Fasciitis
	Compartment syndrome
Skin and subcutaneous tissue	Herpes zoster
	Cellulitis
	Trauma
	Infiltrated IV line
	Restrictive tape or bandages
	"Hair tourniquet" (infants)
Other causes	Benign nocturnal pain
	Behavioral or psychogenic

IV, Intravenous.

MAJOR THREAT TO LIFE

1. Infection

    Either a localized infection (e.g., osteomyelitis, pyomyositis, or septic arthritis) or a systemic infection (e.g., meningococcemia, Rocky Mountain spotted fever, or toxic shock syndrome) may result in significant extremity pain.

2. Malignancy

    Malignancy is not usually an immediate threat unless cell lysis results in severe hyperuricemia, hyperkalemia, and other metabolic disturbances.

3. Sickle cell disease—vaso-oclusive pain crisis

    If the crisis is accompanied by signs and symptoms of infection or acute chest syndrome, it may be life threatening.

4. Compartment syndrome (compromising the vascular supply)

5. Deep venous thrombosis leading to pulmonary embolism

6. Arterial thrombosis leading to peripheral gangrene
7. Vasculitis

    If also involving major organ systems (lungs, heart, central nervous system [CNS], gut, kidneys), vasculitis may threaten life. Kawasaki disease may result in coronary artery aneurysms and a subsequent risk for rupture or myocardial infarction.

8. Rheumatic fever

    If carditis is also present, congestive heart failure may ensue.

9. Guillain-Barré syndrome (may compromise respiratory function)

BEDSIDE

As noted earlier, your primary goal while on call is to determine whether the child has one of the major threats just listed. If you can exclude a life-threatening possibility, a secondary goal should be to narrow the extensive differential diagnosis for extremity pain to a few likely possibilities. Regardless of the cause, improving the comfort of the child should be a priority.

Quick-Look Test

Does the child look well (comfortable), sick (uncomfortable), or critical? Is the child moving the affected extremity or extremities?

If the child appears critically ill, you should immediately suspect a multisystem illness (sepsis, vasculitis). With most causes of extremity pain, the child appears well or only mildly uncomfortable. However, in a young child response to even minimal discomfort may be severe. Note the posture of the child. The child may protect or position the extremity in a way that minimizes discomfort. For example, children with a septic hip usually prefer to hold the hip flexed, externally rotated, and abducted (Fig. 16.1).

Airway and Vital Signs

As with any pain, mild tachycardia and tachypnea may be expected. Severe abnormalities in the heart rate or respiratory rate or abnormal blood pressure should not be expected and may be clues that the extremity pain is only one manifestation of a systemic process. Similarly, a compromised airway suggests a more significant problem affecting the lungs, heart, CNS, and/or abdomen. Fever may indicate infection or any inflammatory condition (e.g., vasculitis, lupus, dermatomyositis, rheumatic fever, malignancy).

Selective History and Chart Review

Where is the pain?

In a young child, this question may not be easy to answer. Young children may not be able to localize pain well or may give

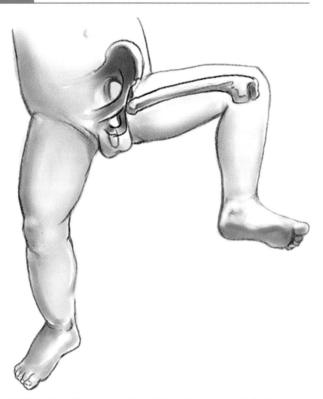

FIGURE 16.1 Posturing of a child with a septic left hip. In an attempt to relax the joint capsule, the child holds the affected hip flexed, externally rotated, and abducted.

inconsistent answers. In many instances, you need to rely on a careful examination to localize the affected area or areas. Remember also that pain may be referred from other sites. Knee or thigh pain may represent a pathologic condition of the hip. Hip pain may be a symptom of lower back or intra-abdominal disease. You should therefore fully examine the joints proximal and distal to the site of pain.

Is the pain felt at a single site or at multiple sites? Is the pain well localized or diffuse?

Osteomyelitis, septic joints, fractures, pyomyositis, osteoid osteomas, hemarthroses, traumatic injuries, primary bone tumors, and cellulitis are most often well localized and at a single site. Isolated, unilateral hip pain (or referred thigh or knee pain) is suggestive of a septic hip, transient synovitis, slipped epiphysis, Legg-Calvé-Perthes disease, avascular necrosis, or a spondyloarthropathy (in an older child), but you should also consider the other localized processes just listed. Pain in multiple sites usually indicates a systemic process.

Has the child been irritable, lost weight recently, or had intermittent fever, malaise, and poor appetite?

These findings should raise suspicion of a systemic inflammatory condition such as infection, rheumatic disease, inflammatory bowel disease, or malignancy.

Is there a history of sickle cell disease or hemophilia, either in the patient or in the family?

Painful vaso-occlusive crises are the most frequent manifestation of sickle cell disease. These patients tend to have recurrences of pain in the same sites; therefore the development of pain in a new site should raise suspicion of an alternative cause. Hemarthrosis may be the initial manifestation of hemophilia, and these patients also tend to have recurrences in the same joints.

Is there a history of recent extremity trauma?

Such a history raises suspicion of a fracture, hematoma, or compartment syndrome.

Has the child undergone prolonged immobilization?

Immobilization may predispose to deep venous thrombosis.

Is there a hypercoagulable state (birth control pills, lupus anticoagulant, protein C or S deficiency, antithrombin III deficiency, nephrotic syndrome, or malignancy)?

A hypercoagulable state is a risk factor for venous or arterial thrombosis.

Has there been a recent upper respiratory infection or pharyngitis?

This may suggest Guillain-Barré syndrome or rheumatic fever.

Selective Physical Examination

Your examination should initially focus on the affected extremity. The source of the pain may often be unclear from the history alone, and your goal should be to determine whether the pain is the result of a problem in the bone, joint, muscle, nerve, vasculature, or skin and soft tissue. You should first inspect and note the position of the extremity and whether the child is willing to move the extremity spontaneously. Look for swelling, erythema, warmth, or deformity at all the joints, as well as over the long bones and the surface of the skin. Without moving the extremity, attempt to palpate over each of the bones and muscles and around the joints and carefully localize any tenderness as best as you can. Osteomyelitis, bone tumors, and bone infarctions should cause discrete point tenderness. A septic joint may also be tender, but the tenderness may not necessarily be severe unless the joint is moved. Because the hips and shoulders are deep joints surrounded by muscle and soft tissue, it is frequently not possible to appreciate tenderness or warmth at these sites, even in the presence of joint inflammation. Compartment syndrome, myositis, and thrombosis (venous or arterial) may all result in exquisite muscle tenderness. Neuropathies may result in dysesthesia, paresthesia, or hyperesthesia. The passive range of motion of all of the joints of the extremity should be evaluated to determine whether limitations suggestive of arthritis are present. Muscle strength testing in the affected extremity should also be performed and the findings compared with strength elsewhere. If pain is in the lower extremity, your examination should include an assessment of the ability to bear weight and an observation of gait. Weakness is a clue that the underlying process may involve muscle and/or nerve. Deep tendon reflexes should also be measured to further evaluate this possibility. Pulses in the extremity should be palpated and tests of distal sensation performed, particularly if compartment syndrome or arterial thrombosis is suspected. Homans sign is suggestive of deep venous thrombosis in the calf and is detected by flexing the knee with the patient supine and then quickly dorsiflexing the ankle to assess whether the patient experiences pain in the calf muscle. However, a negative finding does not rule out the diagnosis.

After your evaluation of the extremities, a general physical examination should be performed to look for signs that may indicate a systemic process. If the child has hip pain, a careful abdominal examination, as well as examination of the spine and lower part of the back, should be performed because pathologic conditions in these sites may result in referred pain (e.g., psoas abscess).

HEENT	Conjunctivitis (Kawasaki disease); pharyngitis (viral, streptococcal, rheumatic fever); oral ulcers (lupus, inflammatory bowel disease); swollen, cracked lips (Kawasaki disease)
Neck	Stiffness (meningitis)
Lungs	Respiratory distress (pulmonary embolism from deep venous thrombosis, acute chest syndrome with sickle cell disease)
Heart	Murmurs of aortic or mitral insufficiency (rheumatic fever)
Abdomen	Tenderness, mass (psoas abscess, appendicitis, vasculitis)

HEENT, Head, Eyes, Ears, Nose, Throat.

Back	Tenderness (diskitis, vertebral osteomyelitis), scoliosis
Skin	Rashes, vesicles, nodules (sepsis, herpes zoster, vasculitis, juvenile idiopathic arthritis, rheumatic fever, dermatomyositis); pustules (disseminated gonococcal infection); erythema, warmth, edema (cellulitis, fasciitis); cyanosis (arterial thrombosis, compartment syndrome); inspection of IV sites for infiltration or restrictive taping; inspection of fingers and toes ("hair tourniquet," foreign body, paronychia)

IV, Intravenous.

Management

Further evaluation and management of major threats to life and other selected causes of extremity pain are discussed here.

Septic Arthritis

A child with fever and a single swollen, painful joint should be considered to have a septic joint until proven otherwise. Septic polyarthritis is also possible but much less common, and other signs and symptoms of sepsis are usually apparent. *Staphylococcus aureus* is the most common cause in young children. *Streptococcus pneumoniae* is also prevalent. In neonates, group B streptococci, *Escherichia coli*, *Listeria monocytogenes*, and *Candida albicans* are likewise common pathogens. *Neisseria gonorrhoeae* infection is an additional consideration in sexually active adolescents. Most septic joints are swollen, erythematous, and warm and have limited range of motion. However, if the affected joint is the hip, pain and limitation of motion may be the only objective signs of arthritis. Remember that the subjective pain may be referred to the thigh or the knee; therefore any patient with fever and pain in these areas needs to undergo a careful evaluation of the ipsilateral hip. Plain radiographs or ultrasound studies of the hip may be helpful when it is unclear from your physical examination whether a hip effusion is present. Once you suspect septic arthritis, the synovial fluid needs to be aspirated immediately, before starting antibiotic treatment. You should proceed as follows:

1. Obtain radiographs of the affected area, a peripheral blood culture, complete blood count (CBC) and differential, C-reactive protein level, and an erythrocyte sedimentation rate. The blood tests may help you monitor the response to treatment. The radiographs should be reviewed to look for evidence of a contiguous osteomyelitis.

2. Aspirate synovial fluid. You may need to consult a rheumatologist, interventional radiologist, or orthopedic surgeon to help with this procedure, and the child may need sedation. The orthopedic surgeon on call should be notified of any potential septic hip because if it is confirmed, open drainage of the hip in the operating room is necessary.

3. The fluid obtained at aspiration should be sent for the following:
   Gram stain
   White blood cell (WBC) count and differential
   Glucose
   Aerobic and anaerobic culture
   Mycobacterial culture (if there are risk factors for tuberculosis)
   Acid-fast staining
   Gonococcal culture (in those who are sexually active)

   The appearance of the fluid should be noted. Septic joints usually result in cloudy or purulent fluid. WBC counts in the fluid are generally greater than 50,000/mm^3, with predominantly neutrophils, and the glucose concentration may be low. Exceptions to these generalizations are common with gonococcal arthritis.

4. After the foregoing procedures have been implemented, intravenous (IV) antibiotics should be empirically started. In children younger than 5 years the combination of nafcillin and cefotaxime provides adequate coverage until culture results are available. In older children, nafcillin alone should be sufficient. If the Gram stain is positive, the choice of antibiotics can be more directed. The use of vancomycin instead of nafcillin should be considered if resistant organisms have been prevalent in the community.

5. A sexually active adolescent should also have throat, rectal, and cervical or urethral cultures obtained before starting antibiotics to further evaluate the possibility of gonococcal infection. The organism is more often cultured from these sites than from synovial fluid.

6. If tuberculosis is suspected from the exposure history, a tuberculin skin test and chest radiographic studies should be performed.

7. If your physical examination (point tenderness) or radiographs suggest osteomyelitis adjacent to the joint, the bone itself should also be aspirated, with any fluid obtained sent for the same studies as listed earlier for synovial fluid. Magnetic resonance imaging (MRI) may also be helpful in distinguishing osteomyelitis from septic arthritis. This distinction is important because a longer duration of antibiotic therapy may be necessary if osteomyelitis is present.

Osteomyelitis

The distal metaphysis of the long bones is a common site for osteomyelitis to develop. Localized point tenderness of a bone in a febrile child should be considered osteomyelitis until proven otherwise. Warmth and soft tissue swelling may be apparent if the periosteum has been penetrated and the infection has spread to adjacent soft tissue. If osteomyelitis is present without contiguous septic arthritis, passive range of motion of the joint is normal. Further evaluation of osteomyelitis is similar to that for septic arthritis, except that bone should be aspirated. MRI may aid in identifying the optimal site to be aspirated and should be considered if physical examination fails to adequately localize the area of maximal tenderness. Plain radiographs are often unhelpful because changes may not be seen within the first week of onset of osteomyelitis. The most common pathogens are the same as those that cause septic arthritis. Salmonella should be considered in children with sickle cell disease, Pseudomonas should be suspected in those with foot osteomyelitis after puncture wounds through shoes, and Kingella should be considered in toddlers or early school-age children with indolent onset. After aspiration of the bone, IV nafcillin and cefotaxime (or ceftazidime if Pseudomonas is suspected) should provide adequate empiric coverage for the most likely pathogens.

Pyomyositis

Localized muscle abscesses containing staphylococci may occur either from hematogenous spread or from penetrating trauma to the muscle (including immunizations). Local warmth, tenderness, and a palpable mass within the muscle should raise suspicion of this disorder. MRI or ultrasonography of the muscle may be helpful. Surgical consultation for drainage is necessary before starting IV antibiotics.

Systemic Infections

Diffuse arthralgias and myalgias may be associated with numerous bacterial and viral systemic illnesses. You need to carefully and thoroughly evaluate the child for other signs of sepsis and potential sources of infection (see Chapter 18). Treatment depends on the specific cause. Influenza A may frequently cause severe pain and tenderness in the calf muscles, often associated with extreme elevations in muscle enzymes (creatine phosphokinase, aldolase). This process is self-limited and usually resolves within a few days. Other viral illnesses, Rocky Mountain spotted fever, or leptospirosis may result in similar findings.

Malignancy

Primary bone tumors (Ewing sarcoma, osteogenic sarcoma), leukemia, and neuroblastoma may all cause extremity pain. The severity may range from mild pain or limping to severe, debilitating pain. Symptoms are often chronic but may be deceptively intermittent. Pain is frequently worse at night, and symptoms may be out of proportion to the objective findings. Plain radiographs may reveal lytic bone lesions, periostitis, or metaphyseal radiolucency. If you suspect malignancy, your goal while on call is to prevent any potential complications until the diagnosis can be confirmed and definitive treatment begun. Potential complications include metabolic disturbances (e.g., hyperuricemia, hyperkalemia), hematologic abnormalities (especially thrombocytopenia or neutropenia), infection (particularly if neutropenia is present), and the effects of space-occupying lesions (e.g., spinal cord compression). You should determine whether the CBC, electrolytes, calcium, uric acid, and phosphate have been checked recently. Consultation with the oncologist on call is necessary, with arrangements made for further diagnostic tests (biopsy, bone marrow aspiration) as soon as possible.

Sickle Cell Crisis

Dactylitis in an infant, also known as hand-foot syndrome, may be the first clinical manifestation of sickle cell anemia. Painful swelling of the hands, feet, and digits is most often symmetric. In a young child, extremity pain is a frequent manifestation of the disease and is due to ischemic necrosis of bone as a result of vaso-occlusion from sickled cells. Affected sites tend to remain the same in the individual child, and the frequency of episodes can vary considerably. Your first goal should be to confirm that the current episode is secondary to vaso-occlusion and not another process. Osteomyelitis may mimic a vaso-occlusive crisis, and if there is any concern regarding infection, you should arrange to aspirate the affected site as described earlier before starting IV antibiotics. Careful evaluation of the child's respiratory status is mandatory to exclude a concurrent acute chest syndrome, and if the child is febrile, a thorough search for sources of infection is necessary. A CBC and reticulocyte count should be obtained, along with appropriate cultures if the child is febrile. If the diagnosis of sickle cell disease has not been confirmed, a peripheral blood smear should be reviewed and hemoglobin electrophoresis performed. Treatment consists of IV hydration and analgesia. Dehydration and acidosis should be corrected when present (see Chapter 15). You need to reevaluate the child frequently, and adjustments to the rate of hydration may be necessary because fluid overload may lead to pulmonary edema and the potential for acute chest syndrome. Oxygen should be administered if the patient is hypoxic. Vaso-occlusive crises often require narcotic analgesics, but acetaminophen and/or nonsteroidal anti-inflammatory drugs may sometimes be sufficient. Ketorolac may be given in a dose of 0.5 mg/kg (maximum of 30 mg) every 6 hours. IV morphine or hydromorphone (Dilaudid) are the most commonly used narcotics. Morphine may be given at 0.1 to 0.2 mg/kg per dose intravenously every 2 to 4 hours and hydromorphone at 0.015 mg/kg per dose every 3 to 4 hours. Alternatively, patient controlled analgesia (PCA) may be used, with a continuous infusion at a basal rate, a bolus amount, and a lock-out interval preprogrammed. A child receiving narcotics also needs frequent reevaluation. Remember that respiratory depression is a serious potential consequence of narcotic administration, and acute chest syndrome may ensue quickly.

Compartment Syndrome

A recent arm or leg fracture or other trauma to an extremity can lead to compartment syndrome. Injury to muscles gives rise to swelling, which if severe enough, becomes limited by the tight-fitting fascia encasing some of the muscle groups in the arm or leg. Increased pressure within this compartment may compress blood vessels and lead to decreased circulation to the muscles and nerves. Pain, tenderness, distal sensory loss and/or weakness, and overlying tension, erythema, or edema may all occur. Pulses are not necessarily affected. If the patient has been placed in a cast for a recent fracture and is experiencing pain, the cast needs to be removed to adequately evaluate the extremity. Immediate surgical consultation and fasciotomy are necessary because irreversible necrosis may occur.

Deep Venous Thrombosis

Deep venous thrombosis is unusual in the pediatric age group but may occur in children who have been immobilized, are on prolonged bed rest, or have a hypercoagulable state. The goals of treatment are to prevent embolization and potential pulmonary infarction. Heparinization should be implemented if the child has any of these risk factors and physical examination reveals tenderness, warmth, edema, distended veins, and/or a positive Homans sign suggestive of thrombosis. After a baseline partial thromboplastin time (PTT) is obtained, an 80-U/kg IV loading dose should be followed by a continuous infusion at 18 U/kg/hour and the dose adjusted to produce a PTT of 1.5 to 2.5 times the control value.

Arterial Thrombosis

Also unusual in childhood, arterial thrombosis or embolism is suggested by the four Ps: pain, pallor, pulselessness, and paresthesias. Hypercoagulable states are the major risk factors in childhood, along with complications of indwelling catheters or attempts at placement of arterial lines. Heparin should be initiated as described earlier for venous thrombosis and vascular surgery consultation obtained immediately.

Vasculitis

Vasculitis may result in extremity pain for a number of reasons, including vaso-occlusion, neuropathy (ischemic as a result of effects on the blood supply to the nerve), myositis, skin and soft tissue involvement, and arthritis. The vasculitis may be life threatening if other organ systems are also involved. Consultation with a pediatric rheumatologist is necessary, with consideration given to treatment with steroids or cytotoxic agents.

Rheumatic Fever

Migratory polyarthritis or arthralgias and a history of recent pharyngitis or known streptococcal pharyngitis should raise your suspicion of rheumatic fever. A careful cardiac examination should be performed to listen for murmurs of aortic or mitral insufficiency. You should also look for signs and symptoms of associated congestive heart failure. A chest radiograph, echocardiogram, and streptococcal antibody tests (antistreptolysin O [ASO], anti-DNAse B) will be useful. The arthritis of rheumatic fever tends to affect large joints; the pain is often severe and disproportionate to objective findings and responds dramatically to salicylates or other nonsteroidal agents. Prednisone (if severe congestive heart failure is present) may also be necessary.

Guillain-Barré Syndrome

Pain and tenderness of muscles may be a feature accompanying the ascending weakness or paralysis of Guillain-Barré syndrome. The deep tendon reflexes should be carefully evaluated if the diagnosis is suspected, as should the airway and respiratory status. Cerebrospinal fluid analysis is necessary, with an albuminocytologic dissociation (protein greater than twice normal with <10 WBCs/mm^3) in a patient with a subacute polyneuropathy being diagnostic for Guillain-Barré syndrome. Consultation with a pediatric neurologist is usually necessary, and consideration should be given to treatment with IV immunoglobulin, steroids, or plasmapheresis.

REMEMBER

When evaluating an inpatient with extremity pain, first isolate the site and then organize your approach: bones, joints, muscles, blood vessels, nerves, skin. Use the opposite extremity as a control for your physical examination. When on call, concentrate on two goals:

1. Exclude a life- or limb-threatening process.
2. Make the child more comfortable.

Eye Problems and Visual Abnormalities

Rose Doolittle, MD

Acute eye problems in children are less common than most of the other problems discussed in this book, and isolated problems of the eye are rarely life threatening. However, any problem involving the eye must be evaluated promptly for two reasons. First, eye and/or visual complaints may herald significant central nervous system (CNS) disease, including meningitis, encephalitis, and increased intracranial pressure (ICP). Second, any process involving the eye may potentially threaten vision.

PHONE CALL

Questions

1. Does the child appear well or sick?
2. How old is the child?
3. Is there drainage from the eye? What is the appearance of the drainage?
4. Is there periorbital swelling and erythema?
5. Is vision affected?
6. Is there pain (pain with eye motion or tenderness to palpation) or photophobia?
7. Is there a sensation of a foreign body? Does the patient wear contacts?
8. What was the reason for admission?

A child who appears ill should be suspected of having a systemic illness with associated eye manifestations. A number of systemic infections (viral, bacterial, rickettsial) may produce conjunctivitis in addition to other signs and symptoms. The age of the child, the appearance of any drainage, the presence of periorbital swelling, and any pain or loss of vision will help you to differentiate the possible causes of eye inflammation. Pain or photophobia in a normal-appearing eye suggests migraine or early uveitis. If the call is regarding a newborn with eye drainage, ophthalmia neonatorum is a major consideration.

Orders

None.

Inform RN

"Will arrive at the bedside in … minutes." Ill-appearing children, those with swelling or erythema around the eye, those with pain or abnormal vision, and newborns all need to be seen immediately.

ELEVATOR THOUGHTS

What causes eye redness, drainage, pain, or swelling?
Conjunctivitis or keratoconjunctivitis
    Bacterial (*Neisseria gonorrhoeae* and *Chlamydia trachomatis* in
        the newborn)
    Viral (herpes simplex in the newborn)
    Chemical (silver nitrate in the newborn)
    Allergic
    Kawasaki disease
    Other infections (e.g., Rocky Mountain spotted fever, leptospirosis)
Periorbital or orbital cellulitis
Uveitis
Traumatic corneal injury (abrasion, foreign body)
Nasolacrimal duct obstruction (infant)
Subconjunctival hemorrhage
Glaucoma
Panophthalmitis
What causes abnormal or acute loss of vision?
    Many of the conditions just listed may lead to abnormalities in vision, but in the absence of any of these causes, you should consider the following:
Migraine
Increased ICP
Posterior reversible encephalopathy syndrome (PRES)
Retinal artery thrombosis
Optic neuritis
Retinal detachment (e.g., traumatic)
Psychogenic

MAJOR THREAT TO LIFE OR VISION

- Infectious conjunctivitis or keratoconjunctivitis in the newborn
- Periorbital or orbital cellulitis

- Panophthalmitis
- Severe trauma
- Increased ICP
- Retinal artery thrombosis (secondary to vasculitis, emboli, or hypercoagulability)
- Meningitis (if photophobia is the primary complaint)

Treatment of each of these conditions should begin as soon as possible after diagnosis. Empiric treatment of *N. gonorrhoeae* conjunctivitis (in a newborn) and periorbital or orbital cellulitis (in an older child) should be considered if these conditions cannot be immediately excluded.

BEDSIDE

Quick-Look Test

Does the child look well (comfortable), sick (uncomfortable or distressed), or toxic (critically ill)?

A child who looks ill needs an immediate, thorough evaluation for a systemic illness.

Airway and Vital Signs

The vital signs should not be affected by a localized eye problem unless the child is also systemically ill. Fever should prompt a search for other potential sources and increase your concern about potential cellulitis or ophthalmitis.

Selective History and Chart Review

When did the eye inflammation begin?

In a newborn, onset within 12 hours of birth suggests chemical conjunctivitis from silver nitrate rather than an infectious cause. You should determine whether the infant received silver nitrate or erythromycin ocular prophylaxis (or neither). Gonococcal conjunctivitis typically begins 2 to 5 days after birth, although it may be delayed by partial treatment with ocular prophylaxis. Conjunctivitis secondary to *C. trachomatis* may not appear for 5 to 14 days.

If the child is a newborn, were there any maternal infections during pregnancy?

A history of gonorrhea, chlamydia, or herpes infection should raise your suspicion of these infections as causes.

Has the child been systemically ill or had a recent infection?

Periorbital and orbital cellulitis, as well as panophthalmitis, may occur secondary to hematogenous spread of bacteria, direct extension from sinusitis, or penetrating trauma and subsequent infection. *Staphylococcus aureus*, pneumococcus, and group A streptococcus are the most common pathogens. Conjunctivitis and uveitis may be associated with a number of systemic illnesses. If there has been sudden visual loss in a child with renal disease or hypertension or in a child recently receiving cytotoxic medications, PRES should be a consideration.

Are there other associated symptoms?

The presence of headache or neurologic symptoms may suggest migraine or CNS disease with increased ICP or associated optic neuritis.

Does the patient wear contacts?

Contact lenses have been associated with bacterial keratitis, especially when improperly worn overnight.

Is there a history of trauma to the eye?

Corneal abrasions may easily occur from trauma that is unrecognized or is thought to be insignificant. If the child has recently undergone surgery, incorrect taping of the eyelids during surgery may lead to eye dryness and/or pain during the recovery period. Cellulitis may also develop after infection of a relatively minor abrasion or laceration of the skin near the eye.

Selective Physical Examination

Look carefully at the eyes and surrounding soft tissues, and note the characteristics of any drainage. Observe the sclerae, conjunctivae, and extraocular movements of the child. The presence of pus (hypopyon) or blood (hyphema) in the anterior chamber may produce a visible fluid level between the inferior pole of the iris and the cornea and suggests infection and trauma, respectively. Visualize the retina as best as you can to look for papilledema, hemorrhages, and venous pulsations. If necessary, dilate the pupils so that you can adequately examine the retina. Remember to tell the nurse and document that you have dilated the pupils, so the dilation will not be misinterpreted.

In an infant who appears well, with clear, thin drainage or small amounts of mucoid drainage from the eye, you should suspect nasolacrimal duct obstruction. Thick, purulent drainage with marked injection and hyperemia of the sclerae and conjunctivae suggests gonococcal conjunctivitis in a neonate and other bacterial causes (*Haemophilus influenzae*, pneumococcus, staphylococcus, or streptococcus) in an older child. *C. trachomatis* may result in similar drainage but is generally less severe than that seen with gonococcus. Swelling and erythema of the soft tissues around the eye suggest periorbital cellulitis, especially if the child is febrile. Proptosis or any abnormalities in extraocular movement should make you very suspicious of orbital cellulitis. Papilledema warrants a computed tomography (CT) scan of the orbits to rule out a mass lesion, hemorrhage, cerebral edema, and hydrocephalus.

An eye that is injected but without mucopurulent drainage in an irritable child should raise your suspicion of uveitis, keratitis, trauma, Kawasaki disease, or glaucoma. Childhood glaucoma is rare and produces the classic triad of tearing, photophobia, and spasm of the eyelids secondary to corneal irritation. Corneal abrasions may be detected by instilling fluorescein dye onto the surface of the cornea and visualizing it with a Wood lamp. If herpes is a consideration, consultation with an ophthalmologist is necessary to determine whether characteristic dendritic lesions of the corneal epithelium are present.

Visual acuity should be tested with a Snellen chart, and visual field testing should be performed if the child is old enough to cooperate. Objective abnormalities in vision should be an indication to consult with an ophthalmologist.

Management

Any eye drainage should be Gram stained and cultured. Additional laboratory evaluation depends on the suspected diagnosis. Urgent ophthalmologic consultation should be obtained if you cannot adequately examine the eyes, if there are abnormalities in vision, or if the diagnosis is unclear. Definitive management of many conditions involving the eye needs the expertise of an ophthalmologist. A few of the most likely diagnoses you may need to address while on call are discussed here.

Ophthalmia Neonatorum

If the Gram-stained drainage reveals gram-negative diplococci characteristic of *N. gonorrhoeae*, give ceftriaxone, 25 to 50 mg/kg intravenously (IV) or intramuscularly (IM) (maximum 125 mg/ dose), along with irrigation of the eye with normal saline solution at 15-minute to 2-hour intervals. Typically a one-time dose of ceftriaxone is sufficient; however, treatment may be continued for 48 to 72 hours if the clinical response appears to be inadequate. Blood should be drawn for culture and additional cultures (such as urine and cerebrospinal fluid [CSF]) considered before instituting systemic antibiotic treatment if the infant appears ill. Chlamydia infection can be treated with oral erythromycin for 14 days. Remember that coinfection with other sexually transmitted diseases must be suspected in an infant with gonococcal or chlamydial infection, including syphilis and human immunodeficiency virus (HIV).

Conjunctivitis in an Older Child

Distinguishing viral from bacterial conjunctivitis may be difficult, and many physicians elect to treat all cases of isolated conjunctivitis that are believed to be infectious. "Pink eye" may be treated with topical antibiotics such as bacitracin–polymyxin B or erythromycin for 5 to 7 days.

Herpetic Keratitis

Intravenous acyclovir should begin immediately in a newborn in whom herpetic keratitis is suspected because the infant may also be at risk for disseminated herpes infection. The addition of topical antiviral therapy should be considered and discussed with an ophthalmologist. Older infants and children may be treated with topical antivirals alone.

Periorbital and Orbital Cellulitis

If periorbital cellulitis is suspected, empiric intravenous antibiotic treatment directed against the most likely pathogens should be initiated. The combination of clindamycin and ampicillin-sulbactam is a reasonable choice to cover skin flora including methicillin-resistant *S. aureus* (MRSA) and the usual bacterial etiologies of sinusitis, respectively. Blood cultures can be considered prior to giving antibiotics; however, these are typically low yield in older children. In an ill-appearing infant, CSF, blood, and urine should be obtained for culture before starting antibiotics. If proptosis or any abnormality or pain with eye movement is noted, an emergency CT scan of the orbits should be obtained to look for orbital cellulitis or a frank orbital abscess. When in doubt, perform the CT scan. Otolaryngologic and ophthalmologic consultations should be obtained immediately and surgical drainage of the infected orbit considered. Orbital cellulitis has potential for severe complications. Pressure within the orbit may affect the optic nerve and lead to visual loss. Alternatively, extension of the infection may result in cavernous sinus thrombosis or epidural or cerebral abscess.

Trauma

Corneal abrasions can be treated with topical antibiotics such as erythromycin or tobramycin applied three times a day. If the abrasion is large, the eye should be patched for 24 hours to promote healing. More severe forms of trauma should be managed by an ophthalmologist.

REMEMBER

1. Eye complaints may indicate a systemic or a CNS process.
2. Infection, trauma, and vascular occlusion of the eye are major threats to vision and should be excluded or appropriately managed.
3. Urgent ophthalmologic consultation may frequently be necessary and should be obtained if you suspect a process that may threaten life or vision.

Fever

Vanessa C. McFadden, MD, PhD

One of the most common and potentially serious problems that the pediatrician manages while on call is fever. Fever can be a symptom of mild self-limited infections, serious infections, malignancies, or inflammatory illness. In a child who has already been hospitalized with appropriate evaluation, fever may be an expected finding that can be anticipated and treated. However, fever should never be ignored.

In general, the accepted temperature that constitutes fever is 38.5°C, which corresponds to approximately 101.5°F. Regardless of age, this temperature is considered above normal. In neonates we often consider 38°C or higher as a fever and an indication for evaluation to rule out sepsis. Therefore fever must be considered in the context of the specific patient's signs and symptoms, the child's age, and the underlying diagnosis that led to the child's admission to the hospital.

Fever is a sign of potentially life-threatening illness and deserves prompt, hands-on evaluation.

PHONE CALL

It is important that the pediatrician obtain accurate information when notified about a child with fever. This allows prioritization of the call. The following questions are suggested:
1. How old is the child?
2. What is the child's admitting diagnosis?
3. What are the child's vital signs?
4. What is the child's appearance? How is the child acting? Is the child alert? Oriented? Distressed? Agitated? Are the extremities well perfused?
5. Has the child been febrile previously during this admission?
6. Are there standing orders for an antipyretic and/or laboratory tests in the event of fever?

7. Does the child have any underlying condition that may compromise the immune system (e.g., cancer, neutropenia, sickle cell disease, rheumatic disease)?

High fevers (>39.5°C) warrant immediate hands-on evaluation in any child younger than 36 months. This is the age group at highest risk for occult bacteremia. Neonates and young infants are at an even higher risk of serious infection and will require a more extensive evaluation, regardless of other signs and symptoms, than older children. Laboratory tests that were to be ordered in the event of a fever should be obtained, and an antipyretic should be ordered immediately over the telephone. The nurse should also be informed of the intent to evaluate the child immediately.

If the child, regardless of age, shows any signs of hemodynamic decompensation, a normal saline intravenous (IV) fluid bolus of 10 to 20 mL/kg should be started. If the child does not have adequate IV access, it is imperative to obtain at least one reliable IV line.

In an older child (>3 years) the same questions should be asked, and the antipyretic should be administered. Confusion occasionally arises regarding the administration of antipyretics. Regardless of whether laboratory tests will be performed, it is important to give the antipyretic to control the febrile response and make the child more comfortable. An antipyretic does not affect a blood culture or a complete blood count, and antipyretics do not cause significant physical findings to disappear.

ELEVATOR THOUGHTS

The approach to fever in children is very age dependent. Neonates are far more susceptible to bacterial illness and have greater vulnerability to morbidity and mortality. In addition, the pathogens most commonly encountered in neonates differ from those found in older children. This difference is caused by two phenomena. The first is passive transmission of immunity via the placenta in the third trimester of pregnancy. This immunity conveys relative protection from viral illnesses such as varicella, rubella, and rubeola. Humoral factors transmitted in breast milk may also be protective and can last up to 2 to 3 months. The second major reason for the difference in pathogenic flora is immunization against both viral and bacterial pathogens, especially *Haemophilus influenzae* type B (HIB), *Bordetella pertussis*, *Clostridium tetani*, and hepatitis B virus.

If the child is a neonate and has been admitted to "rule out sepsis," cultures and other tests must be reviewed. Antibiotics are commonly started empirically in neonates, and it is important to know the antibiotics, the doses, the dosing interval, and their spectrum of antibacterial coverage. Could the antibiotic therapy already begun be inappropriate or inadequate?

It is important to carefully consider the vital signs in infants. Is the child appropriately tachycardic for the fever? Tachypnea must be distinguished from hyperpnea, which may indicate respiratory compensation for metabolic acidosis. Because blood pressure is generally preserved in infants until late in the course of shock, the blood pressure measurement must be viewed in the context of the child's peripheral perfusion, urine output, and mental status. The child's hydration status should also be assessed. Circulatory collapse and shock, with their resultant metabolic acidosis and end-organ failure, must be avoided.

In an older child with any underlying conditions that predispose to infection, the same considerations apply. For example, a child with sickle cell disease who is older than 3 years should be considered functionally asplenic and therefore more susceptible to encapsulated bacteria. These children should be receiving daily antibiotic prophylaxis against such organisms. Many older children have underlying conditions that may directly affect their immune system or their general health and nutrition status. Congenital heart disease, cystic fibrosis, inflammatory bowel disease, short gut syndrome, and neuromuscular disorders are chronic illnesses that can have a profound effect on the immune system of older children and adolescents.

On the way to evaluate the child, consider the child's age and the urgency of the vital signs. Always prioritize to rule out life-threatening conditions first: septic shock and meningitis.

MAJOR THREAT TO LIFE

- Septic shock
- Meningitis

The cascade of humoral factors released in response to fever can cause hemodynamic instability and jeopardize the function of multiple organ systems. Meningitis can compromise central nervous system function and result in altered mental status, seizures, deafness, and permanent disability.

BEDSIDE

Quick-Look Test

Does the child appear well (comfortable or playful), sick (distressed, agitated), or critical (lethargic, unresponsive)?

Appearing sick or critically ill generally reflects hemodynamic instability.

Airway and Vital Signs

What are the heart rate, respiratory rate, and blood pressure?

Bradycardia in a febrile child is an ominous sign of impending circulatory collapse. Likewise, tachycardia out of proportion to the level of fever can be a sign of the child's desperate effort to preserve cardiac output.

Tachypnea and hyperpnea can reflect primary pulmonary disease, as well as respiratory compensation for metabolic acidosis.

Blood pressure must be viewed in the context of the child's perfusion, urine output, mental status, and volume status. Multiple mechanisms in the body interact to preserve blood pressure.

History and Physical Examination I

What is the volume status? Are there signs of shock? What is the child's mental status?

Repeat vital signs, including temperature.

HEENT[*]	Fundi, photophobia, mucous membranes, presence of tears
Neck	Stiffness
Cardiovascular	Heart rate, blood pressure, perfusion, murmurs, pulses (upper and lower)
Lungs	Quality of breath sounds and respiratory effort
Neurologic	Sensorium change
Skin	Turgor

[*]*HEENT,* Head, eyes, ears, nose, throat.

The physical examination begins on first glance or at least simultaneously with obtaining additional history. If it is at night, turn on the lights to adequately see the child as you ask the nurse or other caretaker for additional history. Review the questions asked on the telephone. What has the child's fluid status been for the past 8 to 12 hours? Has the nurse or caretaker noticed any other changes in behavior, mood, or feeding? What laboratory studies were performed at the time of admission, and what are the results? What medications is the child currently receiving (with dose and interval for each)?

Vital signs should be determined again at the time of your evaluation. This is especially critical if any of the initial vital signs were abnormal. Retake the temperature as well, preferably a rectal temperature. Other methods are adequate for screening but lack both the sensitivity and specificity of a rectal temperature. A thorough age-appropriate physical examination should follow, including funduscopic examination, pneumatic otoscopy, and rectal and/or pelvic examination if appropriate. Regardless of the findings of previous examinations, a complete examination must be performed and documented thoroughly. Special consideration should be given to general appearance and mental status, quality and rate of respirations, quality and rate of pulses, capillary refill time, hydration of the mucous membranes, and skin turgor. Remember that the major threat to life is septic shock and/or meningitis.

Management I

What measures need to be taken to prevent septic shock or to recognize meningitis?

Any known source of infection should be reassessed. Such assessment may require laboratory studies in the case of a child with bacteremia, pneumonia, or meningitis. Venous blood should be obtained for culture, from any febrile patient hospitalized for more than 24 hours. Resistance to obtaining blood for culture is encountered among both nurses and parents, but it is necessary to detect occult bacteremia. Frequently, a complete blood count is also obtained and can yield helpful information regarding the white blood cell count and differential, platelet count, and hemoglobin and hematocrit, which can often indicate the presence of underlying chronic illness. The yield of blood culture is greatest in the setting of a patient with fever higher than 39.5°C and a total white blood cell count greater than 15,000.

Any sign of hemodynamic compromise must be addressed immediately. Perfusion, capillary refill, pulses, blood pressure, and heart rate, along with urine output, help to determine the need for fluid resuscitation. Normal saline or lactated Ringer's solution is appropriate, generally in volumes of 10 to 20 mL/kg. If signs of circulatory compromise persist, the patient should be transferred expeditiously to the pediatric intensive care unit (PICU) for inotropic support.

In a neonate or toxic-appearing child, antibiotics should be promptly given as soon as cultures of blood, urine, and cerebrospinal fluid (CSF) have been obtained. If there is difficulty in obtaining samples for culture quickly and the child appears toxic, empiric antibiotics should be started. In a neonate with fever and no known source, ampicillin and either gentamicin or cefotaxime are given. Older children may receive cefotaxime or ceftriaxone alone unless there is a reason to be specifically concerned regarding staphylococcus or resistant gram-positive organisms, in which case vancomycin may be added. The use of aminoglycosides must be accompanied by assessment of peak and trough levels, as well as blood urea nitrogen and serum creatinine levels, to monitor for nephrotoxicity.

If meningitis is suspected, a lumbar puncture is indicated. However, especially in infants, this procedure is not without risk. Be sure that the patient is hemodynamically stable and in no respiratory distress before placing the patient in a compromising position.

(See Appendix A for how to perform a lumbar puncture.) Be sure that oxygen and airway support supplies are readily available. If there are any lateralizing signs on neurologic evaluation or suspicion of a space-occupying lesion, antibiotics should be given and an emergency head computed tomography (CT) scan without contrast obtained before the lumbar puncture. Whenever possible, record an opening pressure as soon as CSF is obtained, especially in an older child.

A chest radiograph should be obtained in any patient with respiratory distress. For a toddler or preschool child with a sore throat and dysphagia, a lateral neck film should be performed to evaluate the retropharyngeal space, as well as the epiglottis, tonsils, and adenoids. Above all, a careful, thorough physical examination of the child will help you to determine what further work-up may be necessary.

Selective Chart Review

If the patient is stable and does not have signs of meningitis, look for localizing clues in the patient's history and physical examination, progress notes and/or consultations, and laboratory results. Additional information that will be helpful includes the following:

Temperature graph since admission

Recent white blood cell count and differential

Evidence of immunodeficiency (e.g., sickle cell disease, asplenia, malignancy, human immunodeficiency virus [HIV] infection, use of steroids)

Allergies to antibiotics

Current medications

Selective Physical Examination II

Target areas suggested by the chart review of the patient's current complaints.

Vital signs	Repeat now
HEENT	
Fundi	Check for papilledema (intracranial abscess), Roth spots (infective endocarditis)
Ears	Otitis media
Nose	Purulent drainage (sinusitis, foreign body)
Mouth	Dental abscess, pharyngitis, peritonsillar abscess
Neck	Stiffness (meningitis), cervical adenopathy (adenitis, retropharyngeal abscess)
Lungs	Crackles, wheezes, friction rub, consolidation (pneumonia, empyema)
Cardiac	New murmur (infective endocarditis)

Abdomen	Localized tenderness
Musculoskeletal	Erythema, swelling, tenderness
Skin	Rash, petechiae, purpura, IV sites
Pelvic	If indicated

Management II

Besides blood, urine, and CSF cultures if indicated, cultures should be obtained from central lines, potentially affected bones and/or joints, bullous skin lesions, the pharynx, or any other site of apparent inflammation or infection. In addition, a Gram stain should be performed on any such culture material. Examination of the Gram stain can be very useful in making decisions regarding antibiotic coverage. In young children, remember to assess for a urinary tract infection in any boy less than 6 months of age, uncircumcised males 6 to 24 months of age, and all females up to 2 to 3 years of age, when fever source has not been identified.

Which patients need antibiotics now?

1. Patients with signs of sepsis, with or without shock, need broad-spectrum antibiotic coverage promptly.
2. Patients who are immunocompromised (i.e., neutropenic patients, patients receiving chemotherapy, HIV-positive patients, and asplenic patients [e.g., sickle cell patients])

Which patients need specific antibiotics now?

1. Patients with meningitis or any other localized infection that is usually associated with specific bacteria will need specific antibiotic therapy.
2. Patients with a known positive culture
3. Patients with specific antibiotic allergies

Which patients do not need antibiotics until a specific pathogen is diagnosed?

Patients older than 60 days who are not toxic, who are immunocompetent, and who have no specific source identified for their fever

What antibiotic should be administered?

In a neonate, ampicillin is chosen to cover *Listeria monocytogenes* and group B streptococci, and gentamicin or cefotaxime is added to cover gram-negative enteric pathogens. Coverage for *Staphylococcus* species is needed in any postoperative patient, patients with indwelling catheters, gastrostomy tubes, or tracheostomies, and young patients with cystic fibrosis. Older children with cystic fibrosis require *Pseudomonas* coverage. Likewise, immunocompromised patients require *Staphylococcus* coverage, as well as gram-negative coverage and potentially additional specific coverage depending on their underlying illness and past history.

REMEMBER

1. Fever requires hands-on assessment and can be an ominous finding in a young child.
2. Noninfectious sources of fever (i.e., drug-associated fever) are diagnoses of exclusion.
3. Antipyretics do not alter the yield of blood cultures or the white blood cell count or differential.
4. Fever in an immunocompromised patient requires consideration of potential infection with unusual pathogens.
5. Any sign of hemodynamic compromise must be treated quickly, and the patient must be reassessed promptly for improvement.
6. Seizures are commonly associated with a rapidly rising temperature in young children and do not, by themselves, suggest meningitis or other more serious infection.
7. Base empiric selection of antibiotics on the probable organisms for that patient's age, underlying illness, and localizing signs, if present.
8. Document your findings thoroughly, explain them to the parent or family, and notify other providers of the patient's condition and your diagnosis and plan.

chapter 19

Gastrointestinal Bleeding

Kent Rosenwald, MD

In the pediatric population, gastrointestinal (GI) bleeding can occur at any age, with many potential causes throughout the GI tract. GI bleeding can be generally categorized into upper and lower GI bleeding. The differential diagnosis will vary substantially depending on the age of the child, the presence or absence of chronic GI or hepatic disorders, and other risk factors.

PHONE CALL

Questions

1. Age, clinical history, and known medical conditions?
2. Attempt to clarify the source and rapidity of bleeding: Is it fresh (bright red blood) or old (melena, "coffee grounds")?
   Upper GI bleeding may manifest as vomiting bright red blood or "coffee grounds," or as melena, whereas bright red blood from the rectum indicates lower GI tract bleeding. (There can occasionally be bright red blood per rectum in the case of rapid upper GI bleeding.)
3. How much blood has been lost?
   Estimates of blood loss may be very inaccurate, but trace blood will be managed differently than grossly bloody output.
4. What are the current vital signs?
   Watch for tachycardia (early sign of hemodynamic instability) before hypotension (late sign).
5. Does the child appear to be in pain? Appear to be ill?
6. Is the bleeding a new problem or issue?
   Acute infectious illnesses (e.g., bacterial enteritis) cause blood in the stool, as do chronic inflammatory conditions such as Crohn disease and ulcerative colitis.

7. What was the patient's last hemoglobin or hematocrit and platelet count?
8. Is the patient receiving an anticoagulant, such as heparin, warfarin (Coumadin), aspirin, nonsteroidal antiinflammatory drug (NSAID), or fibrinolytic therapy?

Orders

In the case of brisk GI bleeding or hemodynamic instability:

1. Establish intravenous (IV) access with at least one IV, as large a line as possible. You may need to consider two peripheral IV lines in situations in which the blood loss is significant and ongoing.
2. If the patient is hypotensive or the volume of blood loss is large, a 20-mL/kg bolus of normal saline or lactated Ringer's solution should be given immediately over a 5- to 10-minute period. Repeat as necessary while obtaining additional support. Consider transfusion if volume resuscitation is still needed after several fluid boluses.
3. Obtain new or repeat complete blood count (CBC). The drop in hemoglobin and hematocrit may lag in a rapid bleed. Obtain prothrombin time/partial thromboplastin time/international normalized ratio (PT/PTT/INR) if concerned about hepatic dysfunction. Make sure a blood specimen is sent to the blood bank for typing and cross matching.

Inform RN

Tell the RN, "I will arrive at the bedside in … minutes." Patients who are hemodynamically unstable (tachycardic, hypotensive, poorly perfused) or in pain must be examined without delay, and the senior resident should be informed immediately.

ELEVATOR THOUGHTS

Upper GI bleeding	Epistaxis or nasal trauma (vigorous suctioning, "picking") Oral or pharyngeal trauma (including dental) Esophagitis Gastritis Esophageal varices (liver disease, portal hypertension) Mallory-Weiss tear, prolapse gastropathy (vomiting) Peptic ulcer disease Swallowed maternal blood (newborn) Hemorrhagic disease of the newborn (confirm that vitamin K was given) Foreign body ingestion

Lower GI bleeding	Anorectal fissure (constipation)
	Colitis (ischemic, infectious)
	Hemorrhoids
	Meckel diverticulum
	Intussusception
	Malrotation with volvulus
	Hemolytic-uremic syndrome
	Inflammatory bowel disease
	Milk protein allergy (infants)
	Necrotizing enterocolitis (premature infants)
	Polyps
	Henoch-Schönlein purpura (and other vasculitides)
	Vascular malformation
	Hirschsprung disease

GI, Gastrointestinal.

MAJOR THREAT TO LIFE

- Hypovolemic shock
- Ischemic bowel with secondary perforation, peritonitis, and sepsis

Blood loss into the GI tract is often insidious and results in anemia, sometimes severe, but it does not usually cause hemodynamic compromise. However, large-volume blood loss can occur, especially with ulcers, which can erode into arteries. Intussusception or bowel ischemia in particular can be associated with circulatory collapse. Likewise, in a premature infant, lower GI bleeding from necrotizing enterocolitis can be accompanied by septic shock. Children with chronic liver dysfunction before or after liver transplantation may have the potentially fatal combination of esophageal varices and coagulopathy.

BEDSIDE

Quick-Look Test

Does the child appear well (comfortable), sick (uncomfortable), or unstable (critical)?

Children who have had significant blood loss appear pale and poorly perfused and frequently have other signs of hypovolemic shock, such as tachycardia, cold clammy extremities (increased sympathetic tone), and tachypnea.

Airway and Vital Signs

Are there postural changes in blood pressure?

Vital signs should be obtained in the supine and sitting positions, when possible. There should be less than a 20-mm Hg fall in systolic blood pressure. Likewise, diastolic blood pressure should not fluctuate with position changes. Such changes suggest significant blood loss or distributive shock secondary to sepsis.

Selective Physical Examination

What is the child's volume status? Is the child in shock?

Cardiovascular	Pulse quality, capillary refill, warmth of extremities
Abdomen	Rigidity, guarding, rebound tenderness, masses, abnormal bowel sounds, rectal examination, look at the emesis or stool (trace vs. frank blood)
Central nervous system	Mental status changes
Skin	Jaundice, spider nevi, petechiae, purpura,

A rectal examination with heme testing of the stool is absolutely necessary regardless of age or suspected cause of GI bleeding.

Management

What must be done immediately to treat shock (or prevent progression to shock)?

If vital signs and examination indicate hypovolemia or shock from other causes, quickly place a reliable and reasonably large IV line, and give a 20-mL/kg bolus of normal saline. Repeat isotonic fluid boluses as needed while escalating care. In premature infants and neonates, 5% albumin is expensive but preferred if readily available. If the amount of blood loss is large, typing and cross matching should be done immediately. Because the magnitude of the blood loss must be assessed, a CBC and platelet count should be obtained, as well as electrolyte, blood urea nitrogen, creatinine, amylase, and liver transaminase levels. In a crisis situation, non–cross-matched type O-negative blood can be given, although this is rarely necessary. If there is any suggestion of sepsis, a bleeding disorder, and/or a hypoxic or ischemic insult, coagulation studies should also be performed (screening for disseminated intravascular coagulation). Also consider blood cultures and empiric broad-spectrum antibiotics if the child appears septic.

What can be done to stop the source of the bleeding?

Active GI bleeding is difficult to localize and treat. You must treat or prevent hypovolemia immediately and then pursue the underlying cause.

When is surgical consultation appropriate?
- Persistent bleeding requiring transfusion
- Presence of signs and symptoms of bowel obstruction (intussusception or volvulus) or ischemia

When can endoscopy be completed to localize the site of bleeding?

Endoscopic assessment is the test of choice for upper and lower GI bleeding. Before endoscopy the child must be kept without oral intake (NPO) and must be hemodynamically resuscitated.

Is there an underlying coagulopathy?

Coagulopathies can result in heme-positive stools or overt bleeding. Correction of the PT or PTT and discontinuation of anticoagulant therapy should be undertaken immediately.

Upper Gastrointestinal Bleeding (Hematemesis or Melena)

Examine the child for sources of bleeding in the nose, mouth, and throat. Keep in mind that small children put all sorts of objects in their mouths and frequently walk around and fall with objects in their mouths, which can result in significant trauma. Pens, pencils, and various sharp implements can cause lacerations and/or puncture wounds to the tongue, lips, or pharynx when children fall with these objects in their mouths. Consider iatrogenic trauma as well, such as suctioning or recent procedures (e.g., tonsillectomy).

Esophageal bleeding can result from caustic ingestion, varices, or Mallory-Weiss tears and prolapse gastropathy associated with vomiting. Gastritis (including cases due to *Helicobacter pylori*) and peptic ulcer disease (may have epigastric pain relieved with meals) can cause upper GI bleeding as well.

Laboratory Data

CBC, platelet count, reticulocyte count

Electrolytes, blood urea nitrogen, creatinine
- Blood urea nitrogen/creatinine (BUN/Cr) ratio >30 supports upper GI bleed

Liver function tests

PT, PTT, INR

Flat, upright, and/or lateral decubitus abdominal films, especially if the child is uncomfortable

Upper GI (malrotation with midgut volvulus)

An Apt test (to distinguish maternal blood from the infant's blood in the newborn period)

Management

Place an nasogastric (NG) tube if large volume hematemesis. Consider upper endoscopy to identify source of bleeding and potentially intervene. H_2 blockers or proton-pump inhibitors (PPIs)

usually help in alleviating esophagitis and gastritis. For rapid upper GI bleeding, start an IV PPI.

Lower Gastrointestinal Bleeding (Hematochezia and Occasionally Melena)

The classic description of a "currant jelly" stool in an infant or toddler with intermittent irritability strongly suggests intussusception. A mass may sometimes be palpable in the right lower quadrant or on rectal examination.

If there is associated diarrhea, evaluation for bacterial enteritis may begin with stool nucleic acid testing or culture for Salmonella, Shigella, Yersinia, Campylobacter, *Escherichia coli*, and other species. A history of frequent health care system encounters or prolonged antibiotic exposure will predispose to *Clostridium difficile* enterocolitis. Stool should be examined for the presence of leukocytes, ova, and parasites, especially *Giardia lamblia*. Eosinophils seen on Wright stain of the stool suggest milk protein allergy in infants. Growth failure may suggest inflammatory bowel disease. Endoscopy or magnetic resonance (MR) enterography should be considered if inflammatory bowel disease is suspected. Painless lower GI bleeding implies a Meckel diverticulum, whereas associated abdominal pain suggests intussusception in infants and toddlers, inflammatory bowel disease in children and adolescents, or infectious causes if associated with diarrhea.

In infants, careful examination of the perineum may reveal estrogen-withdrawal vaginal bleeding in females or the presence of small fissures around the anus. Premature infants (<35 weeks) are at higher risk for necrotizing enterocolitis. Milk protein allergy may present as bloody mucous stools and increased stool frequency. Also in newborns, passage of stools can cause small tears in anorectal tissue and give rise to fissures that result in small amounts of blood coating the stool.

Bismuth compounds (e.g., Pepto-Bismol) and iron supplements can turn stools black. True melena is pitch black, tarlike, and sticky and has an odor that is not soon forgotten. Iron supplements can also make stools test heme positive.

Laboratory Data

CBC, platelet count, reticulocyte count
Electrolytes, blood urea nitrogen, creatinine
- BUN/Cr ratio >30 supports upper GI bleed instead of lower GI bleed

Liver function tests
PT, PTT, INR
Flat, upright, and/or lateral decubitus abdominal films, especially if the child is uncomfortable

Meckel scan
Ultrasound of bowel for intussusception
Stool cultures/nucleic acid amplification testing (NAAT) for bacterial enteritis, Ova and Parasite (O&P) testing
Proctoscopy

Management

Consider colonoscopy to identify source of bleeding and potentially intervene. For suspected intussusception, nonsurgical reduction (e.g., air enema) is frequently both diagnostic and therapeutic.

REMEMBER

1. Give the child NPO orders and document when the last oral intake was in case surgical intervention or endoscopy is indicated.
2. Resuscitate the child before you pursue diagnostic studies.
3. Insertion of a nasogastric tube for upper GI bleeding can be critically important
4. Medications that may result in bleeding or exacerbate GI bleeding include NSAIDs, steroids, heparin, and warfarin.

Genitourinary Problems

James J. Nocton, MD

Several problems related to the genitourinary system may arise while a child is hospitalized and require prompt attention. Some of these problems, such as hematuria (see Chapter 23) and urine output problems (see Chapter 30), are reviewed elsewhere in this book. In this chapter the approach to evaluating dysuria, scrotal pain, and vaginal bleeding while on call is discussed.

Dysuria

PHONE CALL

Questions

1. Is the child febrile?
2. What is the child's diagnosis?
3. How old is the child?
4. Is the child a boy or a girl?
5. Is there gross hematuria?

The answers to these questions will allow you to begin to think about potential explanations for the problem. If fever is present, a urinary tract infection is much more likely. The child's diagnosis or the presence of gross hematuria may suggest specific causes (such as hemorrhagic cystitis related to cyclophosphamide treatment as part of chemotherapy protocols). Likewise, some problems may be more common at different ages (e.g., sexually transmitted diseases) or occur only in boys (balanitis).

Orders

Ask the nurse to collect the next urine for urinalysis and culture. If the child is an infant, the nurse will need to collect the urine by catheter to avoid contamination.

Inform RN

Tell the RN, "Will arrive at the bedside in … minutes." A child with fever, severe discomfort, or gross hematuria should be seen immediately.

ELEVATOR THOUGHTS

What causes dysuria?
Urinary tract infections
   Cystitis (bacterial, adenoviral, drugs)
   Pyelonephritis
Urethritis
   Sexually transmitted infection (STI; gonococcus)
   Inflammatory (reactive arthritis, Kawasaki disease)
Vaginitis
   STI
   Group A streptococcus
   Foreign body
Passage of renal calculi
Passage of a blood clot (trauma)
Urethral irritation
   Girls
      Bubble bath
      Pinworms
      Urethral prolapse
      Sexual abuse
      Hypercalciuria
      Trauma
   Boys
Hypercalciuria
   Urethral stricture
   Balanitis
   Trauma/foreign body insertion

MAJOR THREAT TO LIFE

Few life-threatening problems are associated with dysuria. If infection is present, it may progress to sepsis and shock. If hemorrhage from bleeding along the genitourinary tract is present, it could eventually lead to hypovolemia and shock.

BEDSIDE

Quick-Look Test

Most children will appear well. If they are distressed, lethargic, or unresponsive, shock from sepsis or hemorrhage and hypovolemia may be imminent.

Airway and Vital Signs

Tachycardia, if present, will most likely be secondary to pain or fever. An increased respiratory rate may also be related to pain or may reflect acidosis from infection. Hypotension will indicate potential shock.

Selective Physical Examination

HEENT[*]	Conjunctivitis may be seen with reactive arthritis or with Kawasaki disease, both of which may cause urethritis
Abdomen	Flank tenderness (pyelonephritis), suprapubic tenderness (cystitis)
Genitals	Urethral or vaginal discharge, ulcerations, penile lesions (balanitis), vesicles (herpes simplex)

[*]HEENT, Head, eyes, ears, nose, throat.

Selective History and Chart Review

Is the child at risk for STIs?

If the child is sexually active or has previously had such infections, the potential for an STI to be the cause is increased.

Is the child at risk for renal calculi?

A family history of renal calculi or conditions leading to potential hypercalcemia (see Chapter 34) increase the risk.

Has there been a history of trauma or kidney tumor?

Trauma to the kidney or Wilms tumor can lead to bleeding into the urinary tract and the passage of blood clots.

Has the child received medications that can cause hemorrhagic cystitis?

Review the child's list of medications and potential adverse effects to answer this question.

Management

Your priority while on call is to establish whether infection or hemorrhage is a probable cause of the dysuria because these are the two potential threats to life. Urinalysis should be performed as quickly as possible. A quick dipstick test at the bedside will determine whether there is heme in the urine, potentially from hemorrhage in the urinary tract, or whether leukocytes and nitrites are present, potentially indicative of infection. The presence of nitrites is more specific for bacteria in the urine because leukocytes may be present with noninfectious urethritis, as well as with urinary tract infections.

Microscopic analysis of urine will allow you to determine whether red blood cells are present, indicative of hemorrhage, rather than hemoglobinuria from hemolysis or myoglobinuria from rhabdomyolysis as the cause for heme in the urine. It will also allow quantitation of the number of white blood cells in the urine, with large numbers being more suggestive of infection.

Urinary Tract Infection

If the child has fever, flank pain and tenderness, and large numbers of white blood cells in the urine, pyelonephritis should be suspected. If there is no fever or flank pain and large numbers of white blood cells are found in the urine with positive nitrites, it is more likely to be a lower urinary tract infection (i.e., cystitis). Cystitis is more common in adolescent females, whereas younger children are more likely to have pyelonephritis. In some instances, it is difficult to determine conclusively whether the infection has ascended the urinary tract and led to pyelonephritis. In either case, if the suspicion of infection is strong, empiric antibiotic treatment should be started after ensuring that an adequate specimen for urine culture has been obtained (catheterization, suprapubic aspiration, or clean-catch specimen). *Escherichia coli* and other enteric pathogens will be the most likely cause, and therefore a third-generation cephalosporin is often the best choice. Pyelonephritis should be treated with intravenous antibiotics, whereas cystitis may be treated orally with a third-generation cephalosporin, trimethoprim-sulfamethoxazole, or, in older children, ciprofloxacin.

Hemorrhagic Cystitis

In the absence of a history of administration of medications that can cause hemorrhagic cystitis, hemorrhage in the urine associated with dysuria may be the result of renal calculi, hypercalciuria, or viral hemorrhagic cystitis. Adenovirus is a common cause of hemorrhagic cystitis and requires only supportive treatment, with resolution generally occurring within several days. However, if cyclophosphamide or another medication that can cause hemorrhagic cystitis has been administered, the child is frequently in significant pain and requires prompt attention. Consultation with a urologist will be necessary, and bladder irrigation should be initiated. A Foley catheter should be placed and normal saline irrigation begun. In some instances, cystoscopy or administration of alum or silver nitrate into the bladder may be necessary. These steps should be undertaken only after consultation with a urologist.

Sexually Transmitted Infections

If the patient is an adolescent with dysuria, an STI is possible. Certainly, a history of previous similar infections or the presence of a vaginal or urethral discharge increases the likelihood of an STI. An adolescent female should undergo a pelvic examination, and appropriate cervical specimens for culture or nucleic acid amplification of gonococcus and Chlamydia should be obtained. A wet preparation should be performed with analysis for clue cells and Trichomonas. If there is cervical motion tenderness or adnexal tenderness on examination and/or significant purulent cervical discharge, treatment should be considered before confirmation of infection by culture. In males a urethral swab can be performed to obtain specimens for culture of gonococcus and Chlamydia. Performing polymerase chain reaction (PCR) for gonococcus and

Chlamydia on urine samples is an alternative in both males and females. Treatment regimens for uncomplicated STIs and those for pelvic inflammatory disease are presented in Tables 20.1 and 20.2, respectively.

TABLE 20.1	Treatment of Uncomplicated Sexually Transmitted Infection in Adolescents
Chlamydia trachomatis	Azithromycin, 1 g orally in a single dose or Doxycycline,[a] 100 mg orally twice daily for 7 days
Neisseria gonorrhoeae	Ceftriaxone, 250 mg intramuscularly in a single dose or Cefixime, 400 mg orally in a single dose plus Treatment of *C. trachomatis* if indicated[b]

[a]Eight years of age or older.
[b]The Centers for Disease Control and Prevention recommend treating persons with a positive gonorrhea test result for both gonorrhea and chlamydia unless a negative result has been obtained with a sensitive chlamydia test.
Modified from Workowski KA, Bolan GA: Sexually transmitted diseases treatment guidelines 2015. MMWR Recomm Rep 64(3):1-137, 2015.

TABLE 20.2	Treatment of Pelvic Inflammatory Disease

Parenteral Regimens (One of the Following)
Cefotetan, 2 g IV q12h, or cefoxitin, 2 g IV q6h, plus doxycycline, 100 mg IV or PO q12h
or
Clindamycin, 900 mg IV q8h, plus gentamicin, loading dose (2 mg/kg-body weight) IV or IM followed by maintenance dose (1.5 mg/kg q8h; single daily dosing [3-5 mg/kg] of gentamicin can be substituted).
Parenteral therapy may be discontinued 24-48 hours after clinical improvement and continue doxycycline, 100 mg PO bid, or clindamycin, 450 mg orally qid, continued for 14 days of total therapy
For tubo-ovarian abscess, addition of either metronidazole, 500 mg PO bid, or clindamycin, 450 mg PO qid, to oral doxycycline provides better coverage against anaerobes
Outpatient Regimens (One of the Following)
Ceftriaxone 250 mg IM in a single dose, or cefoxitin 2 g IM—and probenecid 1 g PO in a single dose once, or other parenteral third-generation cephalosporin (e.g., ceftizoxime or cefotaxime), plus doxycycline 100 mg PO bid for 14 days with or without metronidazole 500 mg PO bid for 14 days

bid, Twice daily; *IM*, intramuscularly; *IV*, intravenously; *PO*, per os (orally); *qid*, four times daily.
Modified from Workowski KA, Bolan GA. Sexually transmitted diseases treatment guidelines 2015. MMWR Recomm Rep 64 (3):1-137, 2015.

Scrotal Pain

Questions

1. How long has the pain been present?
2. Has there been any history of injury or trauma?
3. Is there any radiation of the pain?
4. Are there systemic or other symptoms?
5. Is there swelling?

   The sudden onset of pain or pain after minor injury is suggestive of torsion of the testes or the appendix testis. Radiation of the pain may suggest inguinal hernia, and systemic symptoms such as fever and chills might indicate infection. Nausea and vomiting can be associated with testicular torsion, and dysuria may be seen with urinary tract infection or epididymitis.

Orders

Ask the nurse to collect and save a urine sample if possible.

Inform RN

Tell the RN, "Will arrive at the bedside in ... minutes." Scrotal pain is an emergency and should be evaluated immediately.

ELEVATOR THOUGHTS

What causes scrotal pain?
Testicular torsion (adolescent > prepubertal)
Torsion of testicular appendage (prepubertal > adolescent)
Trauma
Incarcerated inguinal hernia
Epididymitis (adolescents)
Orchitis (mumps)
Vasculitis (Henoch-Schönlein purpura, polyarteritis nodosa)
Referred pain (nephrolithiasis, appendicitis)
Malignancy
Fournier gangrene

MAJOR THREAT TO LIFE

Interruption of vascular flow to the testes with risk of subsequent infarction and loss of the testes is the major immediate threat. Testicular torsion results in the greatest risk for infarction, but severe trauma or vasculitis may rarely also place the patient at risk. Fournier gangrene is unusual in children, but it is a life-threatening infection.

BEDSIDE

Quick-Look Test

Does the child appear well (comfortable), sick (distressed, agitated), or critical (lethargic, unresponsive)?

A child with scrotal pain will generally appear very uncomfortable regardless of the cause. Those with torsion of the appendix testis will not be as uncomfortable as those with testicular torsion. In the rare event of Fournier gangrene, the child may be in septic shock.

Airway and Vital Signs

The airway and vital signs should not be compromised, with the exception that tachycardia and mild hypertension may be present secondary to pain. If fever is noted, infection is obviously a consideration.

Selective Physical Examination

The examination will focus on the scrotum, its contents, and the inguinal canal, as well as the abdomen. The abdomen should be inspected and palpated for signs of an acute abdominal process with potential referred pain to the scrotum. Any scars should be noted because they will indicate a possible previous hernia or undescended testes. When examining the scrotum, note the position of the testis. A high-riding, swollen, exquisitely tender testis is suggestive of testicular torsion. The scrotum may be erythematous, and the cremasteric reflex should be absent. If a firm mass is palpated at the upper pole of the testis and the cremasteric reflex is present, torsion of the appendix testis is much more likely. In some instances the "blue dot sign" may be seen in which the twisted appendix testis is visible through the skin. With epididymitis, the epididymis itself will be firm, tender, and swollen.

Attention should be directed to the inguinal area to look for evidence of hernia. Swelling and pain in the scrotum and inguinal canal, especially with additional signs indicative of potential bowel obstruction, may occur with an incarcerated inguinal hernia.

Selective History and Chart Review

If the patient is an adolescent, is there a history of STI or dysuria?

This will increase the likelihood of epididymitis.

Has there been intermittent pain in the scrotum in the past?

Such pain might reflect previous intermittent episodes of testicular torsion.

Are there rashes, abdominal pain, and other systemic features?

Vasculitides such as Henoch-Schönlein purpura and polyarteritis nodosa may cause scrotal pain and swelling secondary to vasculitis within the spermatic cord.

Management

It may be difficult to distinguish testicular torsion, torsion of the appendix testis, and other causes of scrotal pain by the history and physical findings alone. This is critical because testicular torsion is managed surgically and the other conditions may be managed nonoperatively. Imaging studies may help to determine whether blood flow to the testis is reduced, as seen in testicular torsion. A color Doppler ultrasound is quick and often the most readily available imaging study. A radionuclide testicular flow scan can also be performed, but it requires more time and is often less convenient. When testicular torsion is a consideration, prompt consultation with a pediatric urologist is most helpful.

Testicular Torsion

Testicular torsion is a surgical emergency. If there is a reasonable likelihood of testicular torsion, the patient should be taken to the operating room for surgical exploration because time spent on imaging studies may be detrimental. Even if the torsion can be reduced manually by the pediatric urologist, surgical fixation is necessary to prevent recurrence.

Torsion of the Appendix Testis

Torsion of the appendix testis will eventually lead to infarction of the appendix with subsequent resolution of the pain and swelling. Bed rest plus analgesics for several days is usually sufficient. Imaging studies will most often reveal increased blood flow to the testis.

Incarcerated Hernia

If an incarcerated hernia is suspected, immediate pediatric surgical consultation is necessary, with surgical correction performed. Manual reduction of the hernia may be attempted before surgical repair.

Epididymitis

In prepubertal boys, epididymitis is most often secondary to an anatomic abnormality of the lower genitourinary tract and is usually caused by the same organisms that cause urinary tract infections. In these young boys, urinalysis with culture should be performed, appropriate antibiotics administered when indicated, and consultation with pediatric urology obtained. In adolescent boys, epididymitis is most often an STI, with gonococcus and Chlamydia being most common, and should be treated as described earlier in this chapter under "STIs."

Fournier Gangrene

Systemic symptoms of fever, chills, and potentially shock often accompany this severe necrotizing infection of the perineum. Multiple organisms, including staphylococcus, streptococcus, anaerobes, and gram-negative organisms, have been associated with Fournier gangrene. Surgical débridement and broad-spectrum antibiotics should be instituted promptly.

Vaginal Bleeding

Vaginal bleeding is always abnormal in the absence of secondary sexual characteristics and in girls younger than 8 years. The exception is in a newborn, in whom small amounts of vaginal bleeding may occur as a result of withdrawal from circulating maternal estrogens. In adolescents, it may also be the result of irregular menstruation. Vaginal bleeding is rarely an emergency, but you may need to be prepared to evaluate this problem should it begin while you are on call.

PHONE CALL

Questions

1. How old is the child?
2. Has the child been menstruating previously?
3. Has there been any trauma?
4. What medications is the child receiving?
5. Is there bleeding at other sites?

   The age and menarchal status of the child will affect your differential diagnosis, as will a history of trauma, medications, and the presence of bleeding at multiple sites.

Orders

A complete blood count (CBC) with differential, prothrombin time (PT), and partial thromboplastin time (PTT) should be ordered if the bleeding is heavy or persistent and if these laboratory tests have not been performed recently.

Inform RN

Tell the RN, "I will arrive at the bedside in … minutes." Unless the child is unstable or bleeding profusely, vaginal bleeding is rarely an emergency, and if other situations are a priority, the patient can be evaluated when time allows.

ELEVATOR THOUGHTS

What causes vaginal bleeding?

Prepubertal child   Vaginal foreign body (toilet paper)
                                    Infectious vulvovaginitis
                                    Urethral prolapse
                                    Trauma
                                    Lichen sclerosus

	Pinworms
	Hemangioma
	Malignancy
	Precocious menarche
Pubertal child	Foreign body
	Trauma
	Malignancy
	Cervical polyp
	Coagulopathy
	Hemangioma
	Cervicitis
	Endometrial polyp
	Pelvic inflammatory disease

MAJOR THREAT TO LIFE

Massive bleeding with exsanguination is the primary threat to life.

BEDSIDE

Quick-Look Test

Does the child appear well (comfortable), sick (distressed, agitated), or critical (lethargic, unresponsive)?

If the child is distressed or agitated, excessive bleeding, infection, trauma, or an uncomfortable foreign body should be considered.

Airway and Vital Signs

Fever, tachycardia, or hypotension should increase your suspicion of infection or massive hemorrhage.

Selective Physical Examination

The examination will focus on the external genitalia, and in adolescents, consideration will need to be given to performing a pelvic examination if there is considerable bleeding and the cause is not apparent after examining the external genitalia. In addition, the general examination should focus on the mucous membranes of the nasal and oral cavities and the skin in a search for other signs of hemorrhage that might be indicative of a systemic coagulopathy.

The labia should be examined for signs of trauma, such as lacerations. Any discharge from the vagina and any lesions should be noted, such as hemangiomas or urethral prolapse. The presence of a foreign body should be obvious. The Tanner stage of the child should be documented. Lichen sclerosus of the vulva leads to thinning of the epidermis and has a characteristic appearance.

Selective History and Chart Review

Has the child had menarche?

If other signs of pubertal development are apparent, the current bleeding may represent menarche.

If the child has begun menstruating, what has the pattern of the menstrual periods been and when was the last one?

Soon after menarche, menstruation can be very irregular.

Is there a history of bleeding disorders in the family?

Coagulopathies, including von Willebrand disease or a platelet function defect, may cause menorrhagia without necessarily causing bleeding at other sites.

Management

The cause of the vaginal bleeding may be obvious after your physical examination and selective history, particularly if a laceration, vaginal discharge, foreign body, or mass is evident. If signs of vaginal discharge are present, cultures should be obtained and appropriate antibiotics begun. If the cause is not easily discerned, further evaluation will be necessary, but it does not necessarily need to occur in the middle of the night. Checking the results of the CBC, PT, and PTT can help to reassure you that the bleeding is not excessive and that the patient is not at risk for severe bleeding from a coagulopathy. The patient may require frequent evaluation to ensure that the bleeding does not worsen and that her vital signs do not suggest impending hypovolemia. As long as this is the case, further assessment, including evaluation for precocious puberty and potential consultation with a gynecologist, pediatric hematologist, or pediatric endocrinologist, can proceed in a less urgent manner. Remember, your goal while on call is to ensure that nothing will occur immediately to endanger the patient.

Summary

Genitourinary problems are infrequent while on call and are rarely an emergency. However, a few life-threatening and organ-threatening processes can cause dysuria, scrotal pain, and vaginal bleeding and may need to be addressed while on call. Although it is always optimal to make a definitive diagnosis, when this is not possible, evaluating the patient frequently, providing supportive care, and remaining alert for potential life-threatening processes will allow you to keep your patient safe and comfortable while you plan potential further evaluation.

chapter 21

Headache

Susan K. Light, MD

Headache is a frequent complaint of hospitalized children. It may be a symptom secondary to a life-threatening intracranial process, or it may be a relatively benign and self-limited complaint. The goal while on call is not necessarily to definitively diagnose the cause of the headache. Instead, the more immediate goal is to exclude conditions that require urgent attention and treatment. After this is accomplished, headache can be managed symptomatically and expectantly while planning for further diagnostic evaluation when a clear cause cannot be immediately established.

PHONE CALL

Questions

1. How old is the child?
2. Why is the patient in the hospital?
3. How severe is the headache? Can the child rate the pain such as with a pain scale (Fig. 21.1)?
4. Was the onset sudden or gradual?
5. What are the vital signs?
6. Has the child had a headache like this before?
7. Is the headache positional (is it worse when lying down flat)?

Orders

If a recent set of vital signs have not been recorded, ask the nurse to obtain them, including temperature.

Inform RN

Tell the RN, "I will arrive at the bedside in … minutes."

Increased intracranial pressure (ICP) is the most concerning possible explanation for headache and needs to be considered in all patients with this complaint. Headaches related to increased ICP are associated with nausea, vomiting, mental status changes,

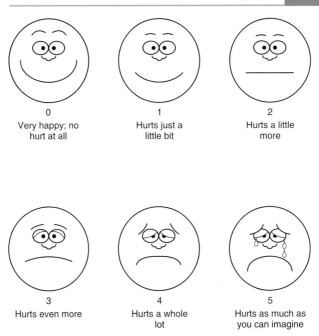

FIGURE 21.1 The Bieri Faces Scale. (Modified from Bieri D, Reeve RA, Champion GB, et al: The faces pain scale for the self-assessment of the severity of pain experienced by children: development, initial validation, and preliminary investigation for ratio scale properties. Pain 41:139-150, 1990.)

and eventually vital sign abnormalities, such as bradycardia and hypertension. Recurrent or chronic headaches should be addressed within a reasonable time but do not warrant an immediate assessment if the vital signs are stable, the pain is not severe, and the child has no other symptoms.

ELEVATOR THOUGHTS

What causes headaches?

Many of the causes are the same as in adults, but the relative frequencies may be very different. For example, brain tumors are the most commonly diagnosed solid tumor of childhood, and many, especially posterior fossa tumors, are associated with characteristic headaches.

Headaches may be a symptom of a disorder outside the nervous system or may arise directly as a result of dysfunction within the nervous system. The **pain-sensitive** structures in the head are as follows:

Intracranial	Cerebral and dural arteries
	Large veins and venous sinuses
	Dura at the base of the brain
	Periosteum of the skull
Extracranial	Cervical roots
	Cranial nerves
	Extracranial arteries
	Muscles attached to the skull
	Periosteum/paranasal sinuses
	Eyes/ears
	Mouth/dental structures
	Skin or soft tissue over the skull

Acute Headache

1. Increased ICP: Headache results from compression and distortion of pain-sensitive dural and vascular structures surrounding the brain. It is worse after a few hours of being recumbent or asleep and decreases after a period of being awake and upright (positional headache). When more severe, it increases with coughing, straining, and bending over and may be associated with visual obscuration. Causes include:
   Brain tumor
   Subdural or epidural hematoma
   Malignant hypertension
   Pseudotumor cerebri
   Trauma (closed head injury)
2. Infectious: Headache results from inflammation of pain-sensitive structures surrounding the brain (meningismus). It is usually generalized, severe, throbbing, and associated with nuchal rigidity and photophobia. Causes include:
   Meningitis
   Encephalitis
   Sinusitis or mastoiditis
   Brain abscess
3. Vascular: Subarachnoid hemorrhage causes an explosive, sudden onset, "worst headache of my life." Pain is followed by meningismus and later by headache secondary to increased ICP. Causes include:
   Intraparenchymal hemorrhage
   Vasculitis
   Migraine
   Arteriovenous malformation with bleeding

Cerebral venous sinus thrombosis: seizures, increased ICP, altered mental status

4. Posttraumatic
   Concussion
   Subdural or epidural hematoma
   Cerebral contusion
5. Other
   Acute angle-closure glaucoma
   Alcohol or drug ingestion

Low-pressure headache: Because of loss of cerebrospinal fluid (such as after a lumbar puncture [LP]), the brain's buoyancy is decreased such that the organ descends when the individual is in the upright position; as a result, traction is exerted on structures at the apex, and structures at the base are compressed. Pain is relieved by lying flat.

Pituitary apoplexy: Acute hemorrhage or infarction of the pituitary gland can cause acute headache referred to the temples/ears, meningismus, visual field changes, and raised ICP-type headache.

CHRONIC (RECURRENT) HEADACHE

Progressive

1. Vascular
   Migraine
   Cluster headaches
   Hypertension
   Subdural hematoma
2. Metabolic
   Hypoglycemia
3. Drugs
   Alcohol
   Nitrates
   Calcium channel blockers
   Nonsteroidal antiinflammatory drugs (NSAIDs)
4. Increased ICP
   Tumor
   Pseudotumor
   Central nervous system vasculitis
   Hydrocephalus
5. Infectious
   Abscess (intracranial, dental)

Nonprogressive

1. Psychogenic
   Tension headaches
   Stress

Depression
Anxiety
2. Other
   Temporomandibular joint disease
   Posttraumatic
   School avoidance/attention seeking

MAJOR THREAT TO LIFE

Headaches caused by increased ICP can be a presenting symptom of the following life-threatening diagnoses:

- Intracranial bleeding: subarachnoid, subdural, epidural hemorrhage
- Meningitis
- Herniation (transtentorial, cerebellar, central)
- Tumor
- Cerebral venous thrombosis
- Acute obstructive hydrocephalus

All of these conditions can progress rapidly and are associated with a poor outcome if unrecognized. Herniation is a significant cause of death secondary to cerebral edema after trauma, intraparenchymal bleeding, or hypoxic-ischemic encephalopathy (Fig. 21.2).

BEDSIDE

Quick-Look Test

Does the patient appear well (comfortable), sick (uncomfortable, distressed), or critical (about to die)?

Most patients with chronic or recurrent headaches are fairly comfortable. Those with migraines, meningitis, subarachnoid hemorrhage, or subdural or epidural hematomas generally appear ill.

AIRWAY AND VITAL SIGNS

What is the temperature?

Fever in the setting of headache should prompt a search for infectious causes, including meningitis, abscess, encephalitis, and sinus disease.

What is the blood pressure?

Significant hypertension of any origin can cause headache.

What is the heart rate?

Cushing triad of hypertension, bradycardia, and respiratory changes is a most ominous and generally very late finding that is accompanied by significant mental status change. Tachycardia would be expected in any child complaining of severe headache.

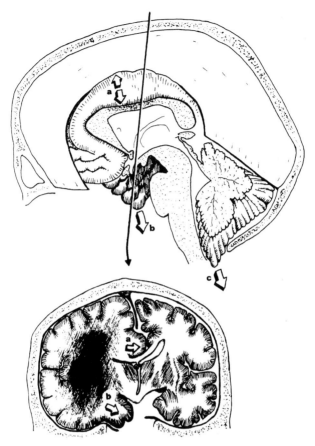

FIGURE 21.2 Central nervous system herniation. *a*, Cingulate herniation; *b*, Uncal herniation; *c*, Cerebellar herniation. (From Marshall SA, Ruedy J: On Call: Principles and Protocols, 4th ed. Philadelphia, Elsevier, 2004, p 122.)

SELECTIVE PHYSICAL EXAMINATION

HEENT   Funduscopic examination is ABSOLUTELY ESSENTIAL for detecting vascular changes, hemorrhages, and papilledema (Fig. 21.3) (loss of the optic nerve margin and lack of venous

HEENT, Head, Eyes, Ears, Nose Throat.

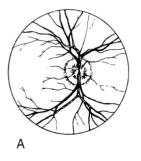

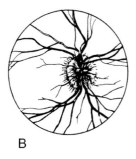

A   B

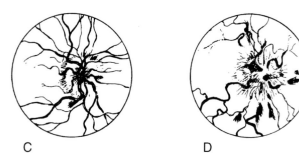

C   D

FIGURE 21.3 Disk changes seen in papilledema. (**A**) Normal.
(**B**) Early papilledema. (**C**) Moderate papilledema with early
hemorrhage. (**D**) Severe papilledema with extensive hemorrhage. (From Marshall SA, Ruedy J: On Call: Principles and
Protocols, 4th ed. Philadelphia, Elsevier, 2004, p 123.)

	pulsations are specific signs of increased ICP); also check visual acuity, symmetry of pupils, photophobia, extraocular movements, ptosis, sinus tenderness, hemotympanum (basilar skull fracture), mastoid tenderness, depressed skull fractures, contusions, jaw pain, or restriction of movement.
Neck	Nuchal rigidity, positive Kernig or Brudzinski sign (Fig. 21.4).
Neurologic	Cranial nerve examination; symmetry of reflexes, tone, and strength; cerebellar function, including balance and gait; mental status examination. MAKE THE CHILD WALK IF AT ALL POSSIBLE!

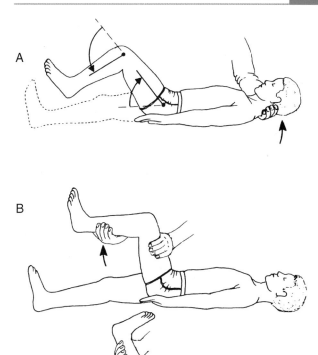

FIGURE 21.4 (A) Brudzinski sign. The test result is positive when the patient actively flexes his hips and knees in response to passive neck flexion by the examiner. **(B)** Kernig sign. The test result is positive when pain or resistance is elicited by passive knee extension from the 90-degree hip-knee flexion position. (From Marshall SA, Ruedy J: On Call: Principles and Protocols, 4th ed. Philadelphia, Elsevier, 2004, p 124.)

MANAGEMENT I

If the patient has a condition associated with hydrocephalus, such as new diagnosis of brain tumor or intracranial bleeding, neurosurgical consultation should be obtained as the patient is being prepared for computed tomography (CT) scan.

In a child with nuchal rigidity, altered mental status, or focal neurologic findings, order an immediate CT scan of the head.

If meningitis is suspected, order an LP tray at the bedside and appropriate intravenous broad-spectrum antibiotics to be given as soon as the CT scan and LP are completed. The CT scan and LP should be completed within 1 hour. If there is to be any delay, give the antibiotics and complete the studies thereafter.

The necessity for a head CT scan is controversial in patients with a completely nonfocal neurologic examination, normal mental status, and no signs of increased ICP, including papilledema. One can proceed either by performing the LP and administering the antibiotics (if you feel comfortable that there is no increase in ICP) or by administering the antibiotics empirically and performing the LP after the head CT scan has been obtained (if increased ICP remains a concern).

In children with nuchal rigidity and signs of increased ICP, LP is absolutely contraindicated because of the risk of brain herniation. Meningitis, subdural empyema, and brain abscess can all produce increased ICP and be manifested as headache. Head CT helps to distinguish among these conditions. In general, when evaluating for acute blood and ventricular size, CT of head without contrast is better than magnetic resonance imaging (MRI). If inflammation is suspected, CT of the head with contrast helps. To evaluate the posterior fossa, order an MRI. When evaluating arteries, order MRI/ magnetic resonance angiography. To evaluate the venous sinuses, order magnetic resonance venography. The empiric antibiotic coverage suggested for children and adolescents is cefotaxime, 50 mg/kg intravenously every 6 hours, along with vancomycin, 15 mg/kg every 6 hours. Vancomycin is a recent addition to the recommended empiric antibiotics because of the alarming increase in resistant *Streptococcus pneumoniae*. Higher doses of antibiotics are needed to allow for meningeal penetration. If abscess or subdural empyema is suspected, clindamycin or metronidazole is added to cover for anaerobes.

In addition to immediate antibiotic treatment, children with a brain abscess or subdural empyema require the expertise of a pediatric neurosurgeon. Moreover, it is prudent to anticipate a therapeutic plan for seizure control (see Chapter 29). If any signs of altered mental status and/or increased ICP are present, therapy should begin immediately (see Chapter 7).

SELECTIVE HISTORY AND CHART REVIEW

If the headache is a new complaint, have the child describe in detail what it feels like, where it hurts the most, and what makes it better or worse. Was there a warning or an aura? Are there associated symptoms? Did it start suddenly or gradually? Has the child ever had a headache like this before?

Characterize the onset, duration, frequency, and pattern of chronic headaches. Do they awaken the child from sleep or keep the child from falling asleep? Are the headaches present as soon as the child awakens in the morning? What time of day does the headache occur? Are there known precipitants, such as foods, change in sleep pattern, trauma, toxins, medications, or psychosocial stressors? Are there any associated symptoms such as an aura, tinnitus, visual changes, mental status changes, seizure activity, nausea, or vomiting?

The chart may contain additional information about past complaints of headache, as well as reports of a family headache history.

A medication history plus a history of head trauma over the past 6 to 8 weeks should be obtained. Headaches secondary to subdural hemorrhage may be delayed for days or even weeks, and therefore the patient and family may not associate the headache with a "distant" head injury.

MANAGEMENT II

Tension Headaches

Also known as stress headaches, muscle tension headaches are the most common headaches in childhood. Frequently described as "bandlike," they are usually bilateral. Pain tends to be mild to moderate, and the duration is highly variable, from 2 to 72 hours. This type of headache is frequently related to undiagnosed refraction defects in school-aged children straining to see the blackboard. Chronic exposure to loud music or noise can also provoke this type of headache. Patients are generally treated conservatively with acetaminophen or ibuprofen and reevaluated in the morning.

Migraine Headaches

Migraine headaches can be incapacitating regardless of the patient's age. Migraines may be preceded by an aura, which can consist of homonymous visual disturbances, unilateral weakness or sensory changes, aphasia or other language disturbances, or the "Alice in Wonderland" syndrome of spatial disorientation. Be aware that these symptoms are similar to those of ischemic stroke. Migraines are frequently unilateral but can be bilateral. Pain intensity is moderate to severe, and the duration is typically approximately 8 hours. Acute therapy should begin with acetaminophen or NSAIDs. Narcotic analgesics should be avoided if possible. The acute administration of vasoconstricting agents such as ergotamine or sumatriptan succinate (Imitrex) should be avoided in children younger than 10 years, if possible. β-Blockers are extensively used for migraine prophylaxis but are of little use as acute therapy.

Posttraumatic (Postconcussive) Headache

Given a history of trauma but no signs of intracranial edema or hemorrhage, postconcussive headaches can occur in the acute posttraumatic phase or at much later times. Mild analgesics such as acetaminophen or NSAIDs, which do not adversely affect the child's mental status or level of consciousness, should be administered. If the headache continues to worsen, consider a CT scan of the head to look for subdural or intraparenchymal blood.

Complicated Migraines

Migraines with brain stem aura, commonly known as basilar migraines, are typically characterized by onset in adolescence and occurrence in females more frequently than males. They are frequently accompanied by visual disturbances, ataxia, vertigo, nausea, vomiting, loss of consciousness, and/or drop attacks. Cranial nerve deficits can be observed. In treatment, avoid sumatriptan because it will constrict vessels in an already ischemic area. Hemiplegic migraine must be distinguished from stroke. There is a slow progression of unilateral weakness and/or sensory changes usually preceding the headache. Symptoms may last hours to days, and in recurrent attacks the alternate side may be affected. Associated symptoms include aphasia, paresthesias, and rarely seizures. Permanent deficits can result from repeated attacks. Ophthalmoplegic migraines generally have an age of onset of less than 10 years. Unilateral eye pain is followed by third nerve palsy, a dilated pupil, and downward and outward deviation of the eye. The fourth and sixth cranial nerves are frequently involved. Ophthalmoplegia resolves in 1 to 4 weeks. Permanent third nerve injury can result from multiple attacks.

Cluster Headaches

Cluster headaches are nonfamilial and tend to afflict males more than females. These headaches are rare before 10 years of age. The headache tends to be rather brief, 30 to 60 minutes, but is severe to excruciating. Often, there is unilateral nasal stuffiness and tearing attributed to histamine release, hence the term histamine cephalgia.

Brain Tumor Headaches

Although headaches can be an initial symptom of a brain tumor, brain tumors are generally an uncommon cause of headache in children. Brain tumor headaches tend to be chronic and progressive, and their onset commonly has a positional component, with maximal pain in the early morning on first rising from bed. The vast majority of children with brain tumors have abnormal findings on neurologic or ophthalmologic examination. A meticulous history and neurologic examination detect most brain tumors, especially in the setting of chronic, progressive headache.

Hemorrhages and Effusions

Subdural, epidural, and subarachnoid hemorrhages can result in headache and are generally diagnosed by CT scan. Therapy may be surgical, with decompression required to avoid herniation. Prompt neurosurgical consultation is warranted. Chronic subdural effusions can occur after meningitis, as well as after trauma, especially child abuse.

Malignant Hypertension

Malignant hypertension is unusual in children. Prompt but careful reduction in blood pressure should be undertaken, as discussed in Chapter 24.

Hydrocephalus

Although more common in younger children than in adolescents, hydrocephalus, like brain tumors, tends to cause recurrent, progressive headache. Therapy requires neurosurgical consultation. Obtaining the opening pressure when performing an LP is very important and may suggest the diagnosis of pseudotumor cerebri if the ventricles are not dilated on CT scan. Pseudotumor is most often seen in obese, adolescent girls but is also associated with several systemic illnesses.

Summary

Headache can be a common complaint in hospitalized children. Most headaches are due to benign causes that require only analgesic therapy. The house officer on call must distinguish these mild headaches from those that are life threatening. Thus headaches warrant prompt evaluation. It is important in the history to distinguish an isolated acute headache from a recurrent acute headache, as well as a pattern of chronic progressive versus chronic nonprogressive headaches. Box 21.1 can be helpful in organizing the differential diagnosis. Key physical examination findings include meningismus, funduscopic irregularities, and abnormal ambulation of the child.

BOX 21.1	Differential Diagnosis of Headache

Acute isolated headache
    Meningitis
    Subarachnoid hemorrhage
    Systemic infection with fever
Acute recurrent headache
    Brain tumor
    Vascular malformation
    Migraine
    Hypertension
    Sinusitis (rare in younger children)
Chronic progressive headache
    Brain tumor
    Hydrocephalus
    Brain abscess
    Subdural hemorrhage
    Pseudotumor cerebri
Chronic nonprogressive headache
    Depression
    Stress, tension headache
    Posttraumatic
    School avoidance or attention seeking

CHAPTER 22

Heart Rate and Rhythm Abnormalities

Daniel Beacher, MD

When evaluating a heart rhythm disturbance, the primary concern is the hemodynamic status of the patient. A patient who is pulseless should be treated according to the Pediatric Advanced Life Support (PALS) cardiac arrest algorithm. A patient who is hemodynamically unstable—weak pulses, poor perfusion, hypotension, altered mental status—requires immediate intervention. Investigations into the underlying etiology should not delay support of blood pressure (BP) and oxygen-carrying capacity and possible cardioversion.

If the patient is hemodynamically stable, there is more time to investigate the underlying etiology and tailor therapeutic interventions accordingly. In this case, it is best to think of rhythm disturbances in general categories: too fast versus too slow, regular versus irregular, and wide complex versus narrow complex. The task for a house officer confronted by a rhythm disturbance is to find a cause, if possible, and to intervene to preserve cardiac output (CO) before damage to vital organs occurs, including the brain, kidney, liver, and heart itself. CO is equal to stroke volume (SV) times heart rate (HR) ($CO = SV \times HR$), and rhythm abnormalities have a profound effect on both factors in that equation. Loss of atrial and ventricular synchrony compromises ventricular filling and adversely affects SV. Likewise, very high HRs decrease ventricular filling time and compromise SV.

In pediatrics, rhythm abnormalities with a rapid HR are far more common than rhythm abnormalities with a slow HR. The abnormality may be in response to an extracardiac disturbance (e.g., hypoxemia causing sinus bradycardia or fever causing sinus tachycardia), an intrinsic electrical problem, or a combination of both. Regardless of the cause, rhythm disturbances can be life threatening and must be evaluated without delay.

Rapid Heart Rates

PHONE CALL

Abnormal heart rhythms provoke an immediate reaction from the nursing staff. Questions should include the following:

1. What are the patient's BP and perfusion status?
2. Are there any associated symptoms (chest pain, palpitations, respiratory distress)?
3. What is the HR?
4. Is the rhythm regular or irregular?
5. Is the QRS complex narrow or wide?
6. How old is the patient?
7. Why is the patient in the hospital?
8. What are the rest of the patient's vital signs (temperature, respiratory rate)?

Orders

1. If the child is hypotensive or has signs of poor perfusion, insert a peripheral intravenous (IV) line and start a bolus of normal saline, 20 mL/kg, run as fast as possible.
2. Ask the nurse to attach the patient to a cardiorespiratory monitor immediately.
3. Call for a stat 12-lead electrocardiogram (ECG) and rhythm strip, if available.
4. Obtain another set of vitals, including BP reading, now.
5. Start the child on supplemental oxygen, 1 to 2 L/min by nasal cannula.

Inform RN

Tell the RN, "I will arrive at the patient's bedside in ... minutes."
Rapid HR with perfusion abnormalities is an emergency.

ELEVATOR THOUGHTS (CAUSES OF RAPID HEART RATES)

Rhythm abnormalities with rapid HRs are best categorized by three features: (1) whether the QRS complex is wide or narrow; (2) the presence and location of P waves; and (3) whether the rhythm is regular or irregular.

A narrow QRS complex is seen when the rhythm originates somewhere above the ventricles (i.e., supraventricular), either in the sinoatrial (SA) node, atria themselves, or atrioventricular (AV) node, and is conducted normally down the His-Purkinje system to the ventricles. P waves preceding narrow QRS complexes suggest an origin in the SA node or the atria (e.g., sinus tachycardia, atrial tachycardia, atrial flutter). Lack of P waves or P waves following narrow QRS complexes suggest either a junctional origin or reentrant rhythm.

A wide QRS complex is seen when the rhythm originates in the ventricles or when there is a supraventricular origin with abnormal conduction to the ventricles (aberrancy). However, distinguishing between these two can be difficult and ventricular arrhythmias pose an immediate threat to life. Therefore a wide complex tachycardia should be assumed to be ventricular tachycardia (VT) unless there is clear and convincing evidence otherwise. The regularity of the rhythm will also help to discriminate between different types of narrow or wide complex rhythms.

MAJOR THREAT TO LIFE

- Hypotension leading to shock
- Congestive heart failure leading to pulmonary compromise and hypoxia

As noted previously, keep in mind the following formulas:

$$CO = HR \times SV$$
$$BP = CO \times SVR$$

Once the HR becomes so high that ventricular filling is compromised, SV and therefore CO fall. The body tries to preserve BP by increasing systemic vascular resistance (SVR) through vasoconstriction, especially in the extremities, thereby resulting in compromised peripheral perfusion.

BEDSIDE

Quick-Look Test

Does the patient look well (comfortable), sick (uncomfortable or distressed), or critical (about to die)?

Tachycardia is uncomfortable and may cause agitation and irritability in infants and toddlers. Older children describe palpitations, pounding of the heart or chest, or racing of the heart. A patient in shock may have mental status changes.

Airway and Vital Signs

What are the HR and rhythm, temperature, and BP?

Hypotension requires immediate action, including a fluid bolus. Fever is a common cause of sinus tachycardia and may be a clue to an underlying etiology (e.g., sepsis causing hypotension). Of note, sinus tachycardia may be a response to hypotension, but it rarely occurs at rates high enough to be a primary cause of hypotension.

Identification of the abnormal rhythm is best accomplished using a 12-lead ECG; however, many rhythms can be identified using the rhythm strip or cardiorespiratory monitor. One should note that the paper speed on the ECG machine and sweep speed on the cardiorespiratory monitor are set to standard speed (25 mm/s). A lower speed (e.g., 12.5 mm/s) makes the QRS complexes narrow and a higher speed (50 mm/s) makes the QRS complexes wide. Recognition of the rhythm disturbance is critical. The following table may be helpful in classification:

	Regular	Irregular
Narrow QRS complex	• sinus tachycardia (Fig. 22.1) • atrial tachycardia (Fig. 22.2) • atrial flutter with regular block (Fig. 22.3) • atrioventricular reentrant tachycardia (AVRT), including Wolff-Parkinson-White (WPW) syndrome (Fig. 22.4) • atrioventricular nodal reentrant tachycardia (AVNRT; Fig. 22.5) • junctional ectopic tachycardia	• atrial fibrillation with rapid ventricular response (Fig. 22.6) • atrial flutter with variable block (Fig. 22.7) • multifocal atrial tachycardia (Fig. 22.8) • sinus tachycardia with premature atrial contractions (Fig. 22.9)
Wide QRS complex	• ventricular tachycardia (Fig. 22.10); the variant torsades de pointes can be seen with long QT syndrome (Fig. 22.11) • any regular narrow complex tachycardia with aberrancy	• sinus tachycardia with premature ventricular complexes (Fig. 22.12) • any irregular wide complex tachycardia with aberrancy

FIGURE 22.1 Sinus tachycardia. (From Marshall SA, Ruedy J: On Call: Principles and Protocols, 4th ed. Philadelphia, Elsevier, 2004, p 137.)

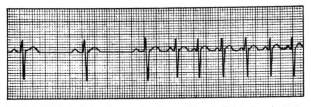

FIGURE 22.2 Atrial tachycardia. (From Marshall SA, Ruedy J: On Call: Principles and Protocols, 4th ed. Philadelphia, Elsevier, 2004, p 138.)

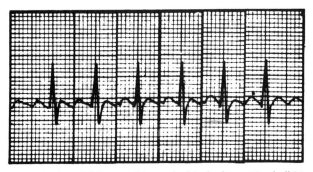

FIGURE 22.3 Atrial flutter with regular block. (From Marshall SA, Ruedy J: On Call: Principles and Protocols, 4th ed. Philadelphia, Elsevier, 2004, p 138.)

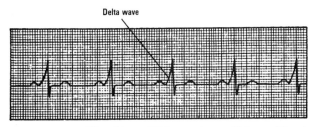

FIGURE 22.4 Wolff-Parkinson-White syndrome. This condition is characterized by a regular rhythm, a PR interval less than 0.12 second, a QRS complex longer than 0.11 second, and a delta wave (i.e., slurred beginning of the QRS). This predisposes to reentrant tachycardia. (From Marshall SA, Ruedy J: On Call: Principles and Protocols, 2nd ed. Philadelphia, WB Saunders Co, 1993, p 121.)

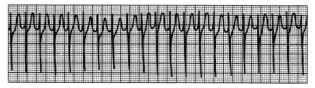

FIGURE 22.5 Atrioventricular nodal reentry tachycardia. (From Marshall SA, Ruedy J: On Call: Principles and Protocols, 4th ed. Philadelphia, Elsevier, 2004, p 138.)

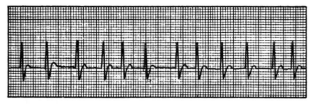

FIGURE 22.6 Atrial fibrillation with rapid ventricular response. (From Marshall SA, Ruedy J: On Call: Principles and Protocols, 4th ed. Philadelphia, Elsevier, 2004, p 136.)

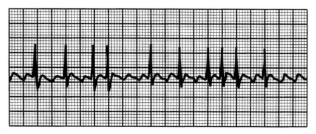

FIGURE 22.7 Atrial flutter with variable block. (From Marshall SA, Ruedy J: On Call: Principles and Protocols, 4th ed. Philadelphia, Elsevier, 2004, p 136.)

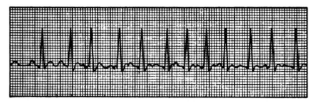

FIGURE 22.8 Multifocal atrial tachycardia. (From Marshall SA, Ruedy J: On Call: Principles and Protocols, 4th ed. Philadelphia, Elsevier, 2004, p 137.)

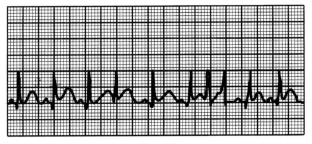

FIGURE 22.9 Sinus tachycardia with premature atrial contractions. (From Marshall SA, Ruedy J: On Call: Principles and Protocols, 4th ed. Philadelphia, Elsevier, 2004, p 137.)

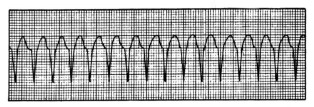

FIGURE 22.10 Ventricular tachycardia. (From Marshall SA, Ruedy J: On Call: Principles and Protocols, 4th ed. Philadelphia, Elsevier, 2004, p 135.)

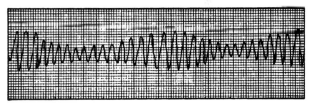

FIGURE 22.11 Torsades de pointes. (From Marshall SA, Ruedy J: On Call: Principles and Protocols, 4th ed. Philadelphia, Elsevier, 2004, p 149.)

Selective History and Chart Review

Identification of sinus tachycardia should prompt investigation into extracardiac causes such as fever, pain, and medications (especially sympathomimetic drugs, such as albuterol, pseudoephedrine, caffeine, and theophylline). A history of heart disease and/or

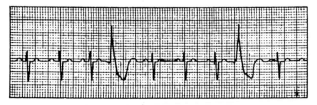

FIGURE 22.12 Sinus tachycardia with premature ventricular contractions. (From Marshall SA, Ruedy J: On Call: Principles and Protocols, 4th ed. Philadelphia, Elsevier, 2004, p 137.)

cardiac surgery is pertinent and may help to narrow the differential. Any previous ECGs are also helpful and may reveal baseline characteristics that predispose to arrhythmia (e.g., Wolff-Parkinson-White syndrome).

Management

Management of Hemodynamically Unstable Patient

Regardless of the cause of the tachycardia, if there are signs of poor perfusion, ventricular filling must be improved by immediately increasing preload (with IV fluids, packed red blood cells, etc.). However, if the patient has significant cardiovascular compromise (especially if the QRS complex is wide), emergency electrocardioversion is indicated. Give the following instructions:

- Page the senior resident and pediatric intensive care unit physician immediately, or call for the "code team."
- Bring the cardiac arrest resuscitation cart to the patient's bedside, and attach the ECG leads of the defibrillator to the child.
- Make sure that the child is receiving oxygen by nasal cannula or mask and that airway management equipment is on hand.
- Ensure that an adequate IV line is in place.
- Select the appropriate energy (begin with 0.5 to 1.0 joule/kg) and synchronize to the patient's R wave (select the monitor lead with the most obvious R wave).
- Clear everyone from contact with the patient, and deliver the shock while recording the ECG.
- If sinus rhythm is obtained, proceed further stabilization.
- Continue to follow the PALS protocol for resuscitation.

Management of Hemodynamically Stable Reentrant Supraventricular Tachycardia

If the patient has no evidence of significant cardiovascular compromise, other methods, such as temporary AV nodal blockade, may be used to convert the rhythm. For atrioventricular reentrant tachycardia (AVRT) or atrioventricular nodal reentrant tachycardia (AVNRT), this may include vagal maneuvers: ice to the face in an infant, having a young child blow through an occluded straw, or eliciting a Valsalva maneuver in an older child. If these are unsuccessful, IV adenosine (0.1 mg/kg, maximum dose = 6 mg) given by rapid push and followed immediately by a large-volume flush is effective in causing the same short-term AV nodal blockade achieved by vagal stimulation. If the initial dose is ineffective, the dose should be doubled, to a maximum of 12 mg. The most common reasons for failure of adenosine is administration in an inadequate IV line or an inadequate flush. The half-life of adenosine in the bloodstream is 6 to 10 seconds; therefore an IV site above the diaphragm is preferable, with at least a 10 mL normal saline flush.

Refractory SVT can be treated with synchronized cardioversion or with IV antiarrhythmic medications. These therapies should not be started without cardiology or critical care input.

Note that the calcium channel blocker verapamil should be avoided in infants and younger children with acute SVT because of its long duration and the possibility of persistent high-grade (life-threatening) AV block.

Management of Hemodynamically Stable Atrial Fibrillation and Atrial Flutter

Atrial fibrillation is a very rare rhythm in children with anatomically normal hearts. It is usually seen in children with congenital heart disease (CHD) and dilated atria (e.g., tricuspid or mitral valve stenosis or regurgitation, pulmonary hypertension, or dilated cardiomyopathy) or as a late complication of corrective surgery. Atrial flutter is more common than atrial fibrillation in children and is also often seen in children with structurally abnormal hearts (although infants with atrial flutter often have structurally normal hearts).

Both atrial fibrillation and flutter become hemodynamically significant if the ventricular response rate is very high or when atrial systole is needed to augment filling of a noncompliant ventricle; both cases result in reduced ventricular filling.

Temporary AV nodal blockade (by vagal maneuver or adenosine) will not terminate atrial flutter or fibrillation but may slow the ventricular response showing fibrillation or flutter waves, thus allowing proper diagnosis. Because of variable ventricular response rates in children, these rhythms are often not well tolerated. They may resolve spontaneously but more often require synchronized cardioversion and/or chemical cardioversion with antiarrhythmic medications. If the patient is hemodynamically stable, these interventions should be performed in consultation with a cardiologist. Particular care should be taken when the abnormal rhythm has been present for more than 24 hours because there is a risk of thrombus formation in the fibrillating or fluttering atria that could be embolized during cardioversion.

Management of Hemodynamically Stable Ventricular Tachycardia

VT is a dangerous rhythm and must be treated immediately. As mentioned previously, any wide complex tachycardia must be assumed to be VT, unless there is clear and convincing evidence otherwise. If the patient is hemodynamically stable, IV amiodarone is an effective treatment for VT; lidocaine is the alternative. Pediatric dosing of amiodarone is 5 mg/kg intravenously infused over a period of 20 to 60 minutes (which may be repeated up to a maximum of 15 mg/kg per day). Synchronized cardioversion may also be used if medical therapy alone does not convert the patient to sinus rhythm.

Once the patient is converted to sinus rhythm, it is important to search for possible causes of the VT, such as myocardial injury or ischemia, hypoxia, electrolyte imbalance (hyperkalemia, hypokalemia, hypomagnesemia, hypocalcemia), cardiomyopathy (arrhythmogenic right ventricular dysplasia), and drugs, including quinidine, disopyramide, tricyclic antidepressants, and phenothiazines

Slow Heart Rates

PHONE CALL

Questions

1. What are the patient's BP and perfusion status?
2. Are there any associated symptoms (respiratory distress, presyncope, or syncope)?
3. What is the HR?
4. Is the rhythm regular or irregular?
5. How old is the patient?
6. What are the rest of the patient's vital signs (temperature, respiratory rate)?
7. Why is the patient in the hospital?
8. What medications is the child receiving?
   Digoxin, β-blockers, and calcium channel blockers can prolong AV nodal conduction and result in bradycardia with a prolonged PR interval; they can also inhibit sinus node automaticity.

Orders

1. If the child is hypotensive or has signs of poor perfusion, insert a peripheral IV line and start a bolus of normal saline, 20 mL/kg, run as fast as possible

2. Ask the nurse to attach the patient to a cardiorespiratory monitor (including a continuous pulse oximeter) immediately.

3. Call for a stat 12-lead ECG and rhythm strip, if available.

4. Call respiratory therapy immediately, administer 100% oxygen, and have a bag-valve mask and intubation supplies at the bedside.

5. Bring the resuscitation "code" cart to the bedside, and attach the patient to the defibrillator monitor.

6. If the HR is less than 60 beats per minute (bpm) in an infant or 40 bpm in a child or adolescent, a dose of 0.02 mg/kg atropine (minimum dose 0.1 mg, maximum dose 0.5 mg in a child and 1 mg in an adolescent) and a dose of 0.01 mg/kg epinephrine should be prepared. If the patient is hypotensive and has an HR < 60 bpm, the code team should be called.

Inform RN

Tell the RN, "Will arrive at the bedside in … minutes."

Bradycardia is an indication of imminent circulatory collapse and must be evaluated immediately.

ELEVATOR THOUGHTS (CAUSES OF SLOW HEART RATES)

Bradycardia in children is often secondary to, or exacerbated by, extracardiac causes, especially hypoxemia and drugs. However, sick sinus syndrome (sinus node dysfunction) and AV block may be secondary to CHD or a consequence of cardiac surgery. With slow sinus rates, one may see junctional (narrow QRS complex) or ventricular (wide QRS complex) escape beats, which may make the rhythm appear irregular. An irregularly slow rhythm may also be seen in atrial fibrillation with a slow ventricular response (Fig. 22.13). Asymptomatic sinus bradycardia is common in well-conditioned athletes and during sleep.

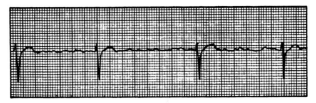

FIGURE 22.13 Atrial fibrillation with slow ventricular response rate. (From Marshall SA, Ruedy J: On Call: Principles and Protocols, 4th ed. Philadelphia, Elsevier, 2004, p 152.)

Rhythm	Drugs	Selected Etiologies	
		Cardiac	Other
Sinus bradycardia (Fig. 22.14)	Digoxin, β-blocker, calcium channel blockers	Neurocardiogenic (vagal) bradycardia, sick sinus syndrome	Hypothyroidism, increased ICP (Cushing triad), respiratory compromise (hypoxemia), anorexia nervosa, electrolyte disturbances
Second-degree AV block, Mobitz type I/Wenckebach (progressively prolonged PR interval until nonconducted P wave and absent QRS complex; Fig. 22.15)	Digoxin, β-blocker, calcium channel blockers	CHD, cardiac surgery, acute myocardial infarction, blunt trauma, myocarditis (including Lyme disease)	Head trauma, electrolyte disturbances
Second-degree AV block, Mobitz type II (normal PR interval with sudden nonconducted P wave and absent QRS complex; Fig. 22.16)	Digoxin, β-blocker, calcium channel blockers	CHD, cardiac surgery, acute myocardial infarction, blunt trauma, myocarditis (including Lyme disease)	Head trauma, electrolyte disturbances
Third-degree/complete AV block (none of the P waves are conducted; QRS complexes are independent of P waves; Fig. 22.17)	Digoxin, β-blocker, calcium channel blockers	CHD, cardiac surgery, acute myocardial infarction, myocarditis (including Lyme disease)	Autoimmune disorders (e.g., infants born to mothers with anti-SSA or anti-SSB antibodies)

AV, Atrioventricular; *CHD,* congenital heart disease; *ICP,* intracranial pressure; *SSA,* Sjögren syndrome antigen A; *SSB,* Sjögren syndrome antigen B.

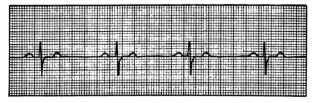

FIGURE 22.14 Sinus bradycardia. (From Marshall SA, Ruedy J: On Call: Principles and Protocols, 4th ed. Philadelphia, Elsevier, 2004, p 150.)

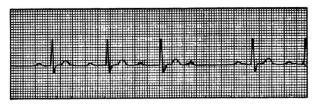

FIGURE 22.15 Second-degree atrioventricular block (type I). (From Marshall SA, Ruedy J: On Call: Principles and Protocols, 4th ed. Philadelphia, Elsevier, 2004, p 151.)

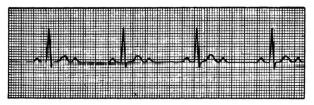

FIGURE 22.16 Second-degree atrioventricular block (type II). (From Marshall SA, Ruedy J: On Call: Principles and Protocols, 4th ed. Philadelphia, Elsevier, 2004, p 151.)

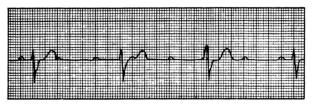

FIGURE 22.17 Third-degree atrioventricular block. (From Marshall SA, Ruedy J: On Call: Principles and Protocols, 4th ed. Philadelphia, Elsevier, 2004, p 152.)

MAJOR THREAT TO LIFE

- Hypotension
- Asystole

Especially in infants, CO is very dependent on HR; consequently, bradycardia significantly decreases CO and thereby leads to end-organ dysfunction. Bradycardia secondary to myocardial infarction (e.g., in those with coronary artery aneurysms from Kawasaki disease) or contusion may deteriorate into a more ominous rhythm, such as ventricular fibrillation or asystole.

BEDSIDE

Quick-Look Test

Does the patient appear well (comfortable), sick (uncomfortable or distressed), or critically ill (about to die)?

Unless the patient is very comfortable without signs of poor perfusion, the "code" cart and other resuscitative measures should be close at hand. Make sure that the patient is attached to a monitor and that the sweep speed of the monitor is set at the standard 25 mm/s and that there is IV access. Make sure that the monitor and the patient's pulse correlate with one another.

Airway and Vital Signs

First, be sure that the patient is ventilating adequately—address airway and breathing first of all.

What is the HR?

Analyze the rhythm strip, and identify the rhythm. Profound bradycardia may require immediate intervention, including the administration of 0.1 mg/kg atropine or 0.02 mg/kg epinephrine (minimum dose 0.1 mg, maximum dose 0.5 mg in a child and 1 mg in an adolescent) via an IV line or endotracheal tube if necessary.

What are the BP and perfusion status?

Regardless of the rhythm, poor perfusion and an HR < 60 means that cardiopulmonary resuscitation must be started, including chest compressions if necessary. Remember: electromechanical dissociation gives a false sense of security because an electrical rhythm is seen despite inadequate contraction. Volume resuscitation is required.

Selective History and Chart Review

Look for a cause or for previous episodes of bradycardia. Remember that the most common causes of bradycardia are related to medications and respiratory compromise.

Does the child have a history of CHD and/or cardiac surgery? Does the child have a past history of Kawasaki disease with coronary artery aneurysms? Has the child been in an area endemic for Lyme disease? Is there a family history of hyperlipidemia?

Was there associated syncope that might point to a vasovagal episode? Was the bradycardia associated with vagal maneuvers, such as straining, micturition, or Valsalva maneuvers?

Selective Physical Examination

Again, look for clues to the cause of the patient's bradycardia (if stable).

Vital signs	Bradypnea (hypothyroidism), hypothermia (hypothyroidism, exposure), hypertension and irregular breathing (ominous in combination, indicating increased ICP, Cushing triad)
HEENT	Coarse facial features, macroglossia, loss of the lateral third of the eyebrows (hypothyroidism); papilledema (increased ICP)
Neck	Goiter, jugular venous distention
Cardiovascular	New S_3 or S_4, mitral regurgitation murmur (myocardial infarction with papillary muscle injury)
Abdomen	Hepatosplenomegaly
Extremities	Poor perfusion and/or peripheral pulses
Neurologic	Mental status changes, evidence of trauma, delayed return phase of deep tendon reflexes (hypothyroidism)
Skin	Annular erythematous papules (neonatal lupus)

HEENT, Head, ears, eyes, nose, and throat; *ICP*, intracranial pressure.

Management
Management of Hemodynamically Unstable Patient

As mentioned previously, regardless of the rhythm, poor perfusion and an HR < 60 means that cardiopulmonary resuscitation must be started, including chest compressions if necessary. The code team should be called, IV access should be obtained, and a defibrillator should be brought into the room. Atropine and epinephrine should be available. Transcutaneous pacing may need to be used.

Hemodynamically Stable Patient
Management of Hemodynamically Stable Sinus Bradycardia

If the child has normal perfusion and BP, no acute intervention is necessary. Search for a cause. If the child has been receiving digoxin, β-blockers, or calcium channel blockers, no further doses should be given until the HR normalizes. Abrupt discontinuation of β-blockers may cause rebound hypertension, angina, or myocardial infarction. The drug should be reinstituted at a lower dose once the HR has normalized.

Management of Hemodynamically Stable Second-Degree Atrioventricular Block Type I

This rhythm does not degenerate into complete heart block. If the patient is hemodynamically stable, no acute intervention is required. Cardiotonic drugs should be withheld until the rhythm normalizes. Continuous monitoring is advisable. If the child is unstable, consider isoproterenol infusion.

Management of Hemodynamically Stable Second-Degree Atrioventricular Block Type II

This rhythm can degenerate into complete heart block. If the patient is hemodynamically stable, no acute intervention is required. If the child is unstable, consider isoproterenol infusion. Given the risk for development of complete heart block, cardiology should be consulted promptly.

Management of Hemodynamically Stable Third-Degree Atrioventricular Block

If the child is hemodynamically stable, no acute intervention is required. If the child is unstable, begin resuscitative measures including atropine and/or epinephrine. Transcutaneous/transvenous pacing and/or isoproterenol may be required. In the setting of acute digoxin ingestion with high blood levels, bradycardia, and second- or third-degree heart block, the digoxin-specific binding antibody Digibind must be given to reduce the toxic effects.

REMEMBER

1. Regardless of the underlying rhythm, if a patient is hemodynamically unstable, initial management should focus on improving CO and oxygen-carrying capacity.
2. Any wide complex tachycardia should be treated as life-threatening VT unless there is clear and convincing evidence otherwise.
3. In a hemodynamically stable patient with narrow complex tachycardia, vagal maneuvers or adenosine may terminate the rhythm or help with diagnosis.
4. Bradycardia is often secondary to respiratory compromise or medications.
5. Proper performance and interpretation of the ECG is essential. You cannot get the answer if you do not get the data!

Hematuria

Anna Schmitz, MD

Hematuria is often described by patients or parents as "red urine" or "brown urine." The first step in evaluating these patients is determining whether the child actually has hematuria, defined as red blood cells in the urine on microscopic urinalysis. Frankly red or pink urine suggests macroscopic hematuria. Tea- or cola-colored urine may reflect hemoglobinuria, myoglobinuria, or excretion of organic dyes, such as those in beets and some confectionery dyes. An orange stain in a diaper is often mistaken for blood when it is more likely to be urate crystals.

Hematuria can be a sign of injury to the lower genitourinary tract, as in trauma or infection, or it may represent glomerular injury as a result of trauma, infection, or an autoimmune condition.

PHONE CALL

Questions

1. How old is the patient?
2. Is the child male or female?
3. Why is the patient in the hospital?
4. Has there been any recent trauma?
5. Are there any associated symptoms, such as frequency, urgency, fever, dysuria, oliguria, or polyuria?
6. If female, is the child menstruating?

Orders

Ask the nurse to obtain a sterile urine specimen for dipstick, microscopic analysis, culture, and Gram stain. For children unable to provide a clean-catch sample, a catheterized specimen should be obtained.

Repeat a full set of vital signs immediately.

Inform RN

Tell the RN, "I will arrive at the bedside in … minutes." Hematuria requires evaluation but rarely is an emergency. In the setting of a trauma patient, it deserves prompt attention because significant kidney injury or pelvic fracture can precipitate internal bleeding and shock.

ELEVATOR THOUGHTS

The differential diagnosis of hematuria (red blood cells in the urine) includes the following:

Infections
    Urinary tract infection
    Viral bladder infection
Trauma
Perineal or meatus irritation
Nephrolithiasis
Glomerular injury
    Postinfectious glomerulonephritis
    Hemolytic-uremic syndrome
    Lupus
    Immunoglobulin A (IgA) nephropathy
    Henoch-Schönlein purpura
    Antineutrophil cytoplasmic antibody-associated vasculitis
    Goodpasture syndrome
Anatomic
    Polycystic kidney disease
    Tumor
Vascular
    Renal artery/vein thrombosis
Exercise induced
Interstitial nephritis
Acute renal tubular injury (shock; medications)
Sickle cell trait
Fictitious
Menses

MAJOR THREAT TO LIFE

Blunt trauma to the flank, back, or abdomen of a child may result in significant renal injury. In addition to hematuria, this may cause intra-abdominal or retroperitoneal bleeding leading to shock. The urine of every trauma victim should be tested for occult blood. Hematuria in the setting of a known bleeding disorder should also be considered an indication of potentially life-threatening coagulopathy.

BEDSIDE

Quick-Look Test

Does the patient appear well (comfortable), sick (uncomfortable or distressed), or critical?

Pain, in the absence of trauma, may be seen with pyelonephritis, nephrolithiasis, cystitis, or perineal irritation. Painless hematuria can be seen in patients with glomerulonephritis, as well as tumor.

Airway and Vital Signs

What are the temperature, heart rate, blood pressure, and respiratory rate?

Hypertension may suggest renal artery stenosis with high renin production or glomerulonephritis. Tachycardia may accompany pain. Respiratory distress can be seen with renal failure and fluid overload. Fever may indicate pyelonephritis.

Selective History and Chart Review

See Table 23.1.

Selective Physical Examination

HEENT	Carefully examine the fundi for signs associated with hypertension; look for periorbital edema
Neck	Check for jugular venous distention and thyromegaly
Lungs	Rales and/or consolidation with hemoptysis suggests Goodpasture syndrome or vasculitis
Cardiovascular	Tachycardia, hypertension, or an S_3 gallop rhythm can imply fluid overload
Abdomen	Flank pain, tenderness, fullness, masses, ascites
Genitourinary	Discharge, edema, erythema, trauma
Skin	Petechiae, purpura
Extremities	Edema

HEENT, Head, Ears, Eyes, Nose, Throat.

Initial Management

The initial step should be to assess the patient's urine output and adjust fluid intake appropriately. Hematuria accompanied by oliguria requires fluid restriction to cover only insensible losses due to the possibility of renal failure with resultant electrolyte disturbances, hypertension, and fluid overload. Hypertension must be managed to avoid complications, and strict dietary protein and potassium restriction may be necessary (see Chapter 24). In renal insufficiency, dialysis may be necessary because of uremia, fluid overload, or severe electrolyte disturbances.

TABLE 23.1 | **History and Chart Review**

Question	Etiology (from History)
Dysuria/frequency/fever?	Urinary tract infection/urethritis
Abdominal or flank pain?	Stones/pyelonephritis
Trauma/exercise?	Direct trauma/exercise induced
Bleeding tendency?	Coagulopathy
Impetigo/pharyngitis?	Postinfectious glomerulonephritis?
Family History	
Kidney disease?	Alport syndrome/polycystic kidneys
Deafness?	Alport syndrome
Stones?	Nephrolithiasis
Other: medications/menses?	Medication induced/fictitious

Laboratory Data

It is important to determine why the urine is colored. Hemoglobin, myoglobin, and red blood cells all can cause red to brown urine, but the differential diagnosis and management differs for each.

If the patient has true hematuria (red blood cells in the urine), reviewing the elements of the urinalysis might provide some clues:

Finding	Possible Diagnosis
Proteinuria	Glomerular disease
White blood cells	Urinary tract infection; interstitial nephritis
Crystals	Stones

At the same time that management initiatives are begun, diagnostic tests should be performed:

Lab Test	Possible Diagnosis
Creatinine/serum K^+	Kidney dysfunction
C3 low (C4 normal)	Postinfectious glomerulonephritis
C3 and C4 low	Lupus
Antistreptolysin O, anti-DNAse B	Postinfectious glomerulonephritis
Urine calcium and urine creatinine	Hypercalciuria (urine calcium/ creatinine ratio >0.2 mg/mg)
Urine culture	Urinary tract infection
Complete blood count	Hemolytic-uremic syndrome
Immunoglobulin A (IgA)	IgA nephropathy
Antinuclear antibody	Lupus
Albumin/cholesterol	Nephrotic syndrome
Hemoglobin electrophoresis	Sickle cell disease

Imaging Test	Possible Diagnosis
CT of abdomen/pelvis	Trauma
Renal ultrasound or CT	Stones
Renal or bladder ultrasound	Anatomic abnormalities, tumor

CT, Computed tomography.

Management

The pediatric nephrologist should be called for:
- Red blood cell casts on microscopic examination (may need biopsy)
- Significant proteinuria (may need biopsy)
- Hypertension, edema
- Abnormal renal function
- Renal structural abnormality
  The pediatric urologist should be called for:
- Traumatic kidney or urethra injury
- Kidney stones with urinary infection or fevers
- Tumors

Summary

Hematuria, although rarely presenting a major threat to life, may occur in a variety of conditions associated with significant morbidity. As with many conditions, a diagnostic work-up should be performed simultaneously with management of any potentially associated problems, such as hypertension or severe edema.

Hypertension

Hema Krishna, MD

Hypertension is a very common problem in adults, but it is relatively rare in children. The normal ranges for systolic and diastolic blood pressure differ based on age and height percentile, thus making the definition of "high blood pressure" variable. Nomograms have been developed by conducting blood pressure screening programs in very large populations of "normal" children. Persistent measurements (three or more) above the 95th percentile have generally been used to define hypertension. It is important to remember that a single measurement recording a high blood pressure does not necessarily indicate hypertension.

Probably the most common "cause" of hypertension in children is the use of an inappropriate cuff size. If the cuff is too small, an artificially high reading is obtained. The cuff width should be two-thirds the length of the upper part of the arm and have a bladder that encircles the arm. Similarly, in obtaining a leg pressure, the cuff should cover two-thirds the length of the thigh. A second common "cause" of high readings is agitation and movement during the blood pressure reading. Even in toddlers, a blood pressure reading can usually be obtained without undue agitation if the child is approached slowly and patiently and reassured that the cuff will squeeze his or her arm for only a short time. Ideally, the child has avoided stimulant drugs or foods, has rested quietly for 5 minutes, and is seated with the back and right arm supported, cubital fossa at heart level. Due to the possibility of coarctation of the aorta resulting in falsely low blood pressure readings, the right arm is the preferred site for obtaining measurements. It is also important to remember that blood pressures obtained in the hospital may be spuriously elevated because of the child's concomitant illness, anxiety or pain, or iatrogenic causes such as medications. As such, an isolated blood pressure reading in this setting should be interpreted with caution.

Approximately 80% to 90% of true hypertension in children results from renal disease, but other treatable causes must also be considered in any evaluation for hypertension.

PHONE CALL

Questions

1. Why is the child hospitalized? What are his or her chronic medical problems?
2. How high is the blood pressure and how was it obtained (manual cuff or Dynemap, arm or leg)?
3. Is this a new finding? What have previous blood pressure readings been?
4. Is the child having any other associated symptoms (chest pain, tachycardia, sweating, shortness of breath, nausea, vomiting, headache, vision/hearing changes, focal numbness or weakness, urine output changes, edema)? Is the child anxious or in pain?
5. If the patient is female, could she be pregnant?
6. What medications has the child received?

Orders

Ask the nurse to have a manual blood pressure cuff of the appropriate size at the patient's bedside.

If the child does not have an intravenous (IV) line, ask the nurse to have IV supplies ready at the bedside.

Inform RN

Tell the RN, "I will arrive at the bedside in … minutes." Situations requiring emergency evaluation include severely elevated blood pressure (in children, systolic pressure above 200 and/or diastolic pressure above 110 mm Hg), hypertension in a pregnant adolescent female, altered mental status, focal neurologic deficits, or pain of any kind.

ELEVATOR THOUGHTS

Major etiologic categories of hypertension include the following:

Renal (glomerulonephritis, vasculitis, tumors, polycystic kidneys, renal scarring, renal artery stenosis)

Coarctation of the aorta (upper extremity pressure > lower extremity pressure)

Increased intracranial pressure (ICP)

Eclampsia

Hyperthyroidism

Drugs (sympathomimetic agents, corticosteroids, oral contraceptives)

Hypercatechol states

Although rare, some life-threatening conditions in children may result in hypertension. Preeclampsia in a pregnant adolescent is accompanied by proteinuria and edema. Headache is frequently associated with the rise in blood pressure.

Catecholamine crisis may be precipitated by a number of conditions:

Drug overdose

Especially common with cocaine, phencyclidine (PCP), and amphetamines; overdose must be suspected regardless of age

Drug interactions

Monoamine oxidase (MAO) inhibitors and indirect-acting catechols (wine, cheese, ephedrine)

Tricyclic antidepressants and direct-acting catechols (epinephrine, norepinephrine, pseudoephedrine)

Pheochromocytoma

Neoplasm overproducing catechols

Burns

Transient hypertension develops in some patients with second- or third-degree burns because of high levels of circulating endogenous catecholamines, renin, and angiotensin II.

Head trauma may result in increased ICP secondary to expanding subdural or epidural hematomas or cerebral edema. The need for the cerebral perfusion pressure to exceed ICP causes the release of endogenous catechols to preserve cerebral blood flow.

The consequences of hypertension include intraventricular hemorrhage in low-birth-weight premature infants. Cerebrovascular accidents are less common in full-term infants and older children but are still a possible complication of extreme hypertension. Hypertensive encephalopathy can include nausea, vomiting, headache, lethargy, confusion, visual disturbances, and seizures.

MAJOR THREAT TO LIFE

The major immediate threat to life is the rapid increase in blood pressure that can occur with eclampsia, drug ingestion, and head injuries, especially with extra-axial hemorrhage and hypertensive encephalopathy.

BEDSIDE

Quick-Look Test

Does the patient appear well (comfortable), sick (uncomfortable or distressed), or critical (about to die)?

A patient having end-organ damage requires immediate action to normalize the blood pressure. Such damage may include neurologic complications such as encephalopathy, focal deficits, or seizures; marked respiratory distress; renal insufficiency, possibly presenting as anuria or oliguria; or cardiac complications such as heart failure or ischemia. Similarly, hypertension caused by suspected aortic dissection (tearing chest pain radiating to the back, possible cocaine use) must be treated rapidly. Patients with surprisingly high blood pressure can appear quite comfortable and in little or no distress.

Airway and Vital Signs

What is the blood pressure?

Check that the appropriate cuff size has been used and then proceed to take the blood pressure yourself from both arms and at least one leg. Coarctation of the aorta is a common source of upper extremity hypertension. The lower extremity blood pressure should always equal or exceed the upper extremity blood pressure. Comparison of upper and lower extremity blood pressures is the definitive diagnostic technique for coarctation of the aorta.

What is the heart rate?

Bradycardia and hypertension in a patient not taking β-blockers may indicate increased ICP. When high blood pressure is accompanied by irregular respirations, it is known as Cushing's triad. Tachycardia with hypertension is consistent with catecholamine-mediated changes.

Is the patient in pain or anxious?

Pain is a very powerful stimulant for catecholamine release, regardless of the source. A patient hospitalized after trauma may have undiagnosed injuries, such as fractures or abdominal injuries, that can be overlooked, especially if he or she is unconscious on arrival and admission.

Selective History and Chart Review

What has the patient's blood pressure been up to this point?

Any previous recorded blood pressure readings are useful to put the patient's current pressure into perspective. Remember, however, that how and where the pressure was obtained are not usually recorded, thus making the previous results less reliable as a comparison. A normal leg pressure may be reassuring except in an infant or child with coarctation of the aorta, whose arm pressure may be significantly higher.

What risk factors does the patient have for high blood pressure?

Does the patient have a history of heart disease?

Could the patient be pregnant? Is a drug ingestion a possibility?

Does the patient have a history of renal disease, especially reflux nephropathy, chronic or recurrent pyelonephritis, nephrotic syndrome, or any of the glomerulonephropathies?

Does the patient have a recent history of sore throat or upper respiratory symptoms?

Postinfectious glomerulonephritis is a common cause of sudden hypertension in children. Probably 80% to 90% of hypertension is a complication of infectious and/or inflammatory renal disease. Primary injury to the renal arteries can occur after umbilical artery cannulation in a newborn and results in altered renal perfusion and high renin production. Proximal tubular disease can result in poor sodium excretion and inappropriate loss of bicarbonate with poor urine acidification.

Selective Physical Examination

Does the patient have evidence of a hypertensive emergency?

HEENT	Assess the fundi for hypertensive changes (generalized or focal arteriolar narrowing, hemorrhages, exudates). Papilledema is an ominous and late finding and is the hallmark of malignant hypertension and hypertensive encephalopathy.
Neck	Jugular venous distention may suggest heart failure; thyromegaly may indicate hyperthyroidism.
Respiratory	Rales, pleural effusion (congestive heart failure [CHF])
Cardiovascular	Increased precordial activity, loud S_2 (pulmonary hypertension), S_3 gallop (CHF), continuous murmur in the back (collaterals secondary to coarctation of the aorta), weak or absent femoral pulses, brachiofemoral delay, diffusely weak or absent pulses (Takayasu arteritis).
Abdomen	Presence of bruits over the kidneys (renal artery stenosis), enlarged kidneys (ureteropelvic junction obstruction, renal vein thrombosis).
Neurologic	Confusion, lethargy, headache, visual disturbances, delirium, agitation, focal neurologic signs.

HEENT, Head, Eye, Ears, Nose, Throat.

Management

Remember, the object is to treat the patient, not a number. Hypertension must be viewed in the context of the entire patient. If the patient is asymptomatic, there is less urgency to normalize the blood pressure than if he or she is encephalopathic. There is a very real risk of overshooting the mark during acute reduction of blood pressure in patients with long-standing hypertension and high levels of auto-regulated cerebral blood flow. Do not treat a blood pressure reading! Treat the condition underlying it or associated with it.

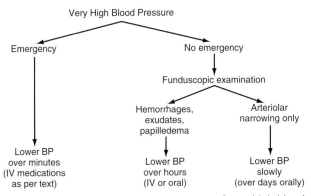

Very High Blood Pressure

Emergency / No emergency

Funduscopic examination

Hemorrhages, exudates, papilledema / Arteriolar narrowing only

Lower BP over minutes (IV medications as per text)

Lower BP over hours (IV or oral)

Lower BP slowly (over days orally)

FIGURE 24.1 Approach to the management of very high blood pressure *(BP)*.

True emergencies require special management. Such emergencies include eclampsia, intracranial hemorrhage, and hypertensive encephalopathy (Fig. 24.1).

It is important to involve your senior resident and an attending physician in such crisis situations and to inform the pediatric intensive care unit (PICU) that your patient requires transfer to a higher level of care and monitoring. No matter how "comfortable" you may feel with managing hypertension, it is important to recognize the critical condition of these patients and the many potential complications inherent in their management.

Hypertensive Encephalopathy

Hypertensive encephalopathy is almost always accompanied by papilledema, retinal hemorrhages, and exudates. Focal neurologic signs, although unusual early on, suggest the presence of a stroke. It is important to remember that lowering the blood pressure precipitously can cause a stroke as well as syncope.

1. Transfer the patient to the PICU for electrocardiographic (ECG) and intra-arterial blood pressure monitoring.
2. While the transfer is being arranged, an initial dose of oral nifedipine can be administered and adequate IV access obtained.
3. If there is evidence of hypertensive encephalopathy, IV infusions of medications such as nitroprusside may be useful because they can be titrated gradually. It is absolutely necessary to have intra-arterial monitoring to use such medications safely.
4. Labetalol, a combination α- and β-blocking agent, may also be administered and can be particularly useful in a patient whose hypertension is mediated by overproduction of endogenous

catecholamines or increased sympathetic tone. Bradycardia may result, and if the patient has a history of reactive airway disease, the respiratory findings must be monitored closely.

5. Once the blood pressure is under control by parenteral means, a suitable oral medication regimen must be initiated in order to discontinue the IV medications and allow the patient to leave the PICU.

Malignant Hypertension

Unless malignant hypertension is accompanied by other emergency conditions such as encephalopathy, control of blood pressure can be accomplished more gradually. Control of blood pressure must often be pursued while a search for the cause is ongoing. As you are gaining control of the blood pressure, begin to arrange the workup to document renal perfusion and function (ultrasonography with Doppler flow study of the renal artery and vein, renal arteriography if necessary, dimercaptosuccinic acid [DMSA] renal scan with or without captopril challenge, blood urea nitrogen, creatinine, urinalysis, creatinine clearance, electrolytes, calcium, phosphate), echocardiogram, serum and urine steroid metabolite levels, and serum renin and angiotensin II levels. Especially if renal disease is suspected, include streptococcal antibody (antistreptolysin-O [ASO], anti-DNAse B) and complement (C3 and C4) studies.

Preeclampsia and Eclampsia

A pregnant adolescent presents a variety of special problems and can be difficult to manage. Hypertension poses a risk to both the adolescent and her unborn fetus. Obviously obstetric consultation is required and, frequently, transfer to a labor and delivery unit.

Intracranial Hemorrhage

Your index of suspicion should be high in the setting of a child with altered mental status, suspicion of child abuse, focal neurologic signs, or associated bradycardia. Subarachnoid bleeding and subdural or epidural hemorrhage can cause increased ICP and secondary hypertension. Intraparenchymal bleeding is a risk in children with known coagulopathies and requires close monitoring and a judicious approach.

Catecholamine Crisis

Pheochromocytoma presents the classic syndrome of pallor, palpitations, and diaphoresis associated with intermittent and alarmingly high blood pressure. Other circumstances that can mimic this syndrome include drug ingestion, especially of cocaine and PCP. Food (cheese), drug (ephedrine), and drink (wine) interactions with MAO inhibitor antidepressant medications can result in similar findings, as can the interaction of tricyclic antidepressants with pseudoephedrine in over-the-counter cold preparations. MAO inhibitors are not widely used in children. Symptoms of catecholamine crisis should prompt immediate transfer to the PICU for close ECG and intra-arterial monitoring. Besides nitroprusside and labetalol, phentolamine mesylate, a powerful direct β-blocker, may be given to decrease systemic vascular resistance (afterload) and venous capacitance by directly relaxing smooth muscle. Alpha blockade is especially important with cocaine and PCP ingestion because of the generalized increase in sympathetic nervous system activity that most children exhibit. When amphetamines have been taken, psychosis and hyperactivity may require the use of chlorpromazine (Thorazine) or haloperidol (Haldol) to control hallucinations and delirium.

Summary

Hypertension is unusual in children and must be taken seriously. Be sure that the correct cuff size has been used and that the conditions for checking the blood pressure have been optimized. Take four-extremity blood pressure readings manually, and carefully record the results to rule out coarctation of the aorta. Acute hypertension implies an intracranial process, drug ingestion or interaction, or another source of catecholamine overproduction. Treat acute hypertension carefully and always in the context of the entire patient. Rapid normalization of blood pressure can itself precipitate problems.

Hypotension and Shock

Amanda A. Wenzel, MD

A variety of disease processes in pediatric patients follow a common pathway of hypotension, decreased tissue perfusion, acidosis, and shock. The physician's task is to quickly assess the magnitude of the problem, intervene to prevent progression of shock, and discover the underlying cause of the hemodynamic compromise. This may seem like a tall order, but remember that fundamentally the blood pressure must be adequate to perfuse the brain, heart, and kidneys. Accordingly, assessment of the child's mental status, pulses and perfusion, and urine output will provide the information needed. Remember too that blood pressure is preserved by a variety of mechanisms and falls only as a late consequence; therefore early recognition of impending hypotension is essential to appropriate management.

PHONE CALL

Questions

1. How old is the patient?
2. Why is the patient in the hospital?
3. What is the blood pressure? What method of measurement was used and from what site on the body was the blood pressure taken?
4. What has been the blood pressure trend over the past several hours?
5. What are the heart rate, temperature, and respiratory rate?
6. What is the child's mental status (agitated, somnolent, unresponsive)?

Orders

1. If the child does not have an intravenous (IV) line, the largest possible IV line should be started immediately. Normal saline

or lactated Ringer's solution, 10 to 20 mL/kg, should be administered over a period of 5 to 10 minutes by IV push if necessary.
2. Oxygen should be administered.
3. If the child is not on a cardiorespiratory monitor, one should be obtained immediately. Request frequent repeat measurements of blood pressure (every 5 minutes).
4. If the child is febrile but alert enough to take medication by mouth, acetaminophen or ibuprofen should be given. Infants or very small children may be given rectal acetaminophen if they cannot take anything by mouth.

Inform RN

Tell the RN, "I will arrive at the bedside immediately."

There should be no delay in seeing a child with impending shock.

ELEVATOR THOUGHTS

Shock is caused by the following conditions:
Sepsis
Hypovolemia
Cardiogenic causes
Anaphylaxis
Adrenal insufficiency
Trauma
Toxins

Two formulas are useful in considering the cause of hypotension:

$$\text{Blood pressure (BP)} = \text{cardiac output (CO)} \times \text{systemic vascular resistance (SVR)}$$

$$\text{Cardiac output (CO)} = \text{heart rate (HR)} \times \text{stroke volume (SV)}$$

Hypotension results from a decrease in either cardiac output or systemic vascular resistance (SVR), and cardiac output is reduced by a decrease in heart rate or stroke volume. Sepsis and anaphylaxis cause hypotension as a result of systemic vasodilatation (decreased SVR) and relative hypovolemia (because of capillary leak), both of which decrease cardiac output. Hypovolemia decreases cardiac filling and lowers stroke volume, thereby leading to tachycardia and ultimately resulting in decreased cardiac output and hypotension. Cardiogenic causes include decreased stroke volume because of decreased ejection fraction, as in dilated cardiomyopathies, dysrhythmias, and cardiac ischemia; decreased heart rate, as in heart block; restriction of cardiac filling (and therefore stroke volume), as in hypertrophic states, mitral stenosis, restrictive cardiomyopathy, and pericardial tamponade; and loss of systemic output via left-to-right shunts when pulmonary vascular resistance is less than SVR.

The most common cause of decreased cardiac output is lack of intravascular volume. This can be caused by external losses, as seen with vomiting and diarrhea, or by internal losses from third spacing, as seen with intestinal obstruction or after major abdominal surgery.

MAJOR THREAT TO LIFE

Shock is the major threat to life. Hypotension becomes life-threatening when there is evidence of inadequate end-organ perfusion. Making the diagnosis of shock or impending circulatory collapse is not usually difficult, but treating shock and its underlying cause can be a challenge. The duty of the on-call physician is to prevent end-organ damage and to find and correct the cause of hemodynamic compromise.

BEDSIDE

Quick-Look Test

Does the patient look well (comfortable), sick (uncomfortable or distressed), or critical (about to die)?

A child who is hypotensive but not in shock appears quite well. However, as soon as perfusion of vital organs is compromised, the patient appears quite ill. The blood pressure may be normal in a child in shock, so attention to end-organ function is of utmost importance.

Airway and Vital Signs

Is the airway clear?

If the child's mental status is compromised, the ability to protect the airway may be impaired. Airway support should be readily at hand for any patient in shock.

Is the child ventilating adequately?

Children in shock are often tachypneic (to blow off accumulated CO_2), grunting (to provide positive end-expiratory pressure and prevent atelectasis), and retracting (to maximize tidal volume). Assess the respiratory rate, aeration, breath sounds, and chest movement. If the work of breathing is excessive, intubation and ventilatory support are indicated.

Assess the Circulation

1. Mild hypotension may be manifested as postural dizziness. Assess for postural hypotension by checking the pulse and

blood pressure in the supine position and again after the patient has been standing for 3 minutes. A postural rise in heart rate of more than 15 beats per minute, a fall in systolic blood pressure of more than 15 mm Hg, or any decrease in diastolic blood pressure suggests hypovolemia.

2. What is the heart rate? Sinus tachycardia is the first response to stress, hypovolemia, sepsis, and decreased myocardial function in infants and children. Nonsinus tachydysrhythmias can lead to circulatory collapse and shock; therefore an electrocardiographic rhythm strip should be checked to rule out a supraventricular tachydysrhythmia (see Chapter 22). Bradycardia in the setting of shock is an ominous, life-threatening sign of circulatory collapse. If bradycardia is present, make sure that the patient is not in heart block and therefore unable to respond to his or her own catecholamine signals (Fig. 25.1). Vagal stimuli can produce profound bradycardia and even asystole in young patients. Episodes are usually short-lived and respond promptly to laying the patient supine with the legs elevated or even in the Trendelenburg position. Prolonged bradycardia should respond to IV atropine (0.02 mg/kg).

Children who are receiving β-blockers or calcium channel blockers or who have ingested such medications accidentally are not able to respond normally to their intrinsic catecholamine signals. Likewise, children with sick sinus syndrome may not respond to $β_1$-chronotropic stimulation and do not compensate with tachycardia in response to stress.

3. Is the child in shock? This should take less than 30 seconds to determine, and shock, if present, requires immediate action regardless of the underlying cause.

Vital signs	Repeat immediately (include urine output)
Cardiovascular	Heart rate, blood pressure, pulse pressure, pulse quality, capillary refill (normal, <2 s)
Neurologic	Mental status

Shock is a clinical diagnosis. No single sign or test establishes the diagnosis. The constellation of low systolic blood pressure for age, cool clammy extremities, poor capillary refill, acrocyanosis, altered mental status (confusion, delirium, lethargy, coma), and decreased urine output (number of wet diapers in infants) indicates progressive circulatory compromise.

4. Is the child febrile? Obviously fever frequently means sepsis, and prompt administration of antibiotics may be indicated. Fever also results in peripheral vasodilation, which decreases SVR and causes decreased cardiac output. A neonate with sepsis may not have significant fever and may indeed be hypothermic.

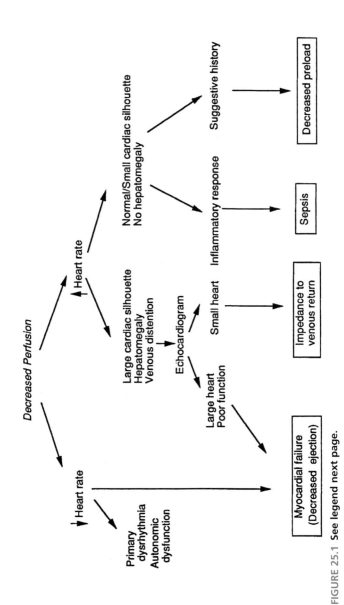

FIGURE 25.1 See legend next page.

Selective Physical Examination

Determine the severity of the hypotension by assessing volume status and end-organ function. Cardiogenic shock may be manifested as volume overload, but in general most shock states include evidence of hypovolemia.

Vital signs	Repeat and document regularly
HEENT	Pupils (narcosis), mucous membranes, tears, fontanelle, periorbital edema, lip edema
Neck	Jugular venous distention (congestive heart failure [CHF], tamponade), deviation of the trachea (tension pneumothorax)
Respiratory	Grunting, retracting, stridor, or wheezing (anaphylaxis); rales (CHF)
Cardiovascular	Displaced point of maximal impulse (dilated cardiomyopathy), distant heart sounds (pericardial effusion, myocarditis), gallop rhythm, holosystolic regurgitant murmurs (ventricular septal defect, mitral or tricuspid regurgitation), loud S_2 (pulmonary hypertension), weak femoral pulses and/or brachiofemoral delay (coarctation of the aorta). Also assess perfusion, skin temperature, and color.

HEENT, Head, Ears, Eyes, Nose, Throat.

Algorithm for discerning the cause of decreased perfusion. Although the heart rate is usually increased in response to poor systemic perfusion, the presence of bradycardia should provoke a search for a primary dysrhythmia (e.g., heart block) or autonomic dysfunction (e.g., spinal cord trauma) or raise concern that there is severe myocardial failure. Alternatively, when the heart rate is increased, one should attempt to determine whether signs of systemic venous engorgement are present. When the heart's silhouette is enlarged and there is venous distention, it is important to distinguish whether the heart is well filled and suffering from poor inotropic function or there is impedance to venous return (e.g., cardiac tamponade or tension pneumothorax). In these circumstances, an echocardiogram is an invaluable tool. When there is tachycardia with no sign of venous distention, inadequate perfusion can be caused by decreased preload and insufficient cardiac filling (e.g., hemorrhage or dehydration) or by diminished effective circulation, as in sepsis (with diffuse inflammation, venodilatation, and maldistribution of blood flow). It is also important to recognize that many of the problems that cause decreased perfusion can do so by more than one mechanism. Sepsis is a good example of a process that can diminish preload and produce myocardial failure simultaneously. (From Behrman RE: Nelson Textbook of Pediatrics, 15th ed. Philadelphia, WB Saunders, 1995, p 248.)

Abdomen	Hepatosplenomegaly, ascites, distention and/or tenderness (ischemia or perforation)
Extremities	Presacral and/or ankle edema (CHF); cold, clammy hands and feet; poor capillary refill
Neurologic	Mental status
Skin	Urticaria (anaphylaxis), skin turgor, burns or wounds, anasarca (capillary leak secondary to sepsis), petechiae or purpura (sepsis and disseminated intravascular coagulopathy)

Selective History and Chart Review

Anaphylaxis has a preceding inciting event, such as food, drug, or radiologic dye exposure, with an abrupt onset and rapidly progressive course. Angioedema and urticaria are often present, as well as wheezing with or without stridor. A neonate with sepsis may have been exposed to an older child with a specific infectious illness. Children with known immunologic compromise—such as HIV infection, sickle cell (SS) disease, asplenia, or neoplasms—may be more susceptible to septic shock. In addition to sepsis or distributive shock, cardiogenic shock may develop in children with known cardiac disorders. A history of significant steroid therapy for autoimmune illnesses or cystic fibrosis increases susceptibility to infection. Rapid withdrawal of steroids may precipitate adrenal crisis and subsequent shock. Recent surgery can result in hemorrhage and hypovolemia. Spinal trauma may lead to neurogenic shock (disturbance in vasomotor tone). Children with dehydration secondary to diarrhea must be assessed carefully. The fact that the patient is hospitalized does not mean that the diarrhea is gone. Children in diapers must be carefully assessed for intake and output. Watery diarrhea can be confused with urine output because modern diapers absorb extremely well. Make sure that the documented urine output is really urine and not watery stool.

Management

What immediate measures must be taken to restore circulatory function and prevent progression of shock and end-organ hypoperfusion?

Normalize intravascular volume. The heart needs preload to function high on the Frank-Starling curve and maximize ejection fraction and therefore stroke volume. Even in some forms of cardiogenic shock, volume expansion is indicated initially. (Children with dilated or hypertrophic cardiomyopathy require high filling volume and pressure to compensate for low ejection fraction and high end-diastolic volume or for poor diastolic compliance with high end-diastolic pressure.)

Volume expansion should start by positioning the patient supine with the legs raised 15 degrees or in the 15-degree head-down Trendelenburg position. In infants, volume replacement should be in the form of either normal saline or other isotonic solution; 10 to 20 mL/kg should be administered over a 5- to 10-minute period by IV push if necessary. Reassess volume status and end-organ function (mental status, heart rate, urine output, perfusion) after each intervention.

Anaphylactic Shock

If the patient is in anaphylactic shock, treat rapidly as follows:

1. Remove inciting antigen if possible (e.g., medication infusion).
2. Epinephrine, 0.01 mg/kg as a 1:1000 solution intravenously immediately (intramuscularly only if necessary)
3. Oxygen via OxyMask
4. 10 to 20 mL/kg of normal saline bolus (repeat as necessary)
5. Diphenhydramine, 1 mg/kg intravenously (maximum 50 mg) administered over 5 minutes
6. Methylprednisolone sodium succinate, 1 to 2 mg/kg intravenously immediately and every 6 hours; steroids have a slower onset of action but may be helpful in mitigating or preventing the biphasic allergic reaction that can occur 6 to 8 hours after the initial reaction.
7. Other adjunctive therapies (H1 or H2 blockers [e.g., ranitidine], β_2 agonists)
8. Note that although adjunctive therapies are helpful, they are not lifesaving; therefore administration of epinephrine takes precedence. Treat signs of hypovolemia and simultaneously assess the magnitude of end-organ damage by obtaining an arterial blood gas reading.

Cardiogenic Shock

Although much less common in pediatric patients, cardiogenic shock can occur because of intrinsic cardiac disease (including structural lesions and dysrhythmias), injury to cardiac muscle (myocardial infarction, trauma, myocarditis), and extrinsic processes such as sepsis. A 12-lead electrocardiogram and chest radiograph obtained promptly will help in assessing the cause and gravity of cardiac failure. It is critical that the physician determine whether the child is preload-dependent to maximize cardiac output, as mentioned earlier. Other clues should exist to suggest congestive heart failure, including jugular venous distention, hepatomegaly, a history of congenital heart disease, and differential pulses. Other conditions, however, can be manifested similarly and result in hypotension and shock. Cardiogenic shock may have to be managed with inotropic support, diuresis, afterload reduction, or

TABLE 25.1	Catecholamines Used for Cardiopulmonary Resuscitation				
	Direct Pressor	Positive Inotrope	Positive Chronotrope	Vasoconstrictor	Vasodilator
Dopamine	++	+	+/−	++[a]	++[b]
Dobutamine	++	+/−	−	−	+
Epinephrine	+++	+++	+++	++[a]	−
Norepinephrine	+++	+++	+++	+++	−

[a]High dose.
[b]Primarily splanchnic and renal in low doses (3 to 5 µg/kg/min).

From Behrman RE, Kliegman R: Nelson Essentials of Pediatrics, 7th ed. Philadelphia, WB Saunders, 2015.

some combination of these. Consultation with a cardiologist may be most helpful. Table 25.1 lists some of the common inotropic agents that may be used.

Acute Pericardial Tamponade

Tamponade physiology results in poor cardiac filling, which compromises stroke volume, elevates right-sided pressure, and causes jugular venous distention and tachycardia (Beck's triad: arterial hypotension, jugular venous distention, and soft or distant heart sounds). Tamponade can be seen in postoperative cardiac patients, children with viral pericarditis, and patients with blunt chest trauma; it can also occur after cardiac catheterization and with inflammatory conditions such as systemic juvenile idiopathic arthritis and systemic lupus erythematosus. Suspect tamponade in patients who appear well hydrated, nonvasodilated, and poorly perfused. They may have a narrow pulse pressure and a pulsus paradoxus of greater than 10 mm Hg during relaxed respirations (Fig. 25.2). If the patient has hypotension that is unresponsive to volume and tamponade is suspected, a code should be called and preparations made for emergent pericardiocentesis. In this procedure, pericardial fluid is removed to relieve the tamponade. The area around the xyphoid process should be prepared in sterile fashion. The skin and subcutaneous tissues should be anesthetized with 1% lidocaine. An 18- or 20-gauge angiocatheter can be placed on a three-way stopcock and attached to a 20-mL syringe. The angiocatheter is then inserted lateral to the xyphoid, aiming for the left shoulder and aspirating as it is inserted and advanced slowly. Once straw-colored fluid is visualized, the catheter can be threaded and the needle withdrawn. The stopcock can be attached directly to the catheter and the fluid aspirated with the syringe.

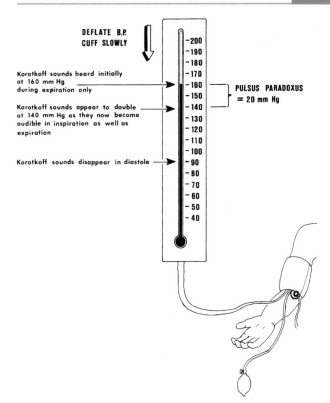

**DEFLATE B.P.
CUFF SLOWLY**

Korotkoff sounds heard initially
at 160 mm Hg
during expiration only

Korotkoff sounds appear to double
at 140 mm Hg as they now become
audible in inspiration as well as
expiration

Korotkoff sounds disappear in diastole

PULSUS PARADOXUS
= 20 mm Hg

FIGURE 25.2 Determination of pulsus paradoxus. *BP*, blood pressure. (From Marshall SA, Ruedy J: On Call: Principles and Protocols, 4th ed. Philadelphia, Elsevier, 2004, p 266.)

Tension Pneumothorax

A rather rare entity, tension pneumothorax precipitates circulatory collapse by inhibiting cardiac filling and therefore stroke volume because of high intrathoracic pressure, which decreases venous return to the heart. The result is jugular venous distention, severe dyspnea, unilateral hyper-resonance, tracheal deviation away from the affected side, and unequal breath sounds. Trauma is the most common cause, but spontaneous pneumothorax can progress to tension pneumothorax as well. Tension pneumothorax is a life-threatening emergency, and there may not be time to wait for a radiograph. If the patient has hypotension that is unresponsive to volume and tension pneumothorax is suspected, a code should be called and preparations made for emergent decompression. Oxygen is then administered immediately and an 18- to 20-gauge needle prepared on a three-way stopcock with a 20-mL syringe. The second intercostal space of the affected side is quickly scrubbed with povidone-iodine (Betadine), alcohol, or chlorhexidine and the needle is inserted at the midclavicular line in a slightly lateral direction, aspirating the while. Insertion should be just above the third rib to avoid damaging any neurovascular structures coursing below the rib. The fifth intercostal space at the midaxillary line may also be used. When air is aspirated, the syringe is filled and flushed out with the stopcock; this is repeated until air is no longer freely aspirated. These maneuvers should rapidly improve the patient's clinical condition. Tension pneumothorax is a true medical emergency and requires prompt, definitive action. Follow-up treatment with a chest radiograph is then mandatory to ensure resolution of the pneumothorax.

Pulmonary Embolism

Though rather unusual, pulmonary embolization can occur in children, especially in adolescents, and is a cause of sudden, severe hypotension and circulatory collapse. Because of the acute obstruction to pulmonary blood flow, left atrial filling decreases, which causes compromised left ventricular filling, decreased stroke volume, acute tachycardia, tachypnea, and chest pain. Cardiac output can rapidly decrease, leading to shock. Preexisting coagulopathy, immobility secondary to trauma or burns, birth control pills, and indwelling central venous catheters may predispose young patients to pulmonary embolization. Fat emboli are a well-known, serious consequence of long-bone fractures, especially of the femur. Embolization or thrombosis and subsequent infarction may also result in the acute chest syndrome of hemoglobin SS disease.

The pathophysiologic consequences of these diverse processes are essentially the same: ventilation/perfusion mismatch, hypoxemia with or without hypercapnia, increased pulmonary vascular resistance, decreased left heart filling, and decreased cardiac output. Secondary decreased perfusion and tissue hypoxemia result in acidemia, which worsens the ventilation/perfusion mismatch (intrapulmonary shunt), and an elevation in pulmonary vascular resistance.

Hypotension from pulmonary embolism is a medical emergency. If it is suspected as the cause of hypotension, immediate therapy can be lifesaving. A code should be activated and evaluation for the use of thrombolytic therapy should begin. Laboratory values should be obtained (complete blood count, prothrombin time, partial thromboplastin time, D-dimers or fibrin split products, and a type and screen) and an emergent computed tomography (CT) of the chest as well as echocardiogram should be performed if available. Acute therapy for pulmonary embolism is largely supportive and includes oxygen with positive-pressure ventilation if necessary, volume and inotropic support as needed, and close monitoring of arterial blood gases for gas exchange and acid-base status. The diagnosis may be suggested by the history and chest radiograph. Definitive diagnosis requires chest CT, pulmonary perfusion scanning, ventilation scintiphotographic studies, and/or pulmonary angiography. Any patient with hypotension from a pulmonary embolism and/or needing thrombolytic therapy requires monitoring in the intensive care unit. Patients with SS disease require at least partial exchange transfusion to lower their percentage of SS hemoglobin.

Hypovolemia

In infants and children, fluid losses from diarrhea, vomiting, excessive sweating, acute blood loss, chronic gastrointestinal bleeding, polyuria, and third-space losses (capillary leak syndromes, including sepsis and systemic inflammatory response syndrome [SIRS]) all can result in hypovolemia and shock. A number of medications—including diuretics, β-blockers, calcium channel blockers, acetylcholinesterase inhibitors, and other antihypertensive medications—can lead to relative or actual hypovolemia. Normal compensatory mechanisms for hypovolemia include increased sympathetic tone with resultant tachycardia, increased myocardial contractility, and peripheral vasoconstriction. Increased myocardial work and oxygen consumption constitute the price paid for this compensation. Therefore the first goal of therapy is to reduce myocardial work by fluid resuscitation.

Practicality, availability, and the type of fluid losses that the child has suffered should guide the choice of fluid for resuscitation. Normal saline and lactated Ringer's solution are readily available and economical; however, crystalloid solutions have a greater propensity for leaking from the tissues; thus colloid solutions are sometimes indicated, as in infants and patients with obvious capillary leak syndromes (Table 25.2). Likewise, a multiple-trauma patient may require whole blood during resuscitation. Children in severe hypovolemic shock may require a fluid bolus of 60 to 80 mL/kg within the first 30 to 60 minutes. However, the risk of fluid overload must be continually reassessed.

Volume expansion may not be enough to sustain cardiac output and perfusion. In this case inotropic and/or vasopressor support is indicated. Table 25.1 lists the inotropic agents used. Dopamine is generally given first; however, epinephrine may be more effective and can be given safely through a peripheral IV or intraosseous (IO) catheter.

The use of inotropic and vasopressor therapy generally requires transfer to an intensive care unit for appropriate, usually invasive

TABLE 25.2	Intravenous Fluids Available for Pediatric Volume Resuscitation

Crystalloids	Colloids
0.9% sodium chloride	5% human serum albumin in 0.9% sodium chloride
Lactated Ringer's solution	25% human serum albumin in 0.9% sodium chloride
Hypertonic saline (3%)	Fresh frozen plasma
	Whole blood

From Behrman RE, Kliegman R: Nelson Essentials of Pediatrics, 2nd ed. Philadelphia, WB Saunders, 1994, p 118.

monitoring. It is important to remember that inotropic support is not a replacement for volume resuscitation.

Sepsis

Sepsis is defined as any life-threatening organ dysfunction resulting from the body's impaired response to infection. Any kind of infection can result in circulatory collapse and shock; therefore early recognition and goal-directed therapy are key to decreasing morbidity and mortality.

As soon as sepsis is recognized by clinical and/or supporting laboratory evidence, IV access should be established (IO access may also be used if an IV cannot be placed). Continuous pulse oximetry is put in place and cardiorespiratory monitoring initiated if not already done. Oxygen supplementation should be applied, and support with respiratory ventilation as appropriate. Once IV access has been established, fluids should be initiated. Boluses of 20 mL/kg isotonic fluid are continued until perfusion improves or signs of fluid overload (rales, hepatomegaly) develop. At the same time, hypoglycemia or electrolyte derangements (potassium, magnesium, and/or calcium), if present, are corrected and empiric broad-spectrum antibiotics are begun. This should all be done rapidly, within the first 15 minutes of recognition.

If the patient requires more than 60 mL/kg of fluid without improvement in hemodynamics, this may indicate a need for the initiation of IV pressors and closer hemodynamic monitoring. A code should be called and the patient should quickly be transferred to the pediatric intensive care unit (PICU) for further evaluation and management.

Adrenal Crisis

Adrenal insufficiency is characterized by hyponatremia, hyperkalemia, acidosis, hypoglycemia, and hypotension or shock. It may occur in combination with other causes of shock (e.g., meningococ-cemia and secondary adrenal infarction, sepsis in a steroid-dependent patient). In addition to fluid resuscitation, if adrenal crisis is suspected, prompt treatment with IV hydrocortisone, 1 to 2 mg/kg, can result in dramatic improvement. Continuation of IV hydrocortisone, 25 to 250 mg/day divided into two or three doses, is usually necessary. Hydrocortisone is preferred to other IV steroid preparations because of its mineralocorticoid effect.

REMEMBER

1. Shock is a clinical diagnosis characterized by inadequate end-organ perfusion and subsequent dysfunction. One must assess its severity by noting the child's mental status (brain), perfusion, heart rate and blood pressure (heart), and urine output (kidney). Blood pressure may be normal and the child may still be in shock. Compensatory mechanisms (tachycardia, vasoconstriction) will maintain blood pressure, but end-organ perfusion will be inadequate.
2. Although the skin is not generally considered a "vital" organ, it can provide valuable information regarding volume status and tissue perfusion. Do not be misled or falsely reassured by a well-perfused patient who has other manifestations of shock. So-called warm shock is no less threatening and frequently precedes circulatory collapse. (Be alert for a patient with tachycardia, wide pulse pressure, and warm extremities.)
3. Hypovolemia is the most common cause of shock in infants and children, with sepsis following close behind.

Lines, Tubes, and Drains

Stephen E. Wilkinson, MD

Nearly every child admitted to the hospital requires an intravenous (IV) line, a catheter, a tube, or a drain of some sort. These devices may be necessary for a variety of reasons, but each may also be a source of trouble. Complications include soft tissue injury (including to vascular and nervous tissues) and pain with placement, blockages, leaks, and full malfunctions. This chapter discusses the placement of a few of these devices, as well as a troubleshooting approach to some of the problems that may arise while you are on call. The placement of IV and intraosseous (IO) lines are discussed in Appendix A. Chest tube placement is not outlined because this will rarely need to be done at the bedside and critical care support will perform or assist you with this procedure if an emergent need arises. Similarly, techniques of central line placement are beyond the scope of this book and are not discussed. Given the risks of complication, placement of lines, tubes, and drains should be supervised by attending physicians or appropriate fellows until competency is recognized by your program and hospital. The *New England Journal of Medicine* maintains an online archive series entitled "Videos in Clinical Medicine"; the video clips there are helpful reviews of procedures. Many hospitals have policies governing lines, tubes, and drains; nursing staff often will be able to locate these quickly.

This chapter is divided into the following sections:

IV lines:
- Infiltrated IV lines
- Medication reactions

Umbilical catheters
- Placement
- Obstructed umbilical arterial or venous catheter

Central lines
- Bleeding at the entry site
- Obstructed central line

Nasogastric (NG) and enteral feeding tubes
- Placement
- Obstructed NG tube and enteral feeding tube
- Displaced NG tube and enteral feeding tube

Urethral catheters
- Placement
- Obstructed urethral catheter
- Gross hematuria in catheterized patients

Chest tubes
- Persistent bubbling in the water seal (air leak)
- Loss of fluctuation of the water seal (tube obstruction)
- Bleeding at the chest tube entry site
- Drainage of blood
- Dyspnea
- Subcutaneous emphysema
- Traumatic or accidental removal of a chest tube

Intravenous Lines: Infiltrated Intravenous

Given their frequency, the most common line issue you will likely face is IV infiltrations. Extravasation of IV fluids or medications into perivascular tissues has variable consequences based on the pH, other redox potentials, osmolality of the infusion, and mechanism of action of the medication being infused; these consequences range from temporary discomfort to permanent tissue damage. In general, nonsevere infiltrates are handled by nursing staff without house staff involvement, so calls regarding infiltration should be treated seriously.

PHONE CALL

Questions

1. What fluid or medication was being infused?
2. What external signs are there of infiltration?

Orders

1. Stop the infusion, if not already stopped, but leave the line in place.
2. Attempt to aspirate as much fluid as possible out of the line and subcutaneous tissues. Do not flush the line.
3. Elevate the extremity above the heart to improve venous flow.

Inform RN

Tell the RN, "I will arrive at the bedside in … minutes." If a nurse feels a need to call about an infiltrated line, the patient should be evaluated as soon as possible.

ELEVATOR THOUGHTS

How noxious is the fluid or medication that infiltrated?
The following lists are helpful, although not exhaustive:
1. Higher-risk medications: Vasopressors/inotropes, chemotherapy, electrolytes (calcium, potassium, sodium bicarbonate, hypertonic normal saline), hypertonic sugars (D12.5 or greater; mannitol; total parenteral nutrition (TPN) with >900 mOsm/L), acyclovir, hydroxyzine.
2. Intermediate-risk medications: Acetazolamide, amikacin, amphotericin B, arginine, D10-D12.5, diazepam, doxycycline, erythromycin, fosphenytoin, ganciclovir, lorazepam, midazolam, morphine, ondansetron, nonionic radiology contrast, pantoprazole, phenobarbital, phenytoin, potassium (60 mEq/L or less), TPN (<900 mOsm/L).
3. Lower-risk medications: Most other fluids and medications.

MAJOR THREAT TO LIFE OR LIMB

- Tissue ischemia due to vasoconstriction.
- Tissue necrosis due to caustic medication-tissue chemical interactions.

BEDSIDE

Quick-Look Test
Does the child appear to be in extreme pain? Is there any hemorrhage at the infusion site?

Airway and Vital Signs
In general, the airway will be stable. Vital signs may be augmented secondary to pain and anxiety.

Management
Again, the infusion should have been stopped and all possible fluid should have been aspirated from the tissue. For medications that are intermediate- or higher-risk medication, calling for rapid response team assistance may expedite some medication availability and administration. For any vasoconstrictive medications, subcutaneous administration of phentolamine should be strongly considered to improve blood flow; a sterile technique should be used if this is done. For other higher-risk fluids and medications, talk with your pharmacist about antidotes. Cold packs may help with pain control (use warm packs for vinca alkaloid chemotherapeutics). The severity of damage from the infiltration should be assessed. Blistering, particularly hemorrhagic blistering, erythema that is not blanchable, and diminished or lost pulses are red flags indicating a need for surgical

evaluation. For intermediate-risk fluids and medications, talk with your pharmacist about hyaluronidase subcutaneous injections to buffer the effects of the infiltrate; sterile technique should be used if this is done. For low severity, lower-risk infusions, warm packs may help to improve circulation and clearance of the infiltrate.

Umbilical Catheters: Umbilical Arterial Catheter Placement

Umbilical arterial catheters (UACs) are placed in critically ill newborns to monitor blood pressure and for easy access for arterial blood gases draws. They may also be used to obtain blood samples for hematologic and chemistry studies, although this is not an indication for placement. For infants with a body weight less than 1500 grams, a 3.5-French (Fr) catheter may be used. For larger infants, a 5-Fr catheter is appropriate. Once in place, the tip of the catheter should rest in one of two places. A "high UAC" will be in the aorta at the approximate level of the diaphragm, at a level between the sixth and ninth thoracic vertebrae on chest radiography. A "low UAC" will be just above the iliac bifurcation of the aorta, between the second and fourth lumbar vertebrae on an abdominal radiography. If the catheter is inserted to a point between these two sites, it may obstruct one or more of the major aortic branches (celiac axis, superior mesenteric artery, renal arteries, inferior mesenteric artery).

Placement should proceed as follows:

1. Place the infant supine on a well-lit, prewarmed warming table.
2. Estimate the length of catheter to be inserted in the following way:
   a. Measure the length of the infant.
   b. For a high UAC, the catheter is inserted one-third the length of the infant.
   c. For a low UAC, the catheter is inserted one-sixth the length of the infant.
   d. Note the marking on the catheter that corresponds to the appropriate length. This mark will be aligned at the orifice of the umbilical stump once the catheter is in place.
3. Restrain the infant's legs by extending a diaper or small blanket across the thighs and securing it to the warming table with tape so that that the infant is not able to raise the legs.
4. Tie a heavy string or umbilical cord tape around the umbilical stump just proximal to where the infant's skin meets the soft tissue of the cord. Ensure this is snug enough to prevent blood from oozing out of the umbilical arteries.
5. Sterile technique should be used throughout the catheter's placement. Apply povidone-iodine to the entire umbilical stump and the cord distally to the point where the cord is clamped. Drape the infant's abdomen so that only the stump and cord are exposed.

6. Prepare the catheter by attaching a three-way stopcock and a 10-mL syringe that is filled with a heparinized solution. Fill the entire length of the catheter with the solution, and then turn the stopcock to the catheter off.

7. Using a scalpel, cut the cord transversely approximately 1 cm above the string or tape-tie and remove the distally clamped cord. This exposes the two umbilical arteries and umbilical vein in cross section so that they can be visualized clearly. Leaving some of the cord itself allows you to shave some off at a later time, should placement be difficult or the distal umbilical arteries become frayed.

8. Grasp the wall of the cord with a hemostat in one hand and pull up gently so that the cord is vertical and perpendicular to the abdomen. (Alternatively, ask a nurse or colleague to do this for you. This procedure is notably easier if a team approach is possible.) With curved forceps in the other hand, insert the tip of the forceps into the lumen of one of the umbilical arteries. These arteries are constricted; therefore the lumen may initially be difficult to visualize. Gently move the tip of the forceps in a circular fashion to gradually dilate the lumen of the artery. Patience is the key to success here, and rushing to dilate the artery may result in fraying and destruction of the distal end of the artery and make it impossible to insert the catheter (Fig. 26.1).

9. Once the lumen is slightly dilated, both tips of the closed forceps may be inserted and the artery dilated further by gently opening the forceps to stretch the walls of the artery. As this is being done, also gradually insert the tips of the forceps deeper and deeper into the lumen to dilate as far as possible.

10. When the artery has been dilated enough to accommodate the umbilical catheter, grasp the catheter near the tip with forceps. While holding the lumen of the umbilical artery open with the other pair of forceps (again, this is much easier if two people work together), insert the catheter tip into the artery and gradually feed the catheter into the vessel with the forceps. Stop when you have reached the estimated length (the marking that you previously noted is positioned where the catheter enters the lumen of the vessel) that places the tip at either a high level (the level of the diaphragm) or a low level (just above the iliac bifurcation of the aorta).

11. With successful catheterization, pulsating blood is usually visible in the catheter. Opening the stopcock and aspirating on the syringe should result in blood being easily drawn into the catheter.

12. While feeding the catheter into the umbilical artery, obstruction may be encountered at the point where the vessels turn at the umbilical wall or because of vasospasm. When obstruction occurs, steady, gentle pressure on the catheter while pulling

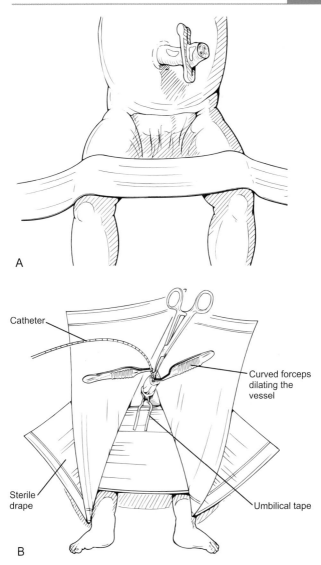

A

Catheter

Curved forceps
dilating the
vessel

Sterile
drape

Umbilical tape

B

FIGURE 26.1 **A**, Position of the infant for umbilical vessel catheterization. **B**, Procedure for inserting an umbilical catheter.

up on the umbilical stump often allows the catheter to pass. If it does not pass, a false tract external to the lumen of the vessel may have been created, and it may be necessary to withdraw the catheter and try again. If, after several attempts, the catheter still cannot be passed, it may be necessary to attempt insertion in the other umbilical artery. Alternatively, shaving the cord again with the scalpel may expose the artery proximal to the false tract and allow you to attempt insertion again.

13. Placement of the catheter should always be confirmed with a radiograph. If the sterility of the field and the catheter is maintained during radiography, the catheter may be adjusted if necessary. Once positioning is confirmed, the catheter should be secured to the cord with a suture and then taped in place.

14. It is common for pallor or cyanosis to appear in a lower extremity after placement of a UAC. This occurs secondary to vasospasm in response to the catheter and is often relieved by warming the opposite leg. Warmth increases blood flow to both extremities as a result of reflex vasodilatation.

Umbilical Catheters: Umbilical Venous Catheter Placement

Umbilical venous catheters (UVCs) are placed for IV access and for monitoring central venous pressures (CVPs). The umbilical vein is a readily available site for IV access in a critically ill newborn. The procedural steps for a UVC are identical to that for an umbilical arterial catheter, although notably easier and faster to perform. UVCs should be placed so that the tip lies within the inferior vena cava, just above the diaphragm. To achieve this, the catheter should be inserted one-sixth the length of the infant. The umbilical vein is thin walled and does not usually require dilatation. Once identified, the lumen is typically easily opened, and the catheter tip may pass freely with gentle pressure. As with a UAC, proper positioning should be confirmed with a radiograph and the catheter secured with a suture and tape.

Umbilical catheters: obstructed umbilical arterial or venous catheter

PHONE CALL

Questions

1. How long has the line been blocked?
2. What are the vital signs? Hypertension or narrowing of the recorded pulse pressure may be a sign of a thrombus at the tip of the arterial catheter.

3. Is there adequate blood flow to the legs (capillary refill, color, distal pulses)?

Orders
None

Inform RN
Tell the RN, "I will arrive at the bedside in … minutes." A blocked umbilical catheter should be evaluated immediately.

ELEVATOR THOUGHTS

What causes an umbilical catheter to be blocked?
1. Thrombus at the catheter tip
2. Kinked or compressed tubing

MAJOR THREAT TO LIFE

- Ischemia of an extremity secondary to thrombosis of an arterial line.
- Pulmonary or cerebral embolism (via a patent foramen ovale, atrial septal defect (ASD), or ventricular septal defect (VSD) secondary to thrombosis of a venous line.

BEDSIDE

Quick-Look Test
If the infant appears ill, suspect a complication such as embolization or distal ischemia.

Airway and Vital Signs
As noted earlier, hypertension or a narrowed recorded blood pressure may be an indication of a thrombus at the tip of an arterial catheter.

Management
Inspect the external portion of the catheter for kinks or compression. Unless there is an obvious kink or compression that can be relieved, the line must be removed. After pulling the line, inspect the tip for a thrombus. Reevaluate the need for the catheter to be replaced before replacing it.

Central Venous Lines: Bleeding at the Entry Site
As previously stated, placement of central venous lines (CVLs) should be directly supervised by an attending or an appropriate fellow.

PHONE CALL

Questions

1. What are the vital signs?
2. What was the reason for admission?
3. Is there bleeding anywhere else?

Orders

Ask the nurse to have a dressing set, sterile gloves, saline flushes or a bottle of saline, and chlorhexidine or povidone-iodine at the child's bedside.

Inform RN

Tell the RN, "I will arrive at the bedside in … minutes." Bleeding at the central line site needs to be evaluated immediately.

ELEVATOR THOUGHTS

What causes bleeding at the entry site?
1. Bleeding from skin capillaries
2. Tracking of venous blood up the line secondary to disordered coagulation
   a. Medications (anticoagulant, antiplatelet, and thrombolytic agents)
   b. Coagulopathy (thrombocytopenia, inherited or acquired factor deficiencies, microangiopathy)

MAJOR THREAT TO LIFE

- Upper airway obstruction secondary to bleeding into the soft tissues of the neck with a jugular catheter.
- Hemorrhagic shock
- Central line–associated bloodstream infection (CLABSI)

BEDSIDE

Quick-Look Test

Does the child appear well (comfortable), sick (uncomfortable or distressed), or critical (about to die)?

The child should appear well unless airway compromise or shock has occurred.

Airway and Vital Signs

Check the airway and the respiratory rate carefully for signs of airway obstruction. Look for hemodynamic changes suggestive of shock.

Selective Chart Review

Review past history for bleeding diatheses. Review labs for last hemoglobin/hematocrit (Hgb/Hct), platelet count, prothrombin time/international normalized ratio (PT/INR), and partial thromboplastin time (PTT). See Chapter 33.

Selective Physical Examination and Management

1. Remove the dressing and try to localize the bleeding.
2. If you cannot localize the site, clean the area with saline where the line enters the skin and reinspect.
3. If possible, elevate the site above the heart as tolerated.
4. Apply, or have the nurse or another team member apply, continuous, firm pressure to the site for 20 minutes (Fig. 26.2).
5. Reinspect. If the bleeding has stopped, clean the area with an antiseptic and secure the line with an occlusive dressing. If bleeding persists, continue to apply pressure for another

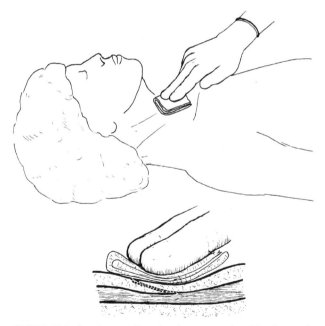

FIGURE 26.2 Continuous firm local pressure for 20 minutes is required to stop oozing of blood from the central line entry site. (From Marshall SA, Ruedy J: On Call: Principles and Protocols, 4th ed. Philadelphia, Elsevier, 2004, p 204.)

20 minutes. If the bleeding has still not stopped, a coagulation defect should be suspected, and blood should be sent for a stat platelet count, PT, and PTT. Refer to Chapter 33 for further evaluation and management of coagulopathies. Review the child's medications for any offending agents.

6. Consider removal of the line if the bleeding is excessive and resistant to the aforementioned measures. Discuss with your team if a smaller catheter line or another location may provide better results. If a line is required, the new line should be placed prior to removing the old line.

Central Venous Lines: Obstructed Central Line

PHONE CALL

Questions

1. How long has the line been obstructed?
2. What was being infused through the line?
3. What are the vital signs, including recent CVP?
4. Are there any changes in flow or vitals with postural changes?

Orders

Ask the RN for a dressing set, sterile gloves, antiseptic (povidone-iodine or chlorhexidine), a 5-mL syringe, and a 21-gauge needle to be placed at the child's bedside. You may need to remove the sterile dressing that is in place, but this should be kept in place until you evaluate the patient.

Inform RN

Tell the RN, "I will arrive at the bedside in … minutes." The child needs to be seen immediately.

ELEVATOR THOUGHTS

What causes a central line to become occluded?
1. Kinked or compressed tubing (Fig. 26.3A)
2. Thrombus at the catheter tip (see Fig. 26.3B)
3. Medication precipitate

MAJOR THREAT TO LIFE

- Loss of access for medication administration
- Inability to titrate medications with loss of CVP monitoring.
- Embolism of thrombi or foreign objects.
- Bacteremia

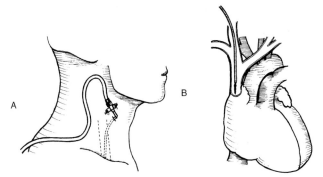

FIGURE 26.3 Causes of blocked central lines. **A,** Kinked tubing. **B,** Thrombus at the catheter tip. (From Marshall SA, Ruedy J: On Call: Principles and Protocols, 4th ed. Philadelphia, Elsevier, 2004, p 200.)

BEDSIDE

Quick-Look Test

Does the child appear well (comfortable), sick (uncomfortable or distressed), or critical (about to die)?

A blocked central line should not cause the child to appear ill unless the obstruction halts administration of vasoactive medications. If the child does appear ill, and no vasoactive medications were being given, search for an alternative explanation for the clinical decline.

Airway and Vital Signs

The airway and vital signs are not affected by a blocked central line unless the line carries a vasoactive or inotropic substance (such as dopamine, dobutamine, epinephrine, norepinephrine, vasopressin, isoproterenol).

Selective Physical Examination and Management

1. Evaluate the need for the line. If the line can be removed without further management, remove it.
2. Inspect the line. Is there obvious kinking or compression? If so, remove the dressing and attempt to straighten the line. If flow is restored, clean the site and secure the line with an occlusive dressing.
3. If there is no compression or kinking, proceed as follows:
   a. Turn the IV line off.
   b. Clean the entry port closest to the insertion site and attach a 5-mL syringe with sterile saline to the central line and clamp the line distal to this site.

   c. Draw back gently on the syringe pulling 3 mL of blood, if possible. This may dislodge a small thrombus and restore flow to the line.

   d. Blocked central lines should never be flushed because flushing may dislodge a clot on the tip of the catheter and produce an embolus.

   e. If no blood will pull back during the previous attempt, a tissue plasminogen activator (tPA) dwell may be put into the line to try to dissolve a presumed thrombus. The volume required will be dependent on the size of the CVL; discuss this with nursing and pharmacy staff.

4. If the preceding measures are unsuccessful, determine the necessity for the central line. If the central line is essential, a new central line needs to be placed at a different site. A new central line should not be reinserted over a guidewire at the same site because this may disrupt any clots leading to embolization.

Nasogastric and Enteral Feeding Tubes: Placement of a Nasogastric Tube

NG tubes are used for controlled feeding and hydration, aspiration of stomach contents, and, less frequently, for gastric lavages. Placement is a relatively simple procedure but may be made more challenging by the child's overall size, his or her willingness to cooperate, and any facial, oral, pharyngeal, esophageal, or gastric anatomic abnormalities. Expert help (such as from an otolaryngologist) should be sought for any child with facial trauma. Small tubes (5 to 10 Fr) may be used in neonates. Larger tubes (12 to 16 Fr) are necessary in older children. In general, smaller tubes are placed for enteral feeding while larger tubes are required for gastric lavage. Generally larger tubes are needed for gastric drainage and are not appropriate for feeding. Nursing staff who will be managing the tube may be helpful in determining the most appropriate size and type of tube to be used.

1. Make sure that you have help to restrain an uncooperative child. Sedation should not ordinarily be necessary unless the child is especially combative or insufficient help is available to provide restraint.

2. Approximate the required length of tubing by holding the tube at the tip of the child's nose, looping it to the tragus of the ear closest to you, and then running it down along the neck and the thorax to the inferior margin of the xyphoid process. This length should be sufficient for gastric placement; mark the length.

3. Examine the nares for any obvious nasal septum deviation or deformities. Choose the naris that appears the most open.

4. Lubricate the end of the tube and the child's external naris.

5. Ask older children to sip some water or juice while the tube is inserted. This closes the epiglottis, protecting the trachea and

easing placement. This should not be attempted in little children or those who may not be able to protect their airway.

6. Quickly and smoothly insert the end of the tube into the naris, directing it toward the child's occiput. Remember that the passage through the nasal cavity is nearly perpendicular to the esophagus; the tube therefore should not be angled superiorly or inferiorly.

7. The tube should be advanced in a smooth, continuous motion. Once through the nasal passage, resistance should be minimal and the tube should advance easily down the posterior of the pharynx, through the esophagus, and then into the stomach. Tilting the head forward slightly opens the esophagus wider, thus making it less likely for the tube to pass into the trachea. Although there may be a gag reflex when the tube touches the oropharynx, notable coughing or choking may indicate passage into the trachea; the tube should be withdrawn and placement should be attempted after the coughing or choking subsides.

8. When the tube is advanced to the point where your marking reaches the external naris, stop advancing and secure the tube in place with tape. A bridle may need to be used to anchor the tube to the nasal septum. These devices have instructions on or in the packaging.

9. Verify the location of the tube within the stomach. This is generally done with an abdominal radiograph. However, it may be clinically evaluated by pushing air through the tube with a syringe (5 mL in neonates; 20 mL in larger children) while auscultating the epigastrum. Alternatively, aspirating the tube with the same syringe may bring up gastric fluid, which may be verified by a low pH on litmus paper.

Nasogastric and Enteral Feeding Tubes: Obstructed Nasogastric Tube or Enteral Feeding Tube

PHONE CALL

Questions

1. How long has the tube been blocked?
2. What type of tube is it?
3. Is the tube dislodged?
4. What are the vital signs and status of the patient?

Orders

Ask the nurse to place several 20- and 50-mL syringes, normal saline solution, and an emesis basin at the bedside.

Inform RN

Tell the RN, "I will arrive at the bedside in … minutes." A blocked tube used for feeding is not an emergent concern, but they should be evaluated as soon as possible in an infant and within several hours in an older child. A blocked tube used for drainage is a greater problem and requires prompt evaluation to avoid complications from the accumulation of gastric fluid or gas.

ELEVATOR THOUGHTS

What causes blocked NG or enteral feeding or draining tubes?
1. External clamps or compression
2. Debris, including blood clots, within the lumen of the tube
3. Failure to irrigate the tube leading to desiccated formula
4. Precipitated medication
5. Suction against mucosa

MAJOR THREAT TO LIFE

- Aspiration: This may happen with any enteral tube, even if functioning properly. If a suction NG tube is blocked, gastric contents may rise around the tube and be aspirated into the lungs, leading to pneumonitis and possibly pneumonia.
- Perforation: Although a rare complication, perforation may happen with excessive suction against an injured mucosa.

BEDSIDE

Quick-Look Test

Does the patient look well (comfortable), sick (uncomfortable or distressed), or critical (about to die)?

Aspiration or perforation may quickly lead to a toxic appearance.

Airway and Vital Signs

The airway and vital signs should not be affected by a blocked tube unless aspiration or perforation has occurred, or if the blocked tube has led to nausea, vomiting, or dehydration.

Management

1. Turn off the pump or suction.
2. Examine the tubing to ensure it is not clamped, kinked, or compressed externally. Also look for visible blockages in the tubing. Very rarely, patients or others may place nonprescribed crushed medications in the tubing; if this is suspected, removed the tube.

3. If the obstruction is due to desiccated formula, a pancrelipase-sodium bicarbonate dwell may dissolve the obstruction. After letting this dwell or if no blockage is seen, irrigate the tube with 5 to 10 mL of normal saline solution for an infant, 20 mL for an older child, and 25 to 50 mL for an adolescent. As you irrigate, listen with a stethoscope over the stomach to ensure proper placement of the tube.

4. If irrigation is unsuccessful, remove the tube and replace it. Blood clots may come from bleeding anywhere in the sinuses, nasal cavity, or the upper alimentary tract. Place the new tube in the contralateral naris. If it is felt that the bleeding is due to esophagitis or gastritis, work that up. If bleeding is felt to be due to varices, get GI to help evaluate the cause and place the tube endoscopically.

Nasogastric and Enteral Feeding Tubes: Displaced Nasogastric Tube and Enteral Feeding Tube

PHONE CALL

Questions

1. How long has the tube been displaced?
2. What type of tube is it?
3. What are the vital signs and the status of the patient?

Orders

Immediately stop using the tube until you have a chance to evaluate the patient.

If a permanent enteral tube (a G-tube or J-tube) is dislodged, have the RN place a red Robinson catheter through the tract to protect it from closure by reepithelialization. The red Robinson tube should be of a small enough caliber that it will not hurt the patient going in. This should be securely taped in place.

Inform RN

Tell the RN, "I will arrive at the bedside in … minutes." As with blocked tubes, infants with dislodged tubes should be evaluated as soon as possible.

ELEVATOR THOUGHTS

What causes an NG or feeding tube to become dislodged?
1. Failure to secure the tube
2. Uncooperative child (normal for infants and young children)

MAJOR THREAT TO LIFE

- Aspiration: Dislodged tubes pose a greater risk of aspiration than a blocked tube, particularly if used for feeding or fluid and medication administration.

BEDSIDE

Quick-Look Test

Does the patient look well (comfortable), sick (uncomfortable or distressed), or critical (about to die)?

Aspiration may cause the patient to appear toxic.

Airway and Vital Signs

If the airway or vital signs are compromised, you should suspect that aspiration has occurred.

Management

1. Inspect the tube. The markings may allow you to estimate the positioning of the tube.
2. Aspirate the tube to determine whether you can obtain gastric fluid. Alternatively, instill a small amount (10 to 20 mL) of air into the tube and listen to the epigastrium with a stethoscope for the rush of air to confirm positioning.
3. If the tube is an enteral feeding tube (e.g., a jejunal tube), it needs to be removed and replaced. It should not be pushed farther down if it has become dislodged.
4. If there are any concerns for a possible aspiration, obtain a chest radiograph; keep in mind that it may take hours of inflammation for imaging to show pneumonitis.
5. Tubes that are in place via a surgically created stoma (G-tube and J-tube) may require replacement under fluoroscopic guidance. Discuss the need for this with a supervising physician.

Urethral Catheters: Placement

Urethral catheters are used to obtain sterile urine specimens, relieve bladder outlet obstructions and retention, prevent incontinent urine from getting into open wounds, and allow accurate measures of urine output in the critically ill. Sterile technique should be ensured when placing a urethral catheter. As with other procedures in pediatric patients, having an experienced "holder" to distract and gently restrain the child during the procedure can be a tremendous help.

1. Have a kit at bedside.
2. Position the child in the supine position. A frog-leg position may help with females. Cleanse the urethral opening thoroughly with a povidone-iodine solution.

3. Lubricate the end of the catheter with petroleum jelly and insert it into the urethral opening; advance the tube with gentle, steady pressure.

4. Once urine flow is visualized in the tube, stop advancing the catheter if this is a one-time catheterization to obtain a sterile urine specimen. If the catheter is to remain in place, advance the catheter farther to ensure that the tip is fully within the bladder; in higher Tanner stage males, advance the catheter to the hub.

5. If a Foley catheter is being used, inflate the balloon on the end of the catheter with a few milliliters of water of saline. This should not hurt the patient. Pain with balloon expansion may be suggestive of placement within the urethra and inflation should immediately stop.

6. Exert gentle traction to make sure that the balloon is against the bladder trigone.

7. Secure the catheter to the medial aspect of the thigh with tape or a clamp (check your kit). Leave a generous portion of the catheter tubing between the anchor point and the urethral opening to allow some slack in the tube as the child moves the leg.

Urethral Catheters: Obstructed Urethral Catheter

PHONE CALL

Questions

1. How long has the catheter been blocked?
2. What are the vital signs?
3. Is the child complaining of suprapubic or abdominal pain?
4. Has there been any hematuria?

Orders

Ask the nurse to try flushing the catheter with 10 mL of normal saline solution if this has not been done already.

Inform RN

Tell the RN, "I will arrive at the bedside in … minutes." If the child is uncomfortable, you should evaluate the child immediately.

ELEVATOR THOUGHTS

What causes blocked urethral catheters?

1. Urinary sediment
2. Blood clots
3. External clamping, kinking, or compression
4. Catheter displacement

MAJOR THREAT TO LIFE

- Bladder rupture
- Progressive renal insufficiency
- Urosepsis (also known as sepsis with a urinary tract infection [UTI])

Bladder rupture may occur if the bladder is unable to drain an increasing volume of urine. Pain may be expected to precede rupture; therefore an uncomfortable child is worrisome. However, some children may be incapable of sensing a distended bladder (e.g., those with spinal cord lesions and comatose or sedated children).

Renal failure may occur secondary to hydronephrosis from chronic urinary tract obstruction. Urinary stasis also increases the risk for infection of the urinary tract, which may potentially progress to sepsis.

BEDSIDE

Quick-Look Test

Does the child look well (comfortable), sick (uncomfortable or distressed), or critical (about to die)?

Most patients look well unless the bladder has been distended enough to cause pain.

Airway and Vital Signs

Unless pain or infection is present, the vital signs are not usually affected by a blocked urethral catheter.

Management

1. Reevaluate the need for the urethral catheter; if no longer needed or if a trial without the catheter is appropriate, remove it.
2. Carefully inspect the catheter and drainage tubing for claps, kinks, compression, or an obvious blockage in the external portion of the tube.
3. Palpate the suprapubic area for fullness suggestive of bladder distention.
4. Aspirate and irrigate the catheter as follows:
   a. Using sterile technique, disconnect the catheter from the drainage tubing.
   b. With a 10- or 30-mL syringe, aspirate the catheter to dislodge and extract any sediment or blood clot that may be obstructing the lumen.
   c. If aspiration does not reveal anything, flush the catheter with 10 to 20 mL of normal saline solution and check for return of flow.

5. If aspiration and flushing fail to relieve the obstruction, remove the catheter and insert a new one, again, only if continued use is indicated.

Urethral Catheters: Gross Hematuria

Discolored urine may be due to bleeding from anywhere in the urinary tract from the glomeruli to the urethral meatus; such bleeding may be secondary to trauma (catheterization, instrumentation, or stones), UTIs, glomerular disease, hemorrhagic cystitis, or even neoplastic processes. Discoloration may also be due to pigmented metabolites (such as with rifampin, beets, and porphyria), myoglobinuria (as a byproduct of rhabdomyolisis), or hemoglobinuria. In catheterized patients, trauma from the catheter and catheter-associated UTIs should be initially suspected with an open mind for other diagnoses.

PHONE CALL

Questions

1. Why does the child have a urethral catheter?
2. How long ago was the catheter placed?
3. Is the child in pain?
4. What are the vital signs?
5. Has the patient received heparin, warfarin, or cyclophosphamide?

Orders

Urine dipstick and urine macro-evaluation/micro-evaluation with reflex urine culture.

Inform RN

Tell the RN, "I will arrive at the bedside in … minutes." Gross hematuria should be evaluated urgently.

ELEVATOR THOUGHTS

What causes gross hematuria in a child with a urinary catheter?
 See earlier. In addition to those causes, keep in mind that coagulopathies and anticoagulant, antiplatelet, and thrombolytic therapies may predispose to bleeding with even small traumatic events from catheterization.

MAJOR THREAT TO LIFE

Perforated bladder or urethra.
Hemorrhagic shock: Although gross hematuria is generally frightening to the child (and often their parents and medical staff), it

is exceedingly rare for any patient to bleed enough from their urinary tract to result in hemodynamic compromise.

BEDSIDE

Quick-Look Test

Does the child look well (comfortable), sick (uncomfortable or distressed), or critical (about to die)?

A perforated urinary tract will make the child look sick or critical and will generally be exquisitely painful. An ascending UTI or pyelonephritis may also make the patient appear sick. Sepsis due to a UTI may make the child appear critical.

Airway and Vital Signs

Vitals are generally normal unless severe pain, fright or anxiety, or infection are present.

Selective History and Chart Review

Has the child received any medication that may cause hematuria or discolor the urine?

Do prior laboratory findings suggest a coagulopathy (particularly abnormal PT, PTT, and platelet levels) or hemolysis (Hgb/Hct with mean corpuscular volume [MCV] and mean corpuscular hemoglobin content MCHC, bilirubin, lactic acid dehydrogenase [LDH], haptoglobin levels)? Reviewing the peripheral smear for evidence of DIC or a microangiopathy may be helpful.

Is there a history of urethral trauma?

Recent surgery, difficulty inserting or removing a urethral catheter, or an obstructed catheter suggests the possibility of trauma.

Management

1. Examine the catheter contents. True hematuria will often, although not always, have red sediment.
2. Physically examine the patient. Evaluate the urethral meatus. Bleeding around the tubing is suggestive of urethral trauma. Evaluation for costovertebral angle tenderness should be performed on every patient with gross hematuria given the possibility of pyelonephritis.
3. If the patient appears ill and trauma is the suspected cause, a period of observation with frequent monitoring of the vital signs and degree of hematuria allows time for the bleeding to spontaneously subside, which it may do. Consultation with a urologist should be considered if the bleeding does not diminish, the vital signs are compromised, or the degree of pain is concerning for a perforation.
4. Review the UA dipstick and macro-/micro-analysis. UTIs are suggested by the presence of white blood cells (WBC), leukocyte

esterase, nitrates, and bacteria on dipstick; however, the presence or absence of these markers varies by the infecting organism and its concentration in the urine. If a UTI is suspected, start empiric antibiotics and ensure a urine culture is obtained. If the patient is very ill, also obtain blood cultures. Other diagnoses that urine studies help with include glomerular disease, for which the presence of red blood cells (RBC) casts has a very high specificity. Myoglobinuria classically shows a positive marker for RBC on dipstick study, whereas none are seen on microscopic evaluation of the urine.

Consider prerenal causes of discolored urine (metabolites, DIC, etc.) and work up and treat appropriately.

Chest Tubes: Placement

Chest tubes are placed in the pleural or mediastinal spaces to evacuate air (pneumothorax, pneumomediastinum), fluid (pleural or pericardial effusions), purulent collections (pleural or pericardial empyemas), or blood (hemothorax, hemomediastinum; Fig. 26.4). They are generally placed by surgeons, although critical

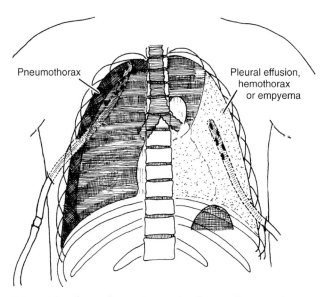

FIGURE 26.4 Chest tubes are inserted to drain air (pneumothorax), blood (hemothorax), fluid (pleural effusion), and pus (empyema). (From Marshall SA, Ruedy J: On Call: Principles and Protocols, 4th ed. Philadelphia, Elsevier, 2004, p 208.)

care or emergency medicine teams or interventional radiologists will place them if needed. These tubes are always connected to an underwater seal, a device that allows for unilateral air movement out of the cavity. With each expiration (similarly with a cough or Valsalva maneuver), increased intrathoracic pressure may expel a small portion of the collected air or fluid. Air, whether from the cavity itself or displaced out of the tubing or collection box by drained fluid, escapes through the water seal. This drainage may be augmented with suction. The seal prevents air from entering back into the system and chest during inspiration (Fig. 26.5). A functioning water seal should have some bubbling with expiration and the water level should oscillate during the respiratory cycle. Thus abnormalities at the water seal may be the first indicator of tube dysfunction. Common drainage setups are depicted in Fig. 26.6; common problems with chest tubes are shown in Fig. 26.7.

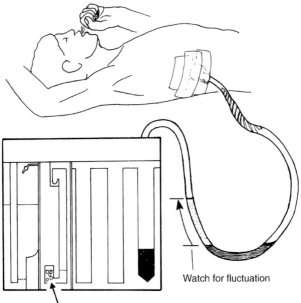

Watch for fluctuation

Watch for bubbling here

FIGURE 26.5 Loss of fluctuation of the underwater seal. Ask the patient to cough, and observe for any fluctuation or bubbling. (From Marshall SA, Ruedy J: On Call: Principles and Protocols, 4th ed. Philadelphia, Elsevier, 2004, p 212.)

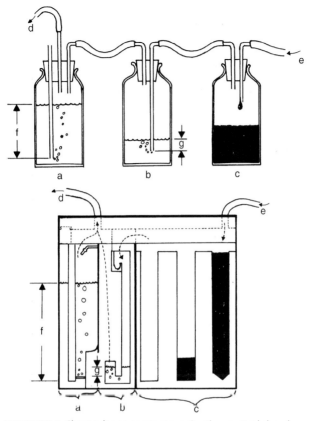

FIGURE 26.6 Chest tube apparatuses. *a*, Suction control chamber. *b*, Underwater seal. *c*, Collection chamber. *d*, To suction. *e*, From patient. *f*, Height equals amount of suction in cm H_2O. *g*, Height equals underwater seal in cm H_2O. (From Marshall SA, Ruedy J: On Call: Principles and Protocols, 4th ed. Philadelphia, Elsevier, 2004, p 209.)

Chest Tubes: Persistent Bubbling in the Water Seal (Air Leak)

PHONE CALL

Questions

1. Is the child in respiratory distress?
2. Why was the chest tube placed?
3. What are the vital signs?

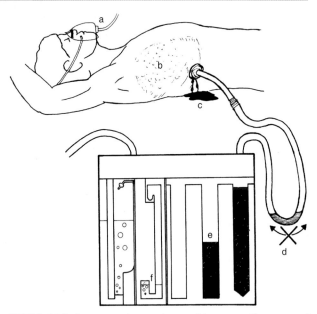

FIGURE 26.7 Common chest tube problems. *a*, Shortness of breath. *b*, Subcutaneous emphysema. *c*, Bleeding at the entry site. *d*, Loss of fluctuation. *e*, Excessive drainage. *f*, Persistent bubbling. (From Marshall SA, Ruedy J: On Call: Principles and Protocols, 4th ed. Philadelphia, Elsevier, 2004, p 210.)

Orders

Two clamps at bedside

Inform RN

Tell the RN, "I will arrive at the bedside in … minutes." The patient needs to be seen as soon as possible and immediately if in respiratory distress.

ELEVATOR THOUGHTS

What causes persistent bubbling in the drainage container?
1. Loose tubing connection
2. Air leaking into the pleural space around the chest tube at the insertion site

3. Traumatic tracheobronchial injury (in children with traumatic pneumothorax, there may be additional injuries)
4. Persistent leak into the pleural space from the bronchoalveolar tree
   a. Postsurgical
   b. Ruptured bleb (spontaneous pneumothorax; seen particularly in patients with asthma, cystic fibrosis)
   c. Bronchopleural fistula
5. Externalization of a proximal side hole on the chest tube (may be visually identified or seen on chest radiography)

MAJOR THREAT TO LIFE

- Tension pneumothorax: If a pneumothorax is not being appropriately evacuated, air may collect and tension may develop leading to hemodynamic collapse (Figs. 26.8 and 26.9).
- Hypoxia: Buildup of air or fluids may lead to lung collapse and a ventilation-perfusion mismatch with severe hypoxia.

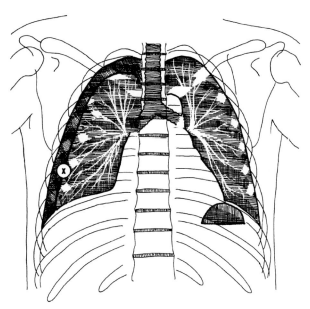

FIGURE 26.8 Pneumothorax. x, Edge of visceral pleura or lung. (From Marshall SA, Ruedy J: On Call: Principles and Protocols, 4th ed. Philadelphia, Elsevier, 2004, p 218.)

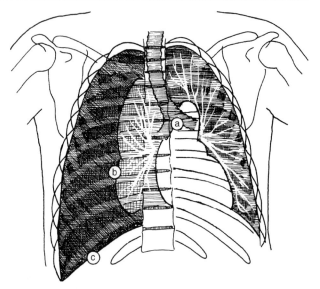

FIGURE 26.9 Tension pneumothorax. *a*, Shifted mediastinum. *b*, Edge of collapsed lung. *c*, Low flattened diaphragm. (From Marshall SA, Ruedy J: On Call: Principles and Protocols, 4th ed. Philadelphia, Elsevier, 2004, p 219.)

BEDSIDE

Quick-Look Test

Does the child appear well (comfortable), sick (uncomfortable or distressed), or critical (about to die)?

A tension pneumothorax may be developing in a child who appears ill. Quickly evaluate the need for a needle thoracotomy decompression or an additional chest tube in an ill-appearing child by listening over the lung fields. If no sounds are heard on the side with the possible tension pneumothorax, treat emergently before getting imaging (see Chapter 10). If the exam is reassuring, obtaining a stat portable chest radiograph may be helpful.

Airway and Vital Signs

If all connections are tight and the chest tube dressing is airtight, a persistent air leak means that the patient has a pneumothorax. As long as air continues to bubble through the collection chamber, the air should drain from the pleural space and not alter the vital signs or compromise the airway. Augmenting air removal with suction should be considered.

Selective History and Chart Review

Why was the chest tube placed?

If the tube was placed for pneumothorax, the collection chamber should be bubbling during expiration unless the lung is fully expanded and the leak into the pleural space has sealed; a continuous bubbling may indicate a worsening pneumothorax.

If the tube was placed to drain fluid (effusion, empyema, or blood) without suction, a new onset of bubbling indicates loose connections external to the chest, air leaking into the pleural space from around the insertion site, or the development of a spontaneous or traumatic pneumothorax.

Selective Physical Examination and Management

1. Inspect the tubing connections and ensure that all seals are airtight.
2. Remove the dressing at the entry site, listen for the sound of air being sucked into the chest while observing the area around the site. If the incision for the tube is inadequately closed to form a seal around the tube, placing sutures to seal the thoracotomy tract may be necessary. If this stops the continuous bubbling, clean the site and reapply the sterile dressing.
3. Inspect the tubing for air leaks along its entire length. Do this by placing a clamp on the tube adjacent to the thoracotomy site. If the bubbling stops, the air leak is coming from within the chest; if the bubbling continues, there is a leak in the line, likely a small hole. If you find the latter to be the case, place a second clamp on the tube 5 to 10 inches away from the first. Continue to move this down in serial increments until the bubbling stops. The leak will be proximal to the patient from the second clamp. Once the spot is found, multiple layers of tape may seal off the leak and allow the tube to continue to be functional. Alternatively, the tubing may be cut and spliced together with a new drainage kit using a connector. Ensure the tubing is clamped close to the patient before cutting any tubing to prevent a pneumothorax via retrograde suction of air into the chest.
4. If the tubing and entry site appear airtight, obtain a chest radiograph to confirm proper chest tube placement. The tube holes should be within the chest, and the tip of the tube should be seen clearly away from the mediastinal and subclavian structures. Comparing this film with the previous film taken after insertion of the chest tube allows you to determine whether a pneumothorax has developed or if an existing one has increased in size. If the pneumothorax is larger or the lung has not reexpanded, the single chest tube may not be adequate to evacuate the air leak. You may need to consider augmenting evacuation of the collection with suction or placing a second chest tube. This

should be discussed with the patient's attending physician. Surgical consultation may also be necessary if the air leak occurred secondary to trauma or surgery.

Chest Tubes: Loss of Fluctuation of the Water Seal (Tube Obstruction)

PHONE CALL

Questions

1. Is the child in respiratory distress?
2. Why was the chest tube placed?
3. What are the vital signs?
4. How long has it been dysfunctional?

Orders

None

Inform RN

Tell the RN, "I will arrive at the bedside in … minutes." You need to evaluate the child immediately.

ELEVATOR THOUGHTS

What causes loss of fluctuation of the underwater seal? Loss of fluctuation means that the tube is not functioning to evacuate air or fluid from the intrathoracic space.

1. External compression or kink in the chest tube
2. Intraluminal chest tube obstruction

MAJOR THREAT TO LIFE

- Tension pneumothorax: If a pneumothorax is not being appropriately evacuated, air may collect and tension may develop leading to hemodynamic collapse (see Figs. 26.8 and 26.9).
- Hypoxia: Buildup of air or fluids may lead to lung collapse and a ventilation-perfusion mismatch with severe hypoxia.

BEDSIDE

Quick-Look Test

Does the child appear well (comfortable), sick (uncomfortable or distressed), or critical (about to die)?

A tension pneumothorax may be developing in a child who appears ill. Quickly evaluate the need for a needle thoracotomy or an additional chest tube in an ill-appearing child by listening over the lung fields. If no sounds are heard on the side with the possible tension pneumothorax, treat emergently before getting imaging (see Chapter 10). If the exam is reassuring, obtaining a stat portable chest radiograph may be helpful.

Airway and Vital Signs

A displaced trachea, tachycardia, tachypnea, hypoxia, and hypotension may all be markers of a tension pneumothorax or lung collapse with a ventilation-perfusion mismatch.

Selective History and Chart Review

- Why was the chest tube placed?
- How long ago did it stop fluctuating?
- What and how much has been drained in the past 24 hours? What was the trend of drainage?

Selective Physical Examination and Management

1. Again, ensure you have examined the trachea and the lung fields to clinically reassure against a tension pneumothorax.
2. Reevaluate the need for the chest tube and remove if possible.
3. Inspect the water seal. Is there any fluctuation? Ask the child to cough, and watch for fluctuation. Poor respiratory effort may lead to minuscule fluctuations. If this is the case, clinically evaluate the child for possible intubation for airway protection.
4. Inspect the tube for external compression or kinks in the tubing. You may need to remove the dressing at the insertion site. If a kink is found, reinspect for fluctuation after repositioning the tube.
5. If the chest tube appears to be clogged, try milking or stripping the tube to relieve obstruction by blood clots or other debris. However, realize that frequent milking may lead to a buildup of negative pressure on the system and should be done minimally and with care. tPA may be used in select circumstances to lyse thrombi, but this should be guided by experts (surgeons, pulmonologists, intensivists).
6. Obtain a portable stat chest radiograph to determine the position of the tube. Reposition the tube if it appears to be close to structures that may be causing an obstruction. Remember that shear force may traumatize intrathoracic vasculature.

Chest Tubes: Bleeding at the Chest Tube Entry Site

PHONE CALL

Questions

1. Is the child in respiratory distress?
2. Why was the chest tube placed?
3. What are the vital signs?

Orders

Ask the RN for sterile gloves, a dressing set, a suture kit, and povidone-iodine at the bedside. You need to remove the sterile dressing around the chest tube site.

Inform RN

Tell the RN, "I will arrive at the bedside in … minutes." You need to see the child immediately.

ELEVATOR THOUGHTS

What causes bleeding around the chest tube entry site?

In general, bleeding around chest tube entry sites (thoracotomy sites) comes from the soft tissues along the tract; even so, intrathoracic bleeding must be considered.

1. Inadequate pressure dressing
2. Inadequate closure of the incision
3. Coagulation disorders
4. Trauma to intercostal or intrathoracic arteries or veins during tube placement or manipulation
5. Blocked chest tube in a child with a hemothorax

MAJOR THREAT TO LIFE

- Hemorrhagic shock: Usually the bleeding is not rapid though direct trauma to any vasculature can lead to shock and exsanguination.
- Hemothorax with subsequent ventilation perfusion defect due to decreased lung volume.
- Sepsis: Active bleeding indicates an opening in the circulatory system. Bacteremia and sepsis may develop; therefore one should watch for signs and symptoms of infection after hemostasis has been achieved.

BEDSIDE

Quick-Look Test

Does the child appear well (comfortable), sick (uncomfortable or distressed), or critical (about to die)?

If the child appears more ill than would be suggested by the volume of extracorporeal blood, a developing hemothorax should be suspected until proved otherwise.

Airway and Vital Signs

The airway is almost always stable. Vital signs are usually stable unless significant hemorrhage (including hemorrhage leading to hemothorax) has occurred. Rapid decompensation indicates massive blood loss, lung collapse, or intrathoracic tension.

Selective History and Chart Review

Why was the chest tube placed?

If it was placed for hemothorax, the main concern is inadequate evacuation of blood from the pleural space. Augmenting drainage with suction may be needed.

Review the patient's personal and family histories with an eye for any coagulopathies, their medications for any anticoagulant, antiplatelet, or thrombolytic therapeutics, and their labs for any coagulation disorders, anemia, or thrombocytopenias.

Selective Physical Examination and Management

1. Do a quick but full chest examination.
2. Remove the dressing and inspect the incision. See if the incision is inadequately closed; if so, additional sutures may tamponade the bleeding. If the incision is adequately closed, reapply a pressure dressing at the site.
3. If the patient's history or medication regimen suggest an etiology, address that after ensuring additional pressure has been placed around the thoracotomy site.
4. If the chest tube appears to be clogged, try milking or stripping the tube to relieve obstruction by blood clots or other debris. However, realize that frequent milking may lead to a buildup of negative pressure on the system and should be done minimally and with care. tPA may be used in select circumstances to lyse thrombi, but this should be guided by experts (surgeons, pulmonologists, intensivists).
5. If bleeding persists in a patient with hemothorax, consider placing a larger chest tube.

6. In those without hemothorax, apply firm pressure by hand over the site for 20 minutes. Repeat this step if necessary. If the bleeding still continues, further evaluation for an unknown coagulopathy may be indicated.

Chest Tubes: Drainage of Blood

PHONE CALL

Questions
1. Is the child in respiratory distress?
2. Why was the chest tube placed?
3. What are the vital signs? Any orthostatic symptoms of changes in vital signs?
4. How much blood has drained?

Orders
None

Inform RN

Tell the RN, "I will arrive at the bedside in … minutes." You need to see the child immediately.

ELEVATOR THOUGHTS

What causes blood to drain from the chest tube?
1. Injury to intercostal or intrathoracic vasculature
2. Pulmonary hemorrhage

MAJOR THREAT TO LIFE

- Hemorrhagic shock: Usually the bleeding is not rapid though direct trauma to any vasculature can lead to shock and exsanguination.
- Respiratory insufficiency secondary to pulmonary hemorrhage: This would usually be due to an underlying condition, not the catheter itself.
- Sepsis: Active bleeding indicates an opening in the circulatory system. Bacteremia and sepsis may develop; therefore one should watch for signs and symptoms of infection after hemostasis has been achieved.

BEDSIDE

Quick-Look Test

Does the child appear well (comfortable), sick (uncomfortable or distressed), or critical (about to die)?

If the child appears more ill than would be suggested by the volume of extracorporeal blood, a developing hemothorax should be suspected until proved otherwise.

Airway and Vital Signs

The airway is almost always stable. Check the heart rate as this is often the first marker of hemodynamic stress. Also review the blood pressure and, if possible, a CVP.

Selective Chart Review and Management

Was the chest tube placed postoperatively? Any recent operations or procedures? Any recent trauma?

If so, determine if the bleeding is within an expected volume range.

What is the trend of volume removed?

An increasing volume over time should raise your suspicions of serious pathology.

What medications has the child received?

Check the list for any anticoagulant, antiplatelet, or thrombolytic medications.

How much blood has been lost?

If the amount of blood loss is small, you may continue to carefully monitor the loss and ask to be informed if the amount lost exceeds 10 mL/hour in an infant or 25 mL/hour in an older child. Increase the frequency of vital sign observations so that the heart rate and blood pressure can be monitored; consider transferring the patient to a critical care unit for close monitoring. In addition and in short order:

1. Order a chest radiograph to evaluate for potential sources of intrathoracic bleeding.
2. Send blood for typing and cross matching for 4 adult units of packed red blood cells.
   Also obtain Hgb, Hct, platelet count, PT, and PTT measurements.
3. Consult cardiothoracic surgery. If the bleeding persists or is excessive, surgical exploration may be necessary to localize and stop the bleeding.
4. If there is any hemodynamic compromise, start aggressive intravenous fluid (IVF) resuscitation until blood products are ready for transfusion.

Chest Tubes: Dyspnea

PHONE CALL

Questions

1. Is the child in respiratory distress?
2. Why was the chest tube placed?
3. What are the vital signs?

Orders

A medical provider should stay with the patient until you arrive. There should be a low threshold for calling for rapid response team or critical care assistance. Ask the nurse for a dressing set, gloves, several sizes of angiocatheters, and povidone-iodine at the bedside. You may need an angiocatheter (one that does not lock after the flash) to evacuate a tension pneumothorax. Ask the nurse to call for an immediate portable chest radiograph.

Inform RN

Tell the RN, "I will arrive at the bedside in … minutes." You need to see the child immediately.

ELEVATOR THOUGHTS

What causes dyspnea in a patient with a chest tube?
1. Tension pneumothorax
2. Expanding pneumothorax
3. Subcutaneous emphysema (see later)
4. Expanding pleural effusion or hemothorax
5. Reexpansion pulmonary edema (after rapid evacuation of the pleural space)
6. Other causes unrelated to the chest tube (see Chapter 28)

MAJOR THREAT TO LIFE

- Tension pneumothorax: If a pneumothorax is not being appropriately evacuated, air may collect and tension may develop leading to hemodynamic collapse (see Figs. 26.8 and 26.9).
- Hypoxia: Buildup of air or fluids may lead to lung collapse and a ventilation-perfusion mismatch with severe hypoxia.

BEDSIDE
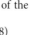

Quick-Look Test

Children with dyspnea usually appear ill.

Airway and Vital Signs

1. Protecting the airway is paramount. Evaluate for stridor or other signs of extrathoracic airway compromise, including subcutaneous emphysema that may be obstructing the upper airway. If needed, call a code to expedite intubation.
2. A displaced trachea, tachycardia, tachypnea, hypoxia, and hypotension may all be markers of a tension pneumothorax or lung collapse with a ventilation-perfusion mismatch.
3. Tachypnea suggests hypercapnia, hypoxia, pain, or anxiety.

Selective Physical Examination

Examine for signs of tension pneumothorax as described previously.

Evaluate the chest tube water seal for bubbling; if the bubbling has stopped, obstruction is suggested (see previous section).

Management

1. Again, if there are any questions about the safety of the airway, call a code to expedite intubation and transfer the patient to a critical care unit.
2. If you suspect tension pneumothorax, it needs to be evacuated (see Chapter 10, Chest Pain).
3. If you suspect an enlarging pneumothorax, look for a correctable cause (blocked or compressed tubing, inadequate suction on the chest tube, or dislodged chest tube). A chest radiograph helps to determine whether the tube is properly positioned.
4. If the chest tube appears to be functioning and no tension or expanding pneumothoraces are present, management should be directed at other causes of dyspnea unrelated to the chest tube (see Chapter 28, Respiratory Distress).

Chest Tubes: Subcutaneous Emphysema

PHONE CALL

Questions

1. Is the child in respiratory distress?
2. Why was the chest tube placed?
3. What are the vital signs?

Orders

Ask the nurse for a dressing set, gloves, and povidone-iodine at the bedside. You need to remove the sterile dressing around the insertion site.

Inform RN

Tell the RN, "I will arrive at the bedside in … minutes." You need to see the child immediately.

ELEVATOR THOUGHTS

What causes subcutaneous emphysema in a patient with a chest tube?

1. Inadequate size of tube
2. Inadequate suction
3. Chest tube aperture in the chest wall
4. Chest tube in the chest wall or abdominal cavity
5. Minor subcutaneous emphysema localized to the insertion site (not uncommon)

MAJOR THREAT TO LIFE

- Upper airway obstruction: Subcutaneous emphysema may extend into the soft tissues of the neck and compress the airway.

BEDSIDE

Quick-Look Test

Does the child appear well (comfortable), sick (uncomfortable or distressed), or critical (about to die)?

If the emphysema is leading to upper airway obstruction, the child will appear ill.

Airway and Vital Signs

1. Inspect and palpate the neck to feel for the crepitus of subcutaneous emphysema. If present, it will feel and may sound like a "crunching" as you palpate.
2. Check the respiratory rate, blood pressure, and heart rate. Subcutaneous emphysema may be associated with a concurrent tension pneumothorax.

Selective Physical Examination and Management

1. If the airway is nearly obstructed (stridor, tachypnea, dyspnea), call for critical care support to expedite intubation to protect their airway.
2. Examine the size of the chest tube. If the tube is too small, air may escape from the pleural space into the chest wall. A new, larger tube may be necessary.
3. Is the suction connected? A tube left only to straight drainage may be inadequate to evacuate a large pneumothorax.

4. Remove the dressing and inspect the insertion site and the chest tube. None of the holes in the tube should be visible. They should all be within the pleural space. If the tube has become misplaced and the holes now lie outside the chest wall, a new tube needs to be inserted. Do not push an extruded tube back into the pleural space, because this increases the risk of infecting the pleural cavity.

Chest Tubes: Traumatic or Accidental Removal of a Chest Tube

PHONE CALL

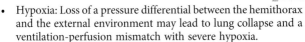

Questions

1. Is the child in respiratory distress?
2. Why was the chest tube placed?
3. What are the vital signs?

Orders

Ask the nurse for occlusive dressing and tape. A medical provider should stay with the patient until you arrive. The RN should also call the provider who will replace the tube (generally the team who initially placed it; if placed in the emergency department (ED) or outside of the hospital, then have general surgery or critical care help). There should be a low threshold for calling for rapid response team or critical care support.

Inform RN

Tell the RN, "I will arrive at the bedside in … minutes." You need to see the child immediately.

MAJOR THREAT TO LIFE

- Hypoxia: Loss of a pressure differential between the hemithorax and the external environment may lead to lung collapse and a ventilation-perfusion mismatch with severe hypoxia.
- Tension pneumothorax: A small opening may lead to air entry into the pleural space and prevent exit therefrom, leading to a buildup of tension. However, if the hole is large, it will act as a decompression tract allowing for air to enter and exit the space. Should this be the case, if the tract is iatrogenically or spontaneously closed, a tension pneumothorax may develop as air from the lung (if perforated) builds up in the space.
- Sepsis: The open tract may lead to infection; therefore one should watch for signs and symptoms of infection after hemostasis has been achieved.

BEDSIDE

Quick-Look Test

Does the child appear well (comfortable), sick (uncomfortable or distressed), or critical (about to die)?

An open tract may lead to collapse of the lung and acute respiratory and hemodynamic collapse.

Airway and Vital Signs

1. If there is any respiratory distress, call for critical care support because an expedited intubation may be required.
2. Continuous cardiorespiratory monitoring and frequent blood pressure measures should be followed.

Selective Physical Examination and Management

1. Quickly examine the patient. Again, if they are in distress, call for critical care support.
2. If the patient is stable from hemodynamically and respiratory standpoints, tape three sides of an occlusive dressing over the thoracotomy tract to protect it until the team responsible for replacing the tube arrives. Do not tape all four sides as this could lead to a tension pneumothorax.

Rashes

Anna Schmitz, MD

Rashes can develop for a wide variety of reasons in a hospitalized child—some very serious and others benign. When you are called by the nurse to evaluate a rash while on call, remember that your goal is not necessarily to arrive at a specific diagnosis or explanation. Instead, excluding illnesses that might be harmful to the child, keeping the child comfortable, and reassuring the patient and family that you have done so may be appropriate immediate goals.

PHONE CALL

Questions

1. How long has the patient had the rash?
2. Is urticaria (hives) present?
3. Is the child wheezing or in any respiratory distress?
4. What are the vital signs?
5. What medications has the child received in the past 12 hours?
6. Does the child have any known allergies?
7. What is the child's age and admitting diagnosis?

Orders

If the rash is associated with signs of anaphylaxis (wheezing, stridor, dysphagia, shortness of breath, periorbital edema, lip swelling, or hypotension), order the following without delay:

1. Place an intravenous (IV) line immediately and start a normal saline bolus.
2. Stop any current infusions (antibiotics, blood products, etc.)

3. Have airway support materials at the bedside, including suction, a laryngoscopy tray, oxygen, and an Ambu bag.
4. Epinephrine, 0.01 mg/kg (0.1 mL/kg of a 1:10,000 solution for IV administration or 0.01 mL/kg of a 1:1,000 solution for sub-cutaneous administration). Do not confuse these doses and routes of administration!
5. IV diphenhydramine (Benadryl), 1 mg/kg and/or IV ranitidine 1 mg/kg
6. IV methylprednisolone, 1 mg/kg

If there are no signs of an acute allergic reaction, instruct the nurse to avoid applying anything to the rash until you have examined the patient.

Inform RN

Tell the RN, "I will arrive at the bedside in … minutes." Evidence of anaphylaxis or acute allergy requires immediate evaluation. A new onset of purpura or petechiae, particularly in a child with fever, also requires immediate evaluation.

ELEVATOR THOUGHTS

Many medications can cause skin eruptions, and such rashes are among the most common that you will be asked to evaluate. The lesions may be urticarial, macular, papular, erythematous, vesicular, bullous, petechial, or purpuric. Most drug rashes are widely distributed over the body. Remember that rashes can evolve, and changes may occur with time. What the nurse observed may not be what you see 2 or 3 hours later. The more common rashes and some of their causes are listed here.

Urticaria (Rare but Potentially Life Threatening)

Histamine-mediated allergic reactions: IV contrast material, antibiotics, opiates, anesthetic agents, vasoactive agents
Drug reactions with an unknown mechanism: aspirin, nonsteroidal antiinflammatory drugs
Food allergies: shellfish, nuts, tomatoes
Physical agents: detergents, perfumes, cold, heat, pressure
Idiopathic

Erythematous, Maculopapular (Morbilliform) Rashes

Infections
    Measles (rubeola)
    Rubella
    Roseola
    Kawasaki disease

Systemic-onset juvenile idiopathic arthritis
> Drug reactions. (Because some drug rashes have a late onset, the
> medication history should include all medications taken in
> the last 4 weeks.)
> Antibiotics
> Antihistamines
> Antidepressants
> Diuretics
> Sedatives

Vesicobullous Rashes

Varicella-zoster (primary, chicken pox; or secondary, herpes zoster)
Erythema multiforme (many viruses and drugs)
Stevens-Johnson syndrome (this is a particularly life-threatening
variant of erythema multiforme characterized by involvement
of at least two mucous membranes, especially the oral mucosa
and eye).
Toxic epidermal necrolysis: Lyell syndrome (sulfonamide, allopurinol)
Antibiotics (sulfonamides, dapsone)
Antiinflammatory agents (penicillamine)
Sedatives (barbiturates)

Petechiae or Purpura

Vasculitis (palpable purpura)
Sepsis or disseminated intravascular coagulopathy (DIC; meningo-
coccemia, *Haemophilus influenzae* sepsis, cytomegalovirus)
Antibiotics (sulfonamides, chloramphenicol)
Diuretics
Antiinflammatory agents (salicylates, indomethacin, phenylbutazone)
Thrombocytopenia

Exfoliative Dermatitis (Erythroderma)

Scarlet fever
Toxic shock syndrome
Antibiotics (streptomycin)
Antiinflammatory agents (gold, phenylbutazone)
Antiepileptics (carbamazepine, phenytoin)

Fixed Drug Reaction

Antibiotics (sulfonamides, metronidazole)
Antiinflammatory drugs (phenylbutazone)
Analgesics (phenacetin)
Sedatives (barbiturates, chlordiazepoxide)
Laxatives (phenolphthalein)
> Certain drugs may produce a skin lesion in a specific area.
Repeated administration of the drug reproduces the skin lesion

in the same location. The lesions are usually dusky red or violaceous patches over the trunk and limbs.

MAJOR THREAT TO LIFE

- Anaphylactic shock
- Septic shock with DIC
- Stevens-Johnson syndrome

Urticarial eruptions indicate histamine release and may be a prodrome to systemic histamine effects, including hypotension and shock. In hospitalized children, drugs and IV contrast materials are the most common causes of anaphylactic reactions.

Sepsis and septic shock can evolve rapidly. The rashes associated with certain conditions, such as meningococcemia and toxic shock syndrome, may develop during the early part of the hospitalization.

Stevens-Johnson syndrome presents a major risk of significant dehydration as a result of oral mucosal involvement, as well as a major threat of permanent visual impairment from uveitis or corneal scarring.

BEDSIDE

Quick-Look Test
Does the child appear well (comfortable), sick (uncomfortable or distressed), or critical?

A patient in impending anaphylaxis appears anxious and hyperalert, usually with progressive respiratory distress.

Airway and Vital Signs
What is the blood pressure?

Hypotension is an ominous sign and requires immediate and aggressive intervention (see Chapter 25).

What is the temperature?

Almost all skin rashes become more apparent when the child is febrile because there is greater perfusion of the skin.

Selective Physical Examination
Is there evidence of impending anaphylaxis, sepsis or DIC, or Stevens-Johnson syndrome?

HEENT	Pharyngeal, periorbital, or facial edema; conjunctivitis or uveitis; oral mucosal lesions
Respiratory	Stridor, wheezing
Skin	Urticarial rash, erythema multiforme rash, purpura, petechiae

HEENT, Head, Eyes, Ears, Nose, Throat.

What is the location of the rash? Is the rash generalized, acral (hands and feet), or localized?

Remember that to evaluate a child for a rash, you must examine the entire child, including the buttocks (a common site for drug eruptions) and the genital region, as well as the scalp.

What is the color of the rash?

Rashes may be erythematous, pale, brown, purple, or pink

Describe the primary lesions (Fig. 27.1):

Macules: flat, with or without a distinct margin (noticeable from the surrounding skin because of the color difference)

Patch: a large macule

Papule: solid, elevated, less than 1 cm

Plaque: solid, elevated, greater than 1 cm

Vesicle: fluid filled, elevated, well circumscribed, less than 1 cm

Pustule: vesicle containing purulent fluid

Bulla: fluid filled, elevated, well circumscribed, greater than 1 cm

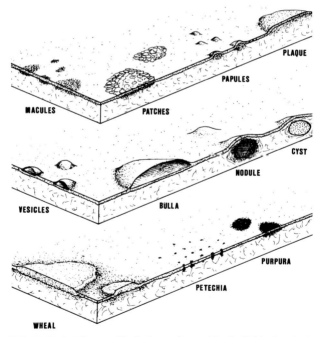

FIGURE 27.1 **Primary skin lesions.** (From Marshall SA, Ruedy J: On Call: Principles and Protocols, 4th ed. Philadelphia, Elsevier, 2004, p 291.)

Nodule: deep-seated mass, indistinct borders, size less than 0.5 cm in both width and depth

Cyst: nodules filled with expressible fluid or semisolid material

Wheal (hives): urticaria; pruritic, well-circumscribed, flat-topped, firm elevation (papule, plaque, or dermal edema) with or without central pallor and with irregular borders

Petechiae: red or purple, nonblanching macules less than 3 mm

Purpura: red or purple, nonblanching macule or papule greater than 3 mm

Describe the secondary lesions (Fig. 27.2):

Scales: dry, thin plates of thickened keratin layers (white color differentiates scales from crusts)

Crust: dried yellow exudate of plasma (results from broken vesicles, bullae, or pustules)

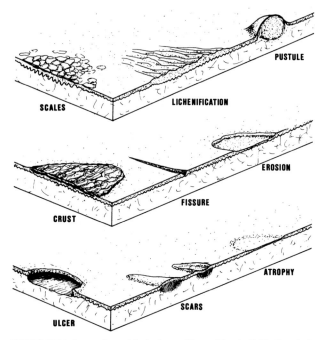

FIGURE 27.2 **Secondary skin lesions.** (From Marshall SA, Ruedy J: On Call: Principles and Protocols, 4th ed. Philadelphia, Elsevier, 2004, p 292.)

Lichenification: dry, leathery thickening; shiny surface with accentuation of skin markings

Fissure: linear, epidermal tear

Erosion: wide, epidermal fissure; moist and well circumscribed

Ulcer: erosion into the dermis

Scar: flat, raised (keloid), or depressed area of fibrosis

Atrophy: depression secondary to thinning of the skin

What is the configuration of the rash?

Annular: circular, well circumscribed

Linear: in lines

Grouped: clusters (e.g., vesicular lesions of herpes zoster or herpes simplex)

Selective History and Chart Review

How long has the rash been present? Is it changing or evolving?

Is it pruritic?

How has it been treated?

Is it a new or recurrent problem?

Which medications was the child receiving before onset of the rash?

Was there previously anything overlying the location of the rash? (i.e., electrocardiogram [ECG] leads, Tegaderm, tape)

Management

1. If the rash is suspected to be a manifestation of an allergy of any kind, it is usually pruritic and should respond to diphenhydramine (Benadryl).
2. If the rash is associated with urticaria and is secondary to a drug reaction, administration of the drug should be withheld until the diagnosis can be confirmed in the morning.
3. If the rash is nonurticarial and thought to be secondary to a drug reaction and the drug is essential to treatment of the child's underlying illness, administration of the drug can be continued with close monitoring of the patient's condition, as long as there is no sign of respiratory compromise or abnormalities in blood pressure and other vital signs.
4. When the rash is not a drug reaction and the diagnosis is clear, the standard recommended treatment of that disorder should be instituted.
5. If the diagnosis of the rash is unclear, describe the lesions thoroughly in your note. If the rash does not cause undue discomfort, no therapy is necessary until the rash evolves or other symptoms or signs develop and a specific diagnosis can be made. Exceptions include the following:

Petechial rash, which can indicate disorders of platelet number or function.

Purpuric rash, which can indicate DIC and sepsis and requires checking a blood culture, prothrombin time, activated partial thromboplastin time, and platelet count, as well as prompt administration of antibiotics.

Vesicular rash secondary to varicella or herpes zoster, which requires immediate isolation of the patient from any potentially immunocompromised children and pregnant women. If the child is immunocompromised or an infant, urgent evaluation and treatment with IV acyclovir is indicated to prevent dissemination of the infection to the central nervous system.

REMEMBER

Your ability to describe the rash is critical to establishing its cause and significance. This will help you to think carefully about the possible explanations and appropriate management when you have been called to make a "rash decision."

CHAPTER 28

Respiratory Distress

Brian Carroll, MD

Respiratory distress is one of the most common complaints that an on-call pediatric house officer is asked to assess. To evaluate a child in respiratory distress, it is necessary to consider the respiratory rate in the context of the age of the child. Neonates typically breathe 35 to 50 times per minute, older infants and toddlers 30 to 40 times per minute, elementary school–aged children 20 to 30 times per minute, and preadolescents and adolescents 12 to 20 times per minute.

In addition to the rate, it is important to observe the quality of the breathing, including depth, use of accessory muscles (e.g., subcostal, intercostal, or supraclavicular retractions), grunting, tracheal tugging, and nasal flaring. Next, you should listen for the presence of adventitious lung sounds such as wheezing, rales, rhonchi, stridor, stertor, or muffled/absent breath sounds. The clinical meaning of these sounds is discussed later in the Physical Examination section. Lastly, you should identify in which phase of the respiratory cycle (inspiratory, expiratory, or both) that these sounds reside because this will help you to identify the location of the pathology. The specific characteristics of the breathing pattern combined with the physical findings and selective laboratory and radiographic tests (when necessary) will allow you to determine the probable cause of the respiratory distress.

PHONE CALL

Questions

1. How old is the patient?
2. Why is the patient in the hospital?
3. How long has the patient been in respiratory distress?
4. Was the onset sudden or gradual?

5. What are the vital signs?
6. Does the child appear cyanotic?
7. Is the child retracting, flaring, wheezing, or coughing?
8. Are oxygen and a pulse oximeter present in the room?

Orders

1. Have the nurse provide oxygen by nasal cannula or mask and obtain a pulse oximeter measurement immediately. Start with 1 to 2 L/min by cannula or 5 to 10 L/min by mask.
2. Set up materials to obtain an arterial blood gas measurement or call the lab to draw blood for arterial blood gas studies.
3. If the child has been admitted for reactive airway disease and/or asthma, have the nurse set up an appropriate dose of a nebulized bronchodilator.
4. Inform the nurse that you are on your way. Respiratory distress deserves immediate evaluation!

ELEVATOR THOUGHTS

Respiratory distress may be a manifestation of several very different pathologic processes. Distress can include depressed respirations, as well as tachypnea.

Pulmonary processes	Pneumonia, bronchospasm, bronchiolitis, pulmonary hemorrhage, or interstitial lung disease
Airway processes	Croup, foreign body aspiration, retropharyngeal abscess, laryngeal edema or spasm, epiglottitis, tracheitis, laryngotracheal malacia, vascular ring, or esophageal masses
Cardiac processes	Congestive heart failure (left-to-right shunt, left ventricular failure), cardiac tamponade, or pulmonary embolism
Space-occupying lesions	Pleural effusion, empyema, pneumothorax, diaphragmatic hernia, massive ascites, or severe scoliosis. Abdominal distention can cause respiratory compromise, especially in infants, who rely on diaphragmatic breathing, or in children with restrictive lung disease (i.e., severe scoliosis).
Neurologic processes	Opiate overdose, increased intracranial pressure, anxiety, or chest wall and/or diaphragmatic weakness. Tachypnea secondary to pain or discomfort.

MAJOR THREAT TO LIFE

Hypoxia resulting in inadequate tissue oxygenation is the most worrisome consequence of any process that results in respiratory distress. In addition, respiratory failure is the most common precipitant of cardiac arrest in children and should be addressed quickly.

BEDSIDE

Quick-Look Test

The first step is to determine if the child appears (1) well (comfortable), (2) sick (uncomfortable or distressed), or (3) critical (about to die).

A child in distress should be placed on a cardiorespiratory monitor immediately and pulse oximetry applied. Oxygen should be administered and airway support supplies, including suctioning and intubation equipment, brought to the bedside. If a child appears critically ill, you should activate the appropriate response team as early as possible to assist you in management.

Airway and Vital Signs

Is the upper airway (including nares) clear, and can the patient protect his or her airway (for example, coughing appropriately and able to swallow secretions)?

An obtunded patient in respiratory distress requires intubation. Upper airway obstruction may make intubation difficult or impossible, such as in a patient with oral or facial trauma, foreign body aspiration, or severe epiglottitis. A surgical airway may thus be necessary via emergency cricothyroidotomy.

What is the respiratory rate and pattern?

Rates less than 20 breaths per minute in most young children reflect central respiratory depression, such as with opiates, barbiturates, or alcohol. Tachypnea suggests hypoxemia, hypercapnia, acidemia, pain, and/or anxiety. Retractions and nasal flaring indicate the use of accessory muscles of respiration because of inadequate tidal volume or airway obstruction. Thoracoabdominal dissociation is a worrisome finding. The chest and abdomen should rise and fall together and not paradoxically.

What is the heart rate?

Increased sympathetic tone secondary to respiratory distress results in sinus tachycardia. Hypercapnia causing acidosis will also cause tachycardia. Bradycardia may herald impending cardiorespiratory collapse, and a normal heart rate may be inappropriate for the level of respiratory distress and a worrisome finding.

Supraventricular tachycardia or nonsinus bradycardia may result in congestive heart failure and subsequent respiratory distress.

What is the temperature?

Fever is accompanied by tachypnea. Obviously, fever suggests infection, and respiratory distress may be due to airway, pleural, or parenchymal lung infection.

What is the blood pressure?

Hypotension in the setting of respiratory distress suggests shock, acidosis, and possible cardiac compromise as a result of tension pneumothorax. In children, pulsus paradoxus, or when inspiration causes a drop in systolic blood pressure of more than the usual 4 to 10 mm Hg, is rarely noted, but it may occur in the setting of respiratory distress and hypotension (pericardial effusion), as well as with obstructive airway disease as a reflection of the degree of airflow obstruction.

Hypertension can occur as a result of increased sympathetic tone from respiratory distress or significant hypercapnia and acidosis.

Selective Physical Examination

Is the patient cyanotic? If yes, see Chapter 13 on Cyanosis.

Vital signs	Repeat now, including pulse oximetry
HEENT	Nasal flaring, cyanotic mucous membranes, oropharyngeal foreign body
Neck	Midline trachea, stridor or stertor
Respiratory	Symmetry of air entry. wheezing, rales, rhonchi, stridor and stertor, decreased breath sounds, dullness to percussion, ability to phonate, retractions, grunting
Neurologic	Mental status, ability to defend the airway (gag reflex)

HEENT, Head, Ears, Eyes, Nose, Throat.

Stridor is a harsh noise usually caused by decreased caliber of a large airway, usually representing obstruction (such as croup) or foreign body. Stertor is a low-pitched "snoring" sound usually representing soft tissue collapse at the level of the larynx or soft palate. Wheezing is a high-pitched "whistling" sound, usually representing small airway obstruction (bronchospasm in asthma). Rhonchi are low-pitched "rattling" noises usually representing secretions in large to medium airways. Rales are a fine "crackling" noise usually representing the popping open of small airways and alveoli that were collapsed due to fluid/exudate collection (pneumonia) or lack of aeration (atelectasis).

After you have identified any adventitious sounds, you should then localize the lesions. A quick rule of thumb is the I/E and E/I rule. If a sound is heard only during *I*nspiration, then the lesion is usually *E*xtrathoracic (above the vocal cords). If heard only in *expiration*, then the lesion is likely *I*ntrathoracic. If a noise is biphasic (heard during both phases), then there is a fixed obstruction such as a foreign body, severe airway narrowing (severe croup), or mass effect. This principle is due to the relative pressure changes during respiration where intraluminal pressure of the upper airway (above the vocal cords) is lower than extraluminal pressure (allowing collapse of the airway) during inspiration but not expiration. Thus, if there is a pathologic narrowing of the upper airway (like croup), that narrowing is worsening during inspiration and the adventitious noise is louder. The opposite is true of the intrathoracic airways, where the intraluminal pressure is higher during inspiration but lower in expiration. Thus airway collapse during expiration will make a pathologic narrowing (like bronchospasm in asthma) worse.

Management

What immediate measures need to be taken to correct hypoxemia?

Administer adequate oxygen. How much oxygen and by what route depend on the age of the child and the amount of distress. Infants may require an oxygen hood because they do not keep a cannula or mask in place easily. Older children may do very well with either a nasal cannula or mask. The amount of oxygen should be just enough to normalize the oxygen saturation (92% to 97%) and/or Po_2. Remember, pulse oximetry does not give any information about the effectiveness of ventilation, such as Pco_2, pH, base excess or deficit, or the alveolar-arterial (A-a) O_2 gradient.

What harm can your treatment cause?

Giving 100% oxygen for a prolonged time can lead to atelectasis because the inert gases that are not absorbed help keep the alveoli inflated. With 100% oxygen, these inert gases are washed out of the alveoli, and collapse can occur as the oxygen is absorbed. Oxygen also has direct toxic effects on the lungs, especially in neonates and infants.

With chronic carbon dioxide retention, the drive for respiration becomes hypoxia, not hypercapnia. Therefore, in patients with chronic, poorly controlled asthma and in patients with cystic fibrosis, it is advisable to not exceed 30% oxygen without checking arterial blood gases carefully.

Is the child dyspneic with effective air movement or with poor air movement?

Children with alveolar disease have distress and hypoxia despite good air movement. This includes children with pneumonia and congestive heart failure. Children with airway disease have diminished air exchange for a variety of reasons.

Management depends on the underlying cause of the respiratory distress. Management of four general categories of respiratory distress is discussed here: pulmonary processes, airway processes, cardiac processes, and space-occupying processes. Management of asthma and respiratory failure is also included.

Pulmonary Processes

Selective History

Is there a history of fever, cough, or upper respiratory infection?
Is the child immunocompromised?
Does the child have a history of pneumonia, aspiration, or bronchospasm?

Selective Physical Examination

Are the breath sounds heard equally in all areas of the chest?
Can areas of consolidation be identified by auscultation or percussion?
Are rhonchi, rales, or wheezing heard (see Physical Examination section earlier)?
In older children, is egophony or whisper pectoriloquy appreciated?

Chest Radiographic Findings

Pulmonary processes vary in their radiographic appearance and include lobar consolidation (bacterial pneumonia), streaky interstitial markings (bronchiolitis), patchy bilateral alveolar infiltrates (mycoplasma), and pleural effusion. Trust your physical examination. Remember that a volume-depleted child with pneumonia may not manifest a full-blown infiltrate until rehydrated. Early in the course of pneumonia, the chest radiograph may also be unimpressive. A two-view chest radiograph (anteroposterior [AP] and lateral) is superior to a single view for evaluating retrocardiac consolidations and pleural effusions but only obtain if the child is able to be safely transported to the radiology department. Otherwise a bedside single-view radiograph is sufficient for most clinical decision-making.

Laboratory Evaluation

Many instances of respiratory distress do not require laboratory evaluation. However, if a patient is ill-appearing or does not respond to treatment as expected, you may obtain laboratory studies. If concerned for infection, obtain a complete blood count and a blood culture before initiating antibiotics. You should obtain a blood gas, preferably arterial sample, to help determine indexes of ventilation not found on bedside monitoring. Sampling sputum is impractical in small children, but in rare cases, you can send sputum for Gram stain and culture. In an immunocompromised child, one must consider *Pneumocystis carinii* pneumonia and other opportunistic pathogens. In infants with bronchiolitis, nasopharyngeal swabs can be obtained for assay for common respiratory viruses such as syncytial virus, influenza, parainfluenza, and adenovirus. However, send only viral swabs if it may change your current management.

Treatment

GENERAL MEASURES

- Oxygen

SPECIFIC MEASURES

Antibiotics. The choice of antibiotic therapy in neonates includes ampicillin and either gentamicin or third-generation cephalosporin to cover both gram-positive *(Streptococcus pneumoniae)* and gram-negative *(Escherichia coli, Haemophilus influenzae)* organisms, as well as *Listeria monocytogenes*. In older children, second- and third-generation cephalosporins are commonly used as monotherapy. Azythromycin is necessary for *Mycoplasma pneumoniae*. If aspiration is suspected, gram-negative and anaerobic coverage is very important so consider adding clindamycin or ampicillin-sulbactam. Hospital-acquired pneumonia may be caused by *Pseudomonas, Enterobacter*, or *Acinetobacter* species, as well as *Serratia*, especially in the cystic fibrosis population.

P. carinii requires intravenous pentamidine or trimethoprim-sulfamethoxazole (Bactrim).

In the setting of significant influenza in the community, an antiviral agent can be started if within the window of efficacy, usually within 4 days of onset of symptoms. However, in the case of significant disease, initiation of therapy is warranted and can be reevaluated.

Bronchodilators. A mainstay of therapy for reactive airway disease, bronchodilators may have some utility in treating lobar bacterial pneumonia but are controversial in bronchiolitis. Nebulizer treatments combined with bronchial hygiene therapy may help loosen inspissated secretions and mucous plugs. Remember that bronchodilators are β_2-agonists but have β_1 activity and result in tachycardia, jitteriness, and sometimes agitation. Albuterol in particular also affects extracellular potassium transport.

Pulmonary Hygiene. Infants are obligate nose breathers and as such are more affected by obstruction of the nasopharynx. Consider nasal or nasopharyngeal suctioning to relieve secretions in a patient with bronchiolitis. If concerned for atelectasis on physical exam or radiograph, consider asking a respiratory therapist to perform chest physiotherapy or positive expiratory pressure (PEP) therapy.

Steroids. Another mainstay in the treatment of reactive airway disease, steroids have limited application in patients with pneumonia. Children with cystic fibrosis or immunocompromised children suspected of having *Pneumocystis* pneumonia may be considered for steroids.

Antituberculosis Regimens. Tuberculosis (TB) must be treated with at least a two-drug regimen and often requires three- or four-drug combinations. Rifampin, isoniazid, ethambutol, pyrazinamide, and streptomycin are recommended in various combinations for extended periods.

Airway Processes

Selective History

Is there any history of a sudden choking or coughing spell preceding the respiratory distress?

Has the child's voice changed?

Can the child phonate?

Is there dysphagia or drooling?

Was the onset of respiratory distress sudden?

Was it associated with sudden high fever, chemical or noxious gas inhalation, or neck trauma?

Selective Physical Examination

Can the child swallow?

Is the child drooling?

Does the child hold his or her head in a particular position or assume a "tripod position"?

Is there evidence of a foreign body in the oropharynx?

Is the neck swollen or mobile, and does the child have any cervical adenopathy?

What is the appearance of the pharynx? (Caution: If acute suppurative epiglottitis is suspected, examination of the pharynx should occur in the operating room with an anesthesiologist and otolaryngologist present.)

Is the trachea in the midline?

Can the child phonate?

Airway Films

A lateral neck film helps to evaluate the integrity of the airway from the nasopharynx to the midtrachea. Significant tonsillar or adenoid enlargement, retropharyngeal abscess or cellulitis, epiglottitis, tracheal pseudomembrane, and foreign bodies may be seen. An anteroposterior airway film may show subglottic steepling in parainfluenza (croup), deviation of the trachea, foreign bodies, or external compression of the trachea.

Laboratory Evaluation

Febrile infants and children must be handled carefully if epiglottitis is suspected. Laboratory studies should include a complete blood count, blood culture, and possibly an arterial blood gas determination but should be postponed until the airway has been visualized and secured. Because not all foreign bodies are radiopaque, otolaryngology and/or general surgical consultation should be obtained for possible rigid bronchoscopy.

Treatment

Disturb a child with suspected epiglottitis as little as possible, and expedite transfer to the operating room for visualization. If concerned for croup, give humidified oxygen and consider nebulized epinephrine with or without steroids for subglottic edema. For suppurative paratracheal processes, broad-spectrum antibiotics should be initiated promptly. Abscesses of the tonsils and retropharynx should be surgically drained as well. In a child with upper airway redundant soft tissue may have positional stertor. Consider repositioning these patients.

Cardiac Processes

Congestive heart failure in infants and children is most often the result of left-to-right shunts as a consequence of congenital heart disease. Because of pulmonary overcirculation, pulmonary edema develops and respiratory distress gradually ensues.

Selective History

Is there a known cardiac defect?
In infants, what is the child's feeding pattern?
How has the child been growing?
Does the child become dyspneic, diaphoretic, and tired with feedings?
What medications does the child take?
Was the onset of symptoms abrupt and associated with pleuritic chest pain?

Selective Physical Examination

General	Assess the child's volume status. Is there fluid overload?
HEENT	Dysmorphic features (high association with congenital heart disease)
Neck	Jugular venous distention (rarely seen in infants and young children)
Chest	Symmetry, precordial activity
Respiratory	Rales, crackles at the bases, pleuritic pain, effusion

Cardiovascular	Location of the point of maximal intensity; abnormal impulses (right ventricular heave, thrills); tachycardia; S_1; S_2, including splitting; S_3; murmurs (systolic and diastolic); clicks, rubs, or gallops; brachial and femoral pulses
Abdomen	Hepatosplenomegaly, hepatojugular reflex, ascites
Extremities	Peripheral edema, thrombophlebitis

The most common congenital defect is a ventricular septal defect, which usually results in a left-to-right shunt and pulmonary overcirculation. Other lesions can cause pulmonary edema, including patent ductus arteriosus, any of the left-sided obstructive lesions (coarctation, aortic stenosis, mitral stenosis), cardiomyopathies (dilated, hypertrophic, or restrictive), and some dysrhythmias.

Chest Radiographic Findings
Cardiomegaly (Fig. 28.1)
Increased pulmonary vascular markings
Right-sided aortic arch

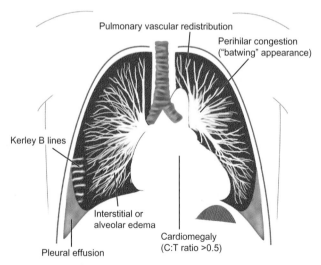

FIGURE 28.1 Chest radiographic features of congestive heart failure. C:T ratio, cardiac diameter to thoracic diameter. (From Marshall SA, Ruedy J: On Call: Principles and Protocols, 4th ed. Philadelphia, Elsevier, 2004, p 270.)

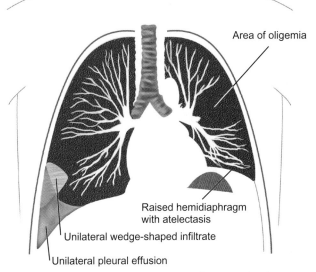

FIGURE 28.2 Variable chest radiographic features of pulmonary embolism. (From Marshall SA, Ruedy J: On Call: Principles and Protocols, 4th ed. Philadelphia, Elsevier, 2004, p 274.)

Kerley B lines
Pleural effusion
Pulmonary embolism findings (Fig. 28.2)

Laboratory Evaluation

A 12- to 15-lead electrocardiogram should be obtained. If the child is desaturated, a hyperoxia test should be performed (see Chapter 13). Definitive diagnosis may require cardiology consultation and an echocardiogram. Serum electrolytes, blood urea nitrogen, and creatinine should be checked to assess hydration status and renal function. If pulmonary embolism is suspected, an arterial blood gas determination is essential. A ventilation-perfusion (V/Q) scan or high-resolution computed tomography (CT) scan is necessary.

Treatment

GENERAL MEASURES

- Oxygen
- Elevate the head of the bed 30 degrees

SPECIFIC MEASURES

Frequently, the first response to a child with apparent cardiogenic respiratory distress is to give intravenous or intramuscular furosemide (Lasix). Although this may be indicated in infants and children with left-to-right shunt lesions, it could be disastrous in a child with cardiomyopathy who depends on a high end-diastolic volume or atrial filling pressure to maximize ventricular volume and maintain cardiac output. Therefore it is imperative to define the child's physiologic features and obtain the cardiac diagnosis underlying the respiratory compromise before empirically treating with a diuretic.

If the child has known cardiac disease and is receiving diuretic therapy, an intravenous dose can be administered to augment diuresis. If a dilated cardiomyopathy is the problem, inotropic support is necessary, and diuretics may initially be contraindicated. Mitral regurgitation may be helped by reduction of systemic afterload.

Pericardial tamponade is a life-threatening emergency that is frequently manifested as respiratory distress with left chest and shoulder pain and coughing. Orthopnea is marked. Drainage of the pericardium, ideally via a catheter placed under echocardiographic guidance, is necessary.

In a crisis, one may acutely decompress the pericardium as follows. First, the area of the xyphoid is prepared in sterile fashion. The skin and subcutaneous tissues should be anesthetized with 1% lidocaine. A No. 18 or 20 angiocatheter can then be placed on a three-way stopcock and attached to a 20-mL syringe. The angiocatheter is inserted lateral to the xyphoid, aiming for the left shoulder and aspirating as it is inserted. Watch the electrocardiographic monitor for signs of ectopy. If straw-colored fluid or thin bloody fluid is obtained, the catheter should be threaded fully and the needle withdrawn. The stopcock can then be attached directly to the catheter and the fluid aspirated. If blood is obtained again, check for ventricular ectopy and for pulsatile flow. If you suspect that you have entered the right ventricle, remove the apparatus and be prepared to give volume replacement. Obviously, placement of sharp objects very close to a beating heart is to be done carefully.

If pulmonary embolism is suspected, anticoagulation therapy must be started immediately. Be certain that the child has no contraindications to anticoagulant therapy, such as a history of a coagulopathy, previous stroke, peptic ulcer disease, or bleeding disorder. A baseline complete blood count, activated partial thromboplastin time (aPTT), prothrombin time, and platelet count must be obtained. Heparin is the mainstay of initial therapy and should be started with a 100-U/kg bolus, followed by an infusion of 15 to

25 U/kg per hour. The aPTT must be monitored closely and the heparin infusion adjusted to maintain the aPTT at 1.5 to 2 times baseline. Thrombolytic therapy is much higher risk and requires transfer to the Pediatric Intensive Care Unit (PICU) and consultation with both cardiology and cardiovascular surgery specialists.

Space-Occupying Processes

Selective History

Does the patient complain of pleuritic pain?
Was the onset gradual or sudden?
Is the patient febrile?
Has the patient ever had symptoms like this before?
In a newborn, could this be a congenital diaphragmatic hernia?

Selective Physical Examination

Is the trachea in the midline?
Do both sides of the chest move together?
Is there obvious splinting?
Is there evidence of ascites or other abdominal processes that are limiting diaphragmatic excursion?
Is there a pleural rub?
Are the breath sounds equal right and left?
Is the abdomen scaphoid?

Chest Radiographic Findings

Pleural effusion
Empyema
Pneumothorax
Intrathoracic masses, including the mediastinum
Severe scoliosis
Massive ascites
Diaphragmatic hernia

Laboratory Evaluation

Thoracentesis may be indicated for diagnosis, as well as therapy. Arterial blood gases should be monitored in children with severe distress. Pleural and/or mediastinal masses require chest CT scanning and/or magnetic resonance imaging after the child's airway and breathing are secure.

Special Section on Asthma

Asthma is one of the most common admitting diagnoses in pediatrics. As a result, there is often a tendency to become complacent regarding the risk for decompensation in these children. Remember, asthma can cause respiratory distress very quickly.

Selective History

Did the child's condition suddenly become worse?
Has the child ever required intubation?
Are there any obvious precipitating triggers?
Is this an anaphylactic reaction?
What are the child's current medications?

Selective Physical Examination

Is there evidence of acute airway obstruction?

Vital signs	Pulsus paradoxus
HEENT	Cyanosis
Neck	Midline trachea, jugular venous distention
Respiratory	Retractions, flaring, prolonged expiration, abnormal inspiratory-expiratory ratio, hyperinflation, wheezing, aeration, consolidation

Chest Radiographic Findings

Hyperinflation
Pneumothorax or pneumomediastinum
Flattened diaphragm
Atelectasis, infiltrates

Laboratory Evaluation

Arterial blood gases are very important in the assessment of an asthmatic patient who has deteriorated acutely. Pulse oximetry studies may be falsely reassuring when the patient's P_{CO_2} has begun to rise, which is indicative of impending respiratory failure.

Treatment

GENERAL MEASURES

- Oxygen
- Intravenous hydration

SPECIFIC MEASURES

The initial response should be nebulizer treatments with β-agonists (albuterol, 2.5 to 10 mg) as often as necessary or even continuously. The anticholinergic agent ipratropium bromide, 0.5 mg, may also be given via nebulizer in conjunction with albuterol. Side effects from either are obviously greater with an increased frequency of treatments.

Intravenous steroids should be given immediately (2 mg/kg methylprednisolone). Steroids should be continued every 4 hours initially at a dose of 1 mg/kg methylprednisolone.

In patients who remain in significant distress, xanthines, such as aminophylline or theophylline, can be used. An initial bolus of 6 mg/kg should be followed by a continuous infusion of 1.0 mg/kg per hour. Serum levels should be monitored closely until a steady state is achieved. Higher levels may cause nausea, vomiting, tachycardia, chest pains, headache, and irritability. Be careful when also giving erythromycin, cimetidine, β-blockers, allopurinol, and other drugs that may potentiate xanthine drug effects or affect serum levels.

Additional treatment may include intubation and mechanical ventilation, intravenous ketamine, and magnesium sulfate. Consultation with the critical care staff and transfer to the PICU will be necessary at the point that these measures are considered.

Warning Signs in Asthma

1. Sudden acute deterioration may signal the development of pneumothorax.
2. A rising P_{CO_2} in the face of maximal therapy portends respiratory failure. Arterial blood gases must be monitored closely.
3. The disappearance of wheezing is not always a good sign. Lack of wheezing may reflect lack of air exchange and indicate respiratory failure. Similarly, not all respiratory noises in asthma are wheezing. Asthmatic children also can get upper airway obstruction and inhaled foreign bodies like other children.
4. A sleepy patient with asthma is a worrisome patient. Because sedatives are contraindicated and both β-agonists and xanthines are stimulants, most patients will be hyperalert or agitated.
5. Rarely, there is a triad of asthma, nasal polyps, and aspirin hypersensitivity. Avoid aspirin and nonsteroidal antiinflammatory drugs whenever possible in patients with asthma because fatal anaphylactoid reactions have been described.

Respiratory Failure

Any of the aforementioned conditions may lead to respiratory failure. Bradypnea (<20 breaths per minute), thoracoabdominal dissociation, CO_2 retention, profound hypoxemia, and profound respiratory acidosis all imply respiratory failure.

1. Ensure that the patient has not received or is not receiving any respiratory depressant, especially narcotics, barbiturates, and benzodiazepines. Do not hesitate to give naloxone hydrochloride (Narcan), 0.2 to 2.0 mg intravenously, if opiates are suspected.
2. Notify the PICU early of a patient in distress. Direct therapy to the underlying causes of the respiratory problem, and assist ventilation and oxygenation as indicated. Acute respiratory acidosis frequently requires mechanical ventilatory support until the underlying cause is addressed.

REMEMBER

1. Abdominal problems may cause significant respiratory distress and compromise.
2. Do not be worried about your inexperience with endotracheal intubation. Unless there is severe upper airway obstruction, most patients can be effectively ventilated for an extended time with a bag-valve mask unit until help and more hands arrive.
3. Even though respiratory distress is a very common cause of calls in the middle of the night, it is essential to monitor patients frequently to make sure that they are responding appropriately to your treatment so that you can make changes in treatment as indicated.

Seizures

Purabi Sonowal, MD

When a seizure unexpectedly develops, the sudden and often dramatic nature of the event has a tendency to create a sense of crisis among parents, other family members, nurses, and house officers. Everyone will feel a need to "do something" and to do it quickly to stop the seizure. The first order of business when you are called is to remain calm and recognize that, although a seizure needs to be addressed immediately, the urgency to "do something" should not lead you to act reflexively or irrationally. There is time to organize your thoughts and develop a plan for further evaluation and treatment that is best for the patient. Remember, almost all seizures are paroxysmal events with abrupt onset, are variable in length but usually brief (minutes), and are generally self-limited. Careful attention to the airway, breathing, and circulation (ABCs) is often all that is initially necessary because this will maintain cerebral blood flow and oxygenation while you consider the need for further treatment or diagnostic tests.

PHONE CALL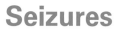

Questions

1. Is the child still seizing?
2. What was witnessed? Ask the nurse to describe what happened. Was it generalized or focal, tonic-clonic, or just tonic? (Was the event actually a seizure and not merely a startle response or myoclonus?)
3. What was the patient's level of consciousness?
4. Was the event associated with apnea, cyanosis, or loss of bladder or bowel control?
5. What is the child's admitting diagnosis?
6. Is the child febrile?

Orders

1. Ask the nurse to see that the child is positioned on his or her side.
2. Ask the nurse to maintain seizure precautions, including suctioning and oxygen supplies at the bedside, padded bedrails, a properly sized oral airway at the bedside, and intravenous (IV) lorazepam readily available.
3. If the child does not have an IV line in place, ask the nurse to have the supplies at the bedside and to have an IV placed.
4. Ask the nurse to also keep ready either nasal midazolam or rectal diazepam because if the child does not have an IV access, then it might be difficult to get an IV access if the child is still seizing and in that case you might need either of these to control the seizure.
5. Ask the nurse to obtain a full set of vital signs immediately and put the patient on continuous pulse oximetry monitoring.
6. Check a point of care blood glucose.

Inform Registered Nurse

Tell the RN, "I will arrive at the bedside in … minutes."

Seizures require immediate evaluation.

ELEVATOR THOUGHTS

Did the child have a seizure?

Remember that several conditions can mimic seizures, including breath-holding spells, syncope, chorea, narcolepsy, benign myoclonus, night terrors, and pseudoseizures. Your first task will be to determine the likelihood that the child experienced a seizure. You should be able to do this after your telephone discussion with the nurse.

What causes seizures?

There are several types of seizures (Table 29.1) and an even longer list of potential causes (Box 29.1).

MAJOR THREAT TO LIFE

• Aspiration
• Hypoxemia

The majority of seizures will have stopped by the time you arrive at the child's bedside. Advise the nurse to try to position the child on his or her side to discourage airway obstruction or aspiration during the postictal state. Patients are rarely apneic

TABLE 29.1	Classification of Epileptic Seizures and Some Epileptic Syndromes

Clinical Seizure Type	Epileptic Syndrome
Partial Seizures	
Simple partial (consciousness not impaired)	Benign focal epilepsy
Motor signs	Juvenile myoclonic epilepsy
Special sensory (visual, auditory, olfactory, gustatory, vertiginous, or somatosensory)	West syndrome
	Lennox-Gastaut syndrome
Autonomic	Acquired epileptic aphasia
Psychic (déjà vu, fear, and others)	Benign neonatal convulsions
Complex partial (consciousness impaired)	
Impaired consciousness at onset	
Development of impaired consciousness	
Generalized Seizures	
Absence	
Typical	
Atypical	
Tonic-clonic	
Atonic	
Myoclonic	
Tonic	
Clonic	
Unclassified	
Neonatal	

From Behrman RE, Kliegman R (eds): Nelson Essentials of Pediatrics, 2nd ed. Philadelphia, WB Saunders, 1994, p 681.

BOX 29.1	Etiology of Seizures

Perinatal Conditions
Cerebral malformation
Intrauterine infection
Hypoxia-ischemia*
Trauma
Hemorrhage*

Infections
Encephalitis*
Meningitis*
Brain abscess

Metabolic Conditions
Hypoglycemia*

Continued

BOX 29.1	Etiology of Seizures—cont'd

Hypocalcemia
Hypomagnesemia
Hyponatremia
Hypernatremia
Storage diseases
Reye syndrome
Degenerative disorders
Porphyria
Pyridoxine dependency (deficiency)

Poisoning
Lead
Drugs
Drug withdrawal

Neurocutaneous Syndromes
Tuberous sclerosis
Neurofibromatosis
Sturge-Weber syndrome
Klippel-Trénaunay-Weber syndrome
Linear sebaceous nevus
Incontinentia pigmenti

Systemic Disorders
Vasculitis (central nervous system or systemic)
Systemic lupus erythematosus
Hypertensive encephalopathy
Renal failure
Hepatic encephalopathy

Other
Trauma*
Tumor
Febrile*
Idiopathic*
Familial

*Common.
From Behrman RE, Kliegman R (eds): Nelson Essentials of Pediatrics, 2nd ed. Philadelphia, WB Saunders, 1994, p 681.

during a seizure. Children can usually withstand status epilepticus for up to 30 minutes with no subsequent neurologic damage. The procedures to follow if the seizure has stopped are discussed subsequently, as are those for status epilepticus.

BEDSIDE

If the Seizure Has Stopped

Quick-Look Test

Does the patient appear well (comfortable), sick (uncomfortable or distressed), or critical (about to die)?

Most children have a period of postictal unresponsiveness after a generalized tonic-clonic seizure. Prolonged depression of mental status is ominous and requires prompt evaluation with head computed tomography (CT) or magnetic resonance imaging (MRI). A child in shock must be stabilized while addressing the seizure.

Airway and Vital Signs

In what position is the child lying?

The patient should be positioned in the left lateral decubitus position to prevent aspiration of vomited gastric contents (Fig. 29.1). Do an immediate oral suctioning if there are secretions in the mouth.

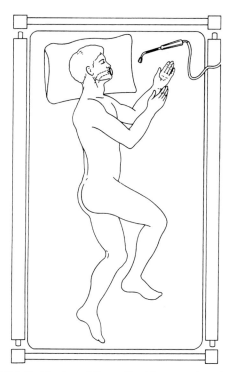

FIGURE 29.1 Positioning of the patient to prevent aspiration of gastric contents. (From Marshall SA, Ruedy J: On Call: Principles and Protocols, 4th ed. Philadelphia, Elsevier, 2004, p 254.)

If the child is unresponsive but adequately ventilating, it is prudent to insert an oral airway. (An awake child does not tolerate an airway, so be prepared to remove it as the child awakens.) Oxygen should be given via nasal prongs or face mask. Have the nurse obtain a repeat set of vital signs, again with a pulse oximeter saturation.

What is the blood glucose result?

Hypoglycemia may be rapidly treated, and raising the serum glucose level may prevent further hypoglycemic seizures.

Management I

After you have established that the event was likely to be a seizure, establish IV access, and draw blood for the following studies: electrolytes, glucose, magnesium, calcium, blood urea nitrogen, creatinine, and serum levels of any anticonvulsant medications that the child may be taking. A toxicology screen and a serum lead level should also be considered. A complete blood count should be obtained, as well as a blood culture if the child is younger than 4 years and has a significant fever. A venous pH determination should be made after any prolonged seizure, and an arterial blood gas determination should be considered and obtained if any respiratory compromise is evident. If encephalitis or meningitis is a consideration because of the presence of fever or other signs and symptoms, a lumbar puncture with cerebrospinal fluid analysis and culture will be necessary.

Selective Physical Examination I

Mental status	Assess the response to verbal, tactile, and painful stimuli. Altered level of consciousness is discussed in Chapter 7, Altered Mental Status
Airway	Check body position, airway patency, and quality of breath sounds

Selective History and Chart Review

Was the event witnessed? Ask witnesses about the characteristics and duration of the seizure.

Was it generalized tonic-clonic or focal?

Did the seizure start focally or was it generalized?

Did the child suffer any injury as a result of the seizure (head trauma, tongue or lip trauma, bruises or lacerations on the extremities)?

Is the child normally receiving anticonvulsants or any other medications that might lower the child's seizure threshold?

What were the child's most recent laboratory results? Quickly review the child's chart before a more complete physical examination.

Selective Physical Examination II

Mental status	Assess whether the child has lost consciousness. Does the child respond to verbal, tactile, or painful stimuli? Is the child in a postictal state?
HEENT	Test the cranial nerves; again assure yourself that the child can defend his or her airway (gag reflex), and check the airway position (Fig. 29.2). Look for a potential source of infection in febrile patients (e.g., otitis, sinusitis). Any children who have had a seizure must have their fundi examined thoroughly,

HEENT, Head, Ears, Eyes, Nose, Throat.

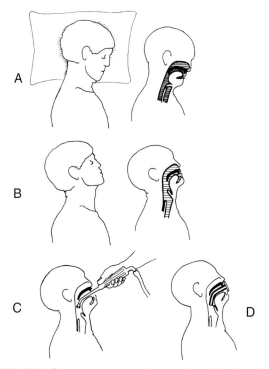

FIGURE 29.2 **Airway management: correct positioning of the head, correct suctioning, and correct insertion of an oral airway. A,** Neck flexion closes the airway. **B,** Neck extension to the sniffing position opens the airway. **C,** Suctioning. **D,** Placement of the airway. (From Marshall SA, Ruedy J: On Call: Principles and Protocols, 4th ed. Philadelphia, Elsevier, 2004, p 255.)

	with dilation of the pupils if necessary, especially in infants (to look for retinal hemorrhages, as well as evidence of papilledema)
Neck	Nuchal rigidity
Lungs	Signs of aspiration (crackles, decreased breath sounds)
Neurologic	Complete neurologic examination within the limits of the child's level of consciousness, including reflexes, motor and sensory function, cerebellar function, visual fields, and short- and long-term memory
Miscellaneous	Check for oral and/or scalp lacerations, passive range of joint mobility, bruising, and other signs of injury incurred during the seizure

Management II

Given the history, one should establish a preliminary or provisional differential diagnosis. Remember that seizures are a symptom, not a diagnosis, and therefore there must be an underlying condition that is manifested by the seizure. Your job is to find and treat the underlying condition. In children, even hospitalized children, fever is a common underlying cause of seizures. It is thought that the rapidity with which the temperature rises precipitates the seizure activity. It may be difficult, however, to determine whether a febrile child with a seizure has simply had a "febrile seizure" or has had a seizure secondary to meningitis, encephalitis, or brain abscess. When this distinction cannot be made, it is necessary to perform a lumbar puncture to rule out meningitis. CT or MRI may be necessary before lumbar puncture to rule out cerebral edema and increased intracranial pressure.

Any child with an abnormal neurologic examination after a seizure should also have an imaging procedure (CT or MRI) performed to rule out tumor, edema, or other space-occupying lesions (arteriovenous malformation, abscess) as a cause of the seizure.

Remember also that there can be complications secondary to seizures, such as aspiration and trauma, especially to the head. Seizure precautions should be ordered immediately whenever an inpatient suffers a seizure.

In a hospitalized child who has a first-time seizure, it is usually prudent to maintain IV access but to withhold anticonvulsant therapy if the seizure is not prolonged and some readily identifiable underlying cause is apparent. Exceptions include a patient with a known seizure disorder who has a subtherapeutic serum anticonvulsant level. This, in fact, is the most common cause of in-hospital seizures in children. Other patients who warrant anticonvulsant therapy are victims of head injuries, children with central nervous system tumors, and those with known cerebrovascular accidents. Remember that benzodiazepines, such as diazepam (Valium) and lorazepam (Ativan), are useful in stopping status epilepticus but have no role in preventing recurrent events. The choice of anticonvulsant depends in part on the type of seizure and the age of the child. Anticonvulsant therapy should be discussed with a child neurologist (see Box 29.1).

If the Child Is Still Seizing

Don't panic! Most seizures resolve spontaneously and last no more than several minutes. (This, of course, is an eternity to the child's parents and often the nurses.) Therefore busy yourself with evaluating the child's ABCs. The child needs the evaluation, and it calms the parents to see that "something" is being done.

Quick-Look Test

Does the child appear well (comfortable), sick (uncomfortable or distressed), or critical (about to die)?

A generalized tonic-clonic seizure is a disconcerting event to witness. However, one should be reassured that a child who is seizing has both a heart rate and a blood pressure. Still, remember your limitations (a seizure is a medical emergency), and have a nurse page your senior resident immediately. You should not deal with a seizure alone if you do not absolutely have to do so. If there is clonic activity of the extremities, gently hold the extremity to see whether you can suppress the activity. If so, it is not seizure activity.

Airway and Vital Signs

In what position is the patient?

If at all possible, the child should be positioned in the lateral decubitus position with suction readily available to prevent aspiration of gastric contents. Be prepared to restrain the child gently but firmly to prevent traumatic injury. Patency of the airway should be the first concern, followed by adequacy of ventilation. Apply oxygen by mask or nasal prongs.

What are the child's vital signs?

Tachycardia is expected with a seizure. It is virtually impossible to obtain an accurate cuff blood pressure reading during a tonic-clonic seizure. The child's perfusion tells as much as a blood pressure reading fraught with inaccuracy. A point of care blood glucose assessment is indicated because hypoglycemia commonly results in seizures (and is easily corrected).

Management I

How long has the child been seizing?

See earlier if the seizure has already stopped. If the seizure has lasted more than 3 minutes, first check the child's ABCs. Closely observe the seizure. Be sure that IV supplies are at hand if the child does not have a working IV line. Do not try to obtain IV access in a seizing patient unless it is absolutely necessary. Remember, the seizure is likely to be over in 2 to 3 minutes. Also remember that the antecubital fossa becomes a less attractive site for IV access in a patient who involuntarily flexes at the elbow. A hand, forearm, or saphenous site will be a better choice.

Medications

Status epilepticus is defined as general or partial seizures lasting longer than 30 minutes without the patient regaining consciousness. Before administering any medication, remember that all anticonvulsants can depress the child's level of consciousness and respiratory drive. It is best to have airway support equipment at hand, including suctioning supplies, Ambu bag, appropriately sized masks, and a laryngoscopy tray. If the child has been seizing for 5 minutes, begin to prepare airway support equipment, check a point of care (finger stick) glucose and administer an IV glucose bolus (5 mL/kg of 10% dextrose in water [$D_{10}W$]) if hypoglycemia is present. Change the IV solution to normal saline, and have anticonvulsant doses readied. Often, this process requires enough time for the seizure to stop spontaneously. In any case, most clinicians agree that treatment should probably be initiated after 10 to 15 minutes of continuous seizure activity. Do not let the presence of a frantic parent or nurse force you into treating the child pharmacologically before you are ready and comfortable doing so. The treatment is not without complications, and the risks of treatment should be considered along with the benefits.

The most important principle of anticonvulsant therapy is to choose a drug and use enough. Small doses of multiple drugs may be ineffective. Use full loading doses and do not administer additional drugs until you have reached the maximum recommended dose.

Diazepam and lorazepam are effective immediately in most children for tonic-clonic seizures. Diazepam has a short half-life, and seizures will tend to recur unless a longer-acting anticonvulsant is also administered. The starting dose of diazepam (see Table 29-2 for dosing). This may be repeated every 10 to 15 minutes to a maximum of three doses. Lorazepam has the benefit of longer duration of action and is less likely than diazepam to result in hypotension and respiratory depression, (see Table 29-2 for dosing).

If an IV line cannot be established, both diazepam and lorazepam can be given rectally. A rectal diazepam gel in standard doses of 2.5, 5, and 10 mg is now available. The rectal and IV doses of lorazepam are identical. Midazolam may be given intranasally if no IV is present. The dose is 0.2 mg/kg to a maximum dose of 10 mg. It is preferable to give via a nasal insufflator, but it can be rapidly given with a syringe as well.

Phenytoin should be used next and is generally begun at a loading dose of 15 to 20 mg/kg at an infusion rate no faster than 1 mg/kg/min. All patients should be on a cardiorespiratory monitor when receiving phenytoin because of the risk for dysrhythmias. If bradycardia or hypotension results, the infusion must be slowed. The prodrug fosphenytoin has been used increasingly because it is more water soluble and less irritating when administered intravenously. The loading dose of fosphenytoin is usually 15 to 20 phenytoin equivalents (PE)/kg. If seizure activity persists, another dose of phenytoin may be given, up to a 25-mg/kg total loading dose. Remember that phenytoin forms a precipitate with glucose solutions and must therefore be administered in saline solution.

Phenobarbital is often the second-line drug for status epilepticus. The loading dose is 5 to 20 mg/kg infused no faster than 1 mg/kg/min. Monitor vital signs, especially respirations and pulse oximetry values. After phenobarbital loading, the child may remain sedated for a period of hours.

Levetiracetam has also been used for status epilepticus with doses of 20 to 60 mg/kg with 50 mg/kg being a common starting point. Table 29.2 has a listing of the drugs used for status epilepticus.

Persistent status seizure activity despite the administration of three anticonvulsants warrants transfer to the intensive care unit for the administration of a continuous infusion of diazepam, propofol, or pentobarbital. Correct any electrolyte abnormalities.

After the child is no longer in status epilepticus, maintenance therapy depends on the type of seizure. Consultation with a pediatric neurologist is recommended, especially to help educate the family about seizure disorders, prognosis, and medication management. Further evaluation, including lumbar puncture, MRI or CT, or electroencephalography, may need to be pursued.

SUMMARY

Seizures are upsetting for all who witness them. The specific characteristics of the episode will help you to determine whether the patient has in fact had a seizure and, if so, what type of seizure occurred. Because most seizures last less than 5 minutes, the most important emergency intervention is to prevent secondary injury, aspiration, and respiratory compromise. Remember to address the

TABLE 29.2	Doses of Commonly Used Antiepileptic Drugs in Status Epilepticus	

Drug[a]	Route	Dosage
Lorazepam	Intravenous	0.1 mg/kg up to 4 mg total, may repeat in 5–10 min
	Intranasal	0.1 mg/kg
Midazolam	Intravenous	0.2 mg/kg up to 10 mg total dose, may repeat in 5–10 min
		0.08–0.23 mg/kg/h maintenance
	Intramuscular	0.2 mg/kg
	Intranasal	0.2 mg/kg
	Buccal	0.5 mg/kg
Diazepam	Intravenous	0.15 mg/kg up to a max total dose of 10 mg, may repeat in 5–10 min
	Rectal	2–5 years: 0.5 mg/kg
		6–11 years: 0.3 mg/kg
		≥12 years: 0.2 mg/kg
Fosphenytoin	Intravenous	20 mg/kg phenytoin equivalents (PE), then 3–6 mg/kg/24 h, loading rate up to 50 mg PE per min
Phenobarbital[b]	Intravenous	5–20 mg/kg
Pentobarbital coma[b]	Intravenous	13.0 mg/kg, then 1–5 mg/kg/hr
Propofol[b]	Intravenous	1 mg/kg (bolus), then 1–15 mg/kg/h (infusion)
Thiopental[b]	Intravenous	5 mg/kg/1st h, then 1–2 mg/kg/h
Valproate[b]	Intravenous	Loading: 25 mg/kg, then 30–60 mg/kg/24 h
Lacosamide[b]	Intravenous	Loading: 4 mg/kg then 4–12 mg/kg/24 h
Levetiracetam	Intravenous	20–60 mg/kg
Topiramate	Enterally	5–10 mg/kg/24 h (loading dose) then same or lower for maintenance

[a]Reflects current trends in use which may not be FDA approved.
[b]May cause PR prolongation.
From Behrman RE: Nelson Textbook of Pediatrics, 20th ed. Philadelphia, Elsevier, 2016, Table 593-18.

ABCs before proceeding to pharmacologic seizure management. In most cases the seizure will end before medications are administered. Status epilepticus is continuous seizure activity without regaining consciousness for 30 minutes. Treatment of status epilepticus should include the following, in order: address the ABCs; administer glucose intravenously; administer diazepam or lorazepam; administer phenytoin or fosphenytoin; administer phenobarbital; and transfer to the pediatric intensive care unit for respiratory support and further management, such as continuous diazepam infusion, pentobarbital, or paraldehyde.

Urine Output Abnormalities

Lea Steffes, MD

Urine output abnormalities can be a challenging problem. There are a wide range of factors that influence urine output including hydration status, cardiac output, intrinsic renal function, and urologic patency to name a few. Urine output is closely measured by the nurses in all pediatric hospitalized patients as a way to monitor the function of multiple organ systems. Therefore, it is common for a pediatric resident to be called with questions regarding too little or too much urine output.

PHONE CALL

Questions

1. How old is the patient?
2. How much does the child weigh?
3. Why is the patient in the hospital?
4. How much urine has the patient produced in the last 24 hours?
5. How much fluid has the child taken in or been given over the last 24 hours?
6. What are the vital signs?
7. What is the child's admitting diagnosis?
8. When did the child last have an electrolyte panel and kidney function checked?

Orders

1. If the child has an indwelling Foley catheter and decreased urine output, ask the nurse to check the catheter for patency and flush the catheter with 10 to 20 mL of normal saline solution if necessary (see Chapter 26).

2. Consider ordering serum electrolyte, blood urea nitrogen (BUN), and creatinine and urinalysis (pH and specific gravity).
3. If the child does not have an intravenous (IV) line, place order to insert peripheral IV and order appropriate fluids based on findings of the electrolyte panel and kidney function.
4. If the child is receiving IV fluids and has decreased urine output with signs of kidney dysfunction on lab results, any potassium in the IV fluid should be removed or at least reduced. The rate of the IV fluids should be adjusted carefully in response to the urine output.

Inform RN

Tell the RN, "I will arrive at the bedside in … minutes."

Decreased urine output deserves fairly prompt evaluation, because it can be a sign of decreased cardiac output, dehydration, or renal failure. Increased urine output also demands evaluation promptly, especially in neonates, infants, and small children. Keep in mind that decreased urine output in neonates may result from congenital anomalies of the genitourinary tract.

ELEVATOR THOUGHTS

Decreased Urine Output
What are the causes?

Reduced cardiac output (prenal)	Heart failure
	Cardiomyopathy
	Congenital heart disease
	Pericardial effusion
	Volume depletion
	Vomiting
	Diarrhea
	Blood loss
Renal causes	Tubulointerstitial problems (acute tubulonecrosis, nephrotoxic drugs)
	Hemolytic-uremic syndrome
	Hemoglobinuria, myoglobinuria
	Acute crystalline nephropathy (oxalosis, hyperuricemia)
	Glomerulonephritis
	Renal artery thrombosis
	Renal artery embolization

Postrenal causes	Ureteropelvic junction (UPJ) obstruction
	Nephrolithiasis
	Bilateral ureteral obstruction
	Bladder outlet obstruction (blocked Foley catheter, urethral trauma, posterior urethral valves)
	Neurogenic bladder
	Syndrome of inappropriate antidiuretic hormone (SIADH) production

Increased Urine Output

What are the causes?
Urinary tract infection
Central diabetes insipidus (DI)
Diuretic use
Distal tubular dysfunction
Nephrogenic DI
High-output phase of acute tubular necrosis
Proximal tubular dysfunction
Aminoaciduria (cystinuria, Hartnup disease)
Familial hypophosphatemic rickets (vitamin D–refractory rickets)
Diabetes mellitus
Psychogenic polydipsia

MAJOR THREAT TO LIFE

- Renal failure
- Hyperkalemia
- Sepsis

Decreased urine output for any cause can become a self-perpetuating situation, with progressive renal insufficiency leading to renal failure. Hyperkalemia is the most serious and life-threatening complication of renal insufficiency because of its high association with cardiac dysrhythmias.

BEDSIDE

Quick-Look Test

Does the patient appear well (comfortable), sick (uncomfortable or distressed), or critical (about to die)?

Critically ill appearing children usually have decreased perfusion with subsequent renal failure. An uncomfortable child may have a distended bladder, flank pain, and/or cramps. Children with serious renal problems frequently appear deceptively well.

Airway and Vital Signs

Check for postural changes and signs of dehydration. A postural rise in heart rate greater than 15 beats per minute, a fall in systolic blood pressure greater than 15 mm Hg, or any decrease in diastolic pressure suggests significant hypovolemia. Baseline tachycardia is frequently a nonspecific indicator of volume depletion and/or stress. Fever suggests an infectious cause. Hypertension is suggestive of a renal artery problem or glomerulonephritis. Hypotension with tachycardia is concerning for hypoperfusion of end organs.

Selective Physical Examination

Approach the physical examination with prerenal, renal, and postrenal causes of decreased renal output in mind. Tachycardia, delayed capillary refill, and dry mucous membranes suggest intravascular depletion and thus a prerenal cause. Edema and hypertension suggest a renal cause. A tender, distended bladder suggests a postrenal cause of decreased urine output.

HEENT	Icterus (hepatorenal syndrome), facial purpura and macroglossia (amyloidosis), periorbital edema (nephrotic syndrome), mucous membranes (dry or moist?)
Respiratory	Crackles, rales, dullness to percussion (fluid overload)
Cardiovascular	Pulse rate and quality, capillary refill
Abdomen	Enlarged kidneys (horseshoe kidney, UPJ obstruction, polycystic kidney), bladder fullness (bladder outlet obstruction), bladder tenderness, flank, or costovertebral angle tenderness
Rectal	Enlarged prostate (rare in children)
Genitourinary	Hypospadias
Pelvic (if indicated)	Cervical and/or adnexal masses (UPJ obstruction)
Skin	Morbilliform rash, purpura, bruising, turgor, jaundice
Extremities	Peripheral edema (nephrotic syndrome, renal failure)

HEENT, Head, Eyes, Ears, Nose, Throat.

Selective Chart Review

Does the child have a past history of urinary tract infection, vesicoureteral reflux, instrumentation, or trauma to the genitourinary tract?
Are there other congenital anomalies?
Does the child have any history of renal failure?
What is the admitting diagnosis?
What medications is the child receiving?
Does the child have a condition that could lead to SIADH?
Has the child had laboratory studies recently that could indicate a prerenal, renal, or postrenal cause of decreased urine output?
What has been the child's fluid intake for the past 48 hours?
What was the urine output trend for the past 48 hours—was the decrease in urine output sudden or gradual?

A BUN-creatinine ratio greater than 20 suggests a prerenal cause, as does a urine specific gravity greater than 1.020 or a urine sodium level less than 20 mmol/L. Table 30.1 illustrates laboratory differences in children with prerenal, renal, and postrenal insufficiency.

If urine output is excessive, DI must be considered. Central DI may result from traumatic head injury, hypoxic-ischemic brain injury, congenital abnormalities. Nephrogenic DI may be primary (a rare X-linked recessive condition) or secondary to acute or chronic renal failure with loss of tubular concentrating ability or insensitivity to antidiuretic hormone at the tubules.

Management I: Decreased Urine Output

Prerenal

In hospitalized children, prerenal causes of decreased urine output are relatively common, and you should be able to conclude whether the cause is prerenal based on the history, the chart review, your examination, and the urinalysis. Euvolemia is the goal. Fluid-resuscitate a dehydrated child and diurese a child in congestive heart failure.

Fluid boluses should always consist of isotonic solutions such as 0.9% saline. Children in acute or chronic renal failure are unable to excrete potassium and are at risk for life-threatening hyperkalemia.

Postrenal

Lower urinary tract obstruction is usually easily managed by placement of a Foley catheter in the bladder.

1. Bladder outlet obstruction in a newborn boy can be secondary to posterior urethral valves and requires urologic surgical intervention. Postobstructive diuresis is often observed once the bladder is decompressed.
2. Obstruction of an indwelling Foley catheter can be relieved by flushing the catheter with 10 to 20 mL of normal saline solution

TABLE 30.1   Laboratory Differential Diagnosis of Renal Insufficiency

	Prerenal		Renal		Postrenal
	Child	Neonate	Child	Neonate	
Urine Na$^+$ (mEq/L)	<20	<20 to 30	>40	>40	Variable, may be >40
FE$_{Na}$ (%)[a]	<1	<2 to 5	>2	>2 to 5	Variable, may be >2
Urine osmolality (mOsm/L)	>500	>300 to 500	≈300	≈300	Variable, may be <300
RFI (%)[b]	<1	<2 to 5	>2	>2 to 5	Variable
Serum BUN-creatinine ratio	>20	≥10	≈10	>10	Variable, may be >20
Response to volume	Diuresis			No change	No change
Response to furosemide	Diuresis			No change	No change or diuresis
Urinalysis	Normal		RBC, WBC, casts, proteinuria		Variable or normal
Comments	Hx: diarrhea, vomiting, hemorrhage, diuretics		Hx: hypotension, anoxia, exposure to nephrotoxins		Hx: poor urine stream or output
	Px: volume depletion		Px: hypertension, edema		Px: flank mass, distended bladder

[a]FE$_{Na}$ = fractional excretion of sodium (%) = (urine sodium/plasma sodium Π urine creatinine/plasma creatinine) × 100.
[b]RFI = renal failure index = (urine sodium/urine creatinine/plasma creatinine) × 100.
BUN, Blood urea nitrogen; *Hx*, history; *Px*, physical signs; *RBC*, red blood cell; *WBC*, white blood cell.
From Behrman RE, Kliegman R (eds): Nelson Essentials of Pediatrics, 2nd ed. Philadelphia, WB Saunders, 1994, p 602.

to displace the catheter from the bladder wall or to dislodge bladder sediment.

3. Successful catheterization of the bladder can help localize the level of obstruction (bladder outlet obstruction and lower urinary tract obstruction). Upper urinary tract obstruction secondary to congenital anomalies or nephrolithiasis is best diagnosed by ultrasonography or computed tomography (CT).

Renal

If prenal and postrenal factors are not causing the patient's poor urine output, it is likely secondary to a renal or glomerular condition.

Are any of the five potentially life-threatening complications or consequences of renal failure present?

Hyperkalemia
Congestive heart failure
Severe metabolic acidosis (pH <7.2)
Uremic encephalopathy
Uremic pericarditis

Hyperkalemia is the most immediately threatening consequence of low urine output. A serum potassium level should be checked and an electrocardiogram should be obtained to check for peaked T waves. Further indications that the serum potassium level is dangerously high are conduction abnormalities, such as PR and QRS prolongation and ST-T wave depression. Potassium-containing intravenous fluids, including parenteral nutrition, should be stopped.

Congestive heart failure is suggested by the presence of jugular venous distention, tachypnea and rales, dependent edema, and an S_3 gallop. Treatment of congestive heart failure usually includes fluid restriction, inotropic support as needed, diuretics, and respiratory support as needed.

Tachypnea may represent pulmonary congestion and/or metabolic acidosis as the child attempts to compensate by reducing PCO_2.

Uremic encephalopathy is generally manifested as a gradual onset of confusion, stupor, or seizures and is almost always an indication for emergency dialysis.

Uremic pericarditis also requires dialysis and is usually manifested as pleuritic chest pain radiating to the shoulder, pericardial friction rub, distant or muffled heart sounds, and diffuse ST-segment elevation on the electrocardiogram.

Is the patient taking any drug that may complicate renal insufficiency?

Potassium supplements
Potassium-sparing diuretics (aldactone, triamterene, amiloride)

Nephrotoxic drugs (nonsteroidal antiinflammatory drugs [NSAIDs], aminoglycosides)

Review the indications for each carefully and consider alternative medications if possible. If aminoglycosides are necessary, serum peak and trough levels should be monitored closely.

Is the child in oliguric renal failure?

If a child produces less than 1 to 2 mL/kg per hour of urine, the child has oliguric renal failure. The first goal of therapy is to convert the patient to nonoliguric renal failure, which has a far better prognosis:

1. Correct prerenal (fluid resuscitation) and postrenal factors (bypass obstruction).
2. Give diuretics to increase urine output. Furosemide, 1 mg/kg per dose, may be given intravenously. If there is no response within 1 to 2 hours, a double dose should be administered. (Larger doses should be administered slowly to avoid ototoxicity.)

Does the child need dialysis?

If the child does not respond to diuretics, the indications for urgent dialysis are any of the five complications of renal failure: hyperkalemia, congestive heart failure with pulmonary edema, metabolic acidosis, uremia, and complications of uremia, including pericarditis and encephalopathy. A nephrology consultation is necessary, and until dialysis can be arranged, it may be necessary to treat the child for the aforementioned conditions with measures that do not involve dialysis.

Hyperkalemia. Glucose with insulin infusion, $NaHCO_3$, and sodium polystyrene sulfonate temporarily reduce the serum potassium level by driving K^+ into intracellular fluid and binding K^+ within the gastrointestinal tract for excretion. Furosemide can also be given to increase potassium excretion in the urine. Calcium gluconate stabilizes the myocardium to help prevent dysrhythmias secondary to hyperkalemia.

Congestive heart failure. Inotropy, afterload reduction, and respiratory support should be provided as needed.

Metabolic acidosis. $NaHCO_3$ provides correction of pH, but it is only temporary. Fluid resuscitation with 0.9% normal saline if concern for hypovolemia/hypoperfusion without congestive heart failure.

Uremia. Uremic pericarditis rarely causes a sizable effusion that requires pericardiocentesis. Conservative measures are recommended, such as the use of NSAIDs, but they need to be used carefully with adequate hydration and close monitoring of renal function. Aspirin and indomethacin are contraindicated, because they may worsen acidosis.

Specific therapy for the renal etiology that caused renal failure, such as glomerulonephritis, frequently depends on the results of renal biopsy. Routine urinalysis, renal ultrasound studies, and 24-hour urine sampling for protein and creatinine should be ordered. The urinalysis should be studied for the following:

Urine dipstick. Hematuria and proteinuria suggest glomerulonephritis. Remember, a positive dipstick result for blood can mean red blood cells, free hemoglobin, or myoglobin. Suspect rhabdomyolysis if the result is positive with few red blood cells by microscopic examination. (In this case, check the creatinine phosphokinase, calcium, phosphate, and urine myoglobin levels.) A positive urine protein test result should prompt investigation of serum albumin, and a 24-hour urine collection for protein and creatinine clearance should be started. When the urine sample is concentrated (specific gravity >1.015), the dipstick may be positive for protein in an otherwise normal child. In this case, a spot urine protein-creatinine ratio may be helpful (a ratio of 0.2 or less suggests normal renal function).

Urine microscopy. Red blood cell casts are diagnostic of glomerulonephritis. Oval fat bodies are suggestive of nephrotic syndrome. White blood cells are characteristic of pyelonephritis and can be seen with nephrolithiasis. Eosinophils are suggestive of acute interstitial nephritis.

Management II: Increased Urine Output

The major threat of any form of DI is dehydration. It is important to match urine output with adequate replacement fluid while searching for the cause. Administration of desmopressin acetate (DDAVP) intravenously or intranasally is both diagnostic (decreased urine output in central DI; no change in urine output in nephrogenic, antidiuretic hormone–insensitive DI) and therapeutic for central DI. If central DI is suspected, an endocrinology consultation is advisable to investigate hypothalamic or pituitary function.

Urinalysis and urine culture should be ordered if there is any suspicion of urinary tract infection or diabetes mellitus resulting in polyuria. Urine and serum electrolytes, creatinine, and osmolarity should also be determined. These tests can help differentiate causes of increased urine output.

Glucose in urine increases suspicion for diabetes mellitus. If glucosuria is present, you should check the serum glucose level, venous pH, and urine for ketones while remembering that diabetes mellitus in childhood is often manifested as diabetic ketoacidosis.

REMEMBER

Many medications are excreted by the kidneys and have effects on kidney function. All medications in an oliguric or anuric child must be scrutinized and discontinued if they are nephrotoxic. Similarly, drugs that require renal metabolism (digoxin, aminoglycosides) must have their doses and dosing schedules modified and levels closely monitored. If this is overlooked, drug levels could reach toxic levels and result in significant problems for the patient.

chapter 31

Vomiting

Alina G. Burek, MD

In hospitalized children, vomiting is often a nonspecific symptom accompanying any illness. A single episode of vomiting or a few instances of intermittent vomiting without additional significant gastrointestinal or neurologic symptoms or signs is unlikely to be indicative of a life-threatening problem. However, as with other problems that arise while on call, it is critical that pediatric house officers consider the potential for life-threatening causes of vomiting and at least assure themselves that such potential causes have been either excluded or evaluated and managed appropriately. It is also important to have an understanding of the complications of vomiting that may arise when vomiting has been excessive.

PHONE CALL

Questions

1. What is the child's age?
2. Has the child been vomiting previously, or is this a new symptom?
3. What is the child's admitting diagnosis? Past medical history?
4. Is fever or diarrhea associated with the vomiting?
5. Is there blood or bile in the vomitus?
6. Does the child have an intravenous (IV) line in place?
7. Does the child appear to be in pain or complaining of pain?
8. Does the child have a headache or other neurologic symptoms?
9. What are patient's most recent vital signs?
10. Any concerning changes on RN's assessment?

Orders

1. The nurse should obtain a new full set of vital signs.
2. If the RN report is concerning, make the patient NPO until you assess (see list of concerning symptoms/signs later).

3. Ask the nurse to hold on to the vomitus for direct observation (this will provide you with great information!)

Inform RN

Tell the RN, "I will be at the bedside in ... minutes."

Vomiting in a neonate or very young infant can frequently be a sign of a surgical problem and deserves evaluation promptly. In older children, one may adjust the urgency of evaluation according to the presence or absence of concerning signs/symptoms such as:

Bilious vomiting

Projectile vomiting

Hematemesis

Hematochezia

Neurologic symptoms (headache, altered consciousness, seizures, etc.)

Severe hypertension

Reported physical examination findings such as abdominal distention, bulging fontanelle, etc.

ELEVATOR THOUGHTS

A brief review of the common causes of vomiting is best organized by age.

Neonatal vomiting	Anatomic
	Gastroesophageal reflux
	Esophageal duplication cyst
	Duodenal atresia or stenosis
	Ileal atresia
	Ladd bands
	Hirschsprung disease
	Tracheoesophageal fistula (esophageal atresia)
	Pyloric stenosis
	Annular pancreas
	Malrotation
	Meconium ileus
	Anal atresia or imperforate anus
	Metabolic
	Inborn errors of metabolism
	Adrenogenital syndrome
	Toxic exposure
	Perinatal drug exposure
	Therapeutic drug overdose/side effects)
	Intracranial (increased intracranial pressure [ICP])

Hydrocephalus

Subdural or subarachnoid hemorrhage
(e.g., nonaccidental trauma)

Infectious

Urinary tract infection

Necrotizing enterocolitis

TORCH (toxoplasmosis, other agents, rubella,
cytomegalovirus, herpes simplex) infection

Others

Dietary protein intolerance or allergy (e.g.,
milk-protein intolerance)

Infant and childhood vomiting

Anatomic

Congenital anomalies of the gastrointestinal
tract

Hirschsprung disease

Intussusception

Malrotation

Swallowed foreign body (bezoar)

Intracranial

Brain tumor

Subdural hematoma

Hydrocephalus

Brain abscess

Metabolic

Inborn errors of metabolism

Uremia

Adrenogenital syndrome

Toxic ingestion

Diabetic ketoacidosis

Infectious

Gastroenteritis (viral vs. parasitic)

Hepatitis

Appendicitis

Bacterial colitis

Mesenteric adenitis

Urinary tract infection

Pancreatitis

Pneumonia

Acute otitis media

Streptococcal pharyngitis

Meningitis

Others

Lactose intolerance

Gluten intolerance

Postconcussive

Preadolescent and adolescent vomiting	Anatomic
	Malrotation
	Incarcerated hernia
	Adhesions
	Intracranial
	Brain tumor
	Cerebrovascular accident
	Subdural hemorrhage
	Metabolic
	Uremia
	Toxic ingestion (including toxic effect of therapeutic medication)
	Diabetic ketoacidosis
	Adrenal crisis
	Infectious
	Gastroenteritis (viral, parasitic)
	Bacterial colitis
	Hepatitis
	Pancreatitis
	Pneumonia
	Urinary tract infection
	Meningitis
	Psychogenic
	Bulimia
	School avoidance
	Anxiety
	Others
	Pregnancy
	Gastroparesis
	Peptic ulcer
	Postconcussive
	Cyclic vomiting

MAJOR THREAT TO LIFE

- Increased ICP
- Surgical abdominal emergencies (intussusception, bowel obstruction, necrotizing enterocolitis)
- Diabetic ketoacidosis
- Adrenal crisis

The differential diagnosis of vomiting is best approached initially by the age of the child. In newborns and neonates, congenital malformations of the gastrointestinal tract must be considered, including duodenal or ileal atresia (associated with Down syndrome), pyloric stenosis, malrotation and midgut volvulus, tracheoesophageal fistula, annular pancreas, meconium ileus, and Hirschsprung disease. In a preterm infant, especially one younger than 32 weeks' gestation and/or under 1500 g, vomiting may be a sign of necrotizing enterocolitis, which can progress rapidly to a perforated viscus, peritonitis, septic shock, and death. Nongastrointestinal diseases of the very young, including urinary tract infection, inborn errors of metabolism, adrenal crisis, and increased ICP (hydrocephalus or subdural hematoma), can produce significant vomiting.

In older infants, infectious gastroenteritis becomes more common, including gastroenteritis secondary to rotavirus and influenza A. In toddlers and older children, toxic ingestion, bacterial food poisoning, hepatitis, and inflammatory bowel diseases are added to viral gastroenteritis. Nongastrointestinal disorders include urinary tract infection, as well as brain tumors, other causes of increased ICP, and postconcussive vomiting. Diabetic ketoacidosis should always be considered in a child with vomiting even if no history of diabetes mellitus, because this could be the first presentation.

BEDSIDE

Quick-Look Test

Does the child appear well (comfortable), sick (uncomfortable or distressed), or critical (about to die)?

All children appear acutely uncomfortable when they are actively vomiting. They are anxious, tachycardic, and frequently diaphoretic. In infectious processes, nausea and vomiting tend to come in waves, with periods of relative calm and comfort in between, and almost invariably occur with fever. Acute surgical vomiting is usually accompanied by abdominal pain, which may or may not be well localized (see Chapter 6, Abdominal Pain). Vomiting associated with intracranial processes often appears early in the day and lessens as the day progresses, often with lack of nausea.

Airway and Vital Signs

What are the temperature, pulse, and blood pressure?

Hypotension associated with vomiting is a late and ominous sign of hypovolemia and shock. Fever implies infectious or inflammatory processes and can worsen dehydration. Hypertension and bradycardia imply severe increased ICP. Remember the Cushing triad: irregular respirations, elevated systolic blood pressure with large pulse pressure, and bradycardia!

Selective History and Chart Review

Is abdominal pain associated with the vomiting?

This is difficult to ascertain in infants but is quite helpful in older children. Although pain can occur with infectious gastroenteritis, it is unusual.

When did the vomiting start?

Vomiting can result from some medications, such as chemotherapeutic agents, as well as overdoses of a variety of other medications. Vomiting after closed head injury can indicate a concussion or more serious complication, such as subarachnoid or subdural hemorrhage. Persistent or recurrent vomiting can represent cyclic vomiting, bulimia, or metabolic-endocrine disorders.

Is the vomiting forceful or effortless?

All babies spit up. All babies have some gastroesophageal reflux. Reflux is normal and is a medical problem only if (1) the volume of reflux is such that the child does not gain weight or (2) the child aspirates. Otherwise, all reflux does is create dirty laundry (the child's as well as the parents'). Reflux should be distinguished from vomiting. Reflux is effortless regurgitation in small infants and can occur immediately after feeding or 2 to 3 hours later. The child is not distressed; in fact, the child may be quite happy and content. Vomiting is forceful and uncomfortable. An infant with pyloric stenosis is often described as having "explosive or projectile" vomiting ("across the room"). Projectile vomiting may also be seen with increased intracranial pressure and it is usually in the absence of nausea or retching.

What is the nature of the emesis?

Bilious, brown, or feculent emesis is pathognomonic of bowel obstruction, either paralytic or mechanical. Frank blood implies upper gastrointestinal bleeding, especially a Mallory-Weiss tear, variceal bleeding, vascular anomalies, vasculitis, esophagitis, or gastric ulcer disease, except in a newborn, in whom it may reflect swallowed maternal blood. Vomiting food after fasting is consistent with gastric outlet obstruction and/or delayed gastric emptying.

Is there associated diarrhea?

Viral and/or bacterial enterocolitis is very common in children. Viral gastroenteritis tends to be seasonal, with specific causes common to summer (enteroviruses) and winter (rotavirus, influenza). Food poisoning with *Staphylococcus* or *Salmonella* can cause a particularly sudden onset of acute vomiting that tends to be followed by diarrhea. The absence of diarrhea and fever should always lead you to consider intracranial causes for the vomiting.

What medications is the child taking?

Emesis is a well-described side effect of certain cancer chemotherapeutic medications, including cyclophosphamide, doxorubicin, and vincristine. Vomiting is also well known with toxic levels of other numerous drugs.

Selective Physical Examination

HEENT	Mucous membranes, dilated pupils, ketotic breath, nystagmus, and cranial nerve deficits may imply a nongastrointestinal cause of vomiting. In infants the fontanelles should be checked
Neck	Nuchal rigidity
Respiratory	Left lower lobe pneumonia and/or empyema may cause vomiting
Abdomen	Quality and activity of bowel sounds, distention, localized or diffuse tenderness, masses, hepatosplenomegaly, costovertebral angle tenderness, rebound tenderness, rigidity. Olive-like mass may indicate pyloric stenosis.
Rectal	Small rectum (Hirschsprung disease), bleeding (occult blood testing positive)
Genitourinary	Hernia, scrotal masses, scrotal pain
Neurologic	Mental status, focal findings, visual fields, funduscopic examination, Romberg sign

HEENT, Head, Eye, Ear, Nose, Throat.

Management

Management of vomiting depends on the underlying cause (Fig. 31.1). In many cases the vomiting is mild, self-limited, and not a sign of serious life-threatening problems, such as increased ICP or a surgical abdomen. After you have excluded these possibilities, you may not need to do any more initially than ensure that the child remains hydrated and frequently reevaluate the child via serial abdominal examinations. Remember that intra-abdominal processes may begin with isolated vomiting and lead to additional signs and symptoms over time. If there are signs of bowel obstruction, rapid gastrointestinal bleeding, or peritonitis, surgical consultation will be necessary. If there are signs of increased ICP, neuroimaging will be necessary, and transfer to the pediatric intensive care unit with institution of measures to decrease ICP may be required (see Chapter 7, Altered Mental Status).

Vomiting in a newborn should be distinguished from reflux. Forceful or persistent vomiting deserves diagnostic evaluation and may require intervention. Flat and upright abdominal films may confirm the presence of intestinal obstruction with a double bubble (duodenal atresia), air-fluid levels (small bowel obstruction), or megacolon (meconium ileus or Hirschsprung disease).

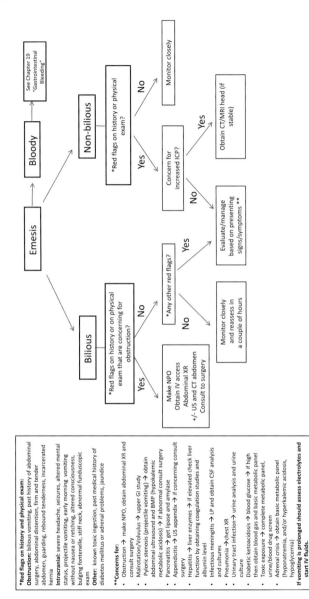

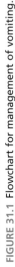

*Red flags on history and physical exam:
Obstruction: bilious vomiting, past history of abdominal surgery, abdominal distention, firm and tender abdomen, guarding, rebound tenderness, incarcerated hernia

Intracranial: severe headache, seizures, altered mental status, projectile vomiting, early morning vomiting without nausea or retching, altered consciousness, bulging fontenelle, stiff neck, abnormal funduscopic exam

Other: known toxic ingestion, past medical history of diabetes mellitus or adrenal problems, jaundice

**Concerns for:
- Obstruction → make NPO, obtain abdominal XR and consult surgery
- Malrotation/Volvulus → upper GI study
- Pyloric stenosis (projective vomiting) → obtain abdominal ultrasound and BMP (hypokalemic metabolic acidosis) → if abnormal consult surgery
- Pancreatitis → get lipase and amylase
- Appendicitis → US appendix → if concerning consult surgery
- Hepatitis → liver enzymes → if elevated check liver function by obtaining coagulation studies and albumin level
- Infectious meningitis → LP and obtain CSF analysis and cultures
- Pneumonia → chest XR
- Urinary tract infection → urine analysis and urine culture
- Diabetic ketoacidosis → blood glucose → if high then obtain blood gas and basic metabolic panel
- Toxic exposure → complete metabolic panel, urine/blood drug screen
- Adrenal crisis → obtain basic metabolic panel (hyponatremia, and/or hyperkalemic acidosis, hypoglycemia)

If vomiting is prolonged should assess electrolytes and start IV fluids.

FIGURE 31.1 Flowchart for management of vomiting.

Plain films may also confirm the presence of a radiopaque foreign body. (Remember, many of the things that children swallow are not radiopaque.) Ultrasound studies are useful in neonates with hypochloremic, hypokalemic metabolic acidosis caused by hypertrophic pyloric stenosis and in older children with suspected appendicitis. Prompt surgical consultation should be obtained if there is a suggestion of bowel obstruction. Bowel obstruction in older children can result from an incarcerated hernia, volvulus, intussusception, or adhesions from previous abdominal surgery.

Dehydration should be addressed as discussed in Chapter 15, Diarrhea and Dehydration. Obviously, the usefulness of oral rehydration may be limited by severe vomiting. For this reason, IV access is very important and should be made a priority.

If the child has been vomiting excessively, keep in mind that electrolyte abnormalities may be developing, particularly hypokalemia. Checking the electrolytes and correcting abnormalities may be necessary (see Chapter 34, Electrolyte Abnormalities).

The use of antiemetic medications is controversial. When the cause of vomiting is clear, such as after chemotherapy, antiemetic medications may and should be used for symptomatic relief. However, in patients with vomiting of unknown cause, antiemetics must be used cautiously. Vomiting may become persistent in children with hepatitis, pancreatitis, and gastroenteritis, especially when there is an element of dehydration. The use of promethazine (Phenergan), chlorpromazine (Thorazine), prochlorperazine (Compazine), or trimethobenzamide (Tigan) may be accompanied by significant extrapyramidal side effects. Ondansetron and granisetron, serotonin antagonists, are effective treatment of a variety of causes of refractory vomiting, including the vomiting associated with chemotherapy.

REMEMBER

The most critical elements when evaluating a hospitalized child with vomiting are to rule out the surgical causes unique to each age group, consider the possibility of intracranial causes of the vomiting, and support the child's hydration status and electrolyte balance while keeping the child comfortable. Oral rehydration can be accomplished in most cases by giving small amounts frequently, such as ice chips. Consider the need for antiemetics very cautiously, especially in children with infectious causes of vomiting. Do not forget that all forms of infectious vomiting are highly contagious. Do yourself and your next patient a big favor and wash your hands very well before and after evaluating every patient. Consider placing patient on contact isolation.

Laboratory-Related Problems

Acidosis and Alkalosis

Corinne Swearingen, MD

Multiple clinical conditions can affect a child's acid-base status. For example, profuse diarrhea may result in a metabolic acidosis because of loss of bicarbonate-rich intestinal fluid in stool. Likewise, vomiting may lead to a metabolic alkalosis from loss of hydrogen ions in gastric fluid. Chronic derangements of a child's acid-base status can interfere with normal growth and development, whereas acute derangements can be potentially fatal. Therefore it is critical for the body to be able to regulate its acid-base status within a certain pH. This is made possible through interactions between the lungs, kidneys, and intracellular and extracellular buffers.

NORMAL ACID-BASE BALANCE

A normal pH is between 7.35 and 7.45. In a healthy individual, normal metabolism produces acids, which must then be buffered. The main buffering system of the body is the bicarbonate buffer system; other effective buffers include proteins (e.g., albumin, hemoglobin), phosphate, and bone.

The bicarbonate buffer system is based on the relationship between CO_2 and bicarbonate:

$$H^+ + HCO_3^- \leftrightarrow H_2CO_3 \leftrightarrow CO_2 + H_2O$$

Acids react with extracellular HCO_3^-, which is then converted to CO_2 and eliminated through the lungs. P_{CO_2} is sensed centrally, and ventilation is adjusted (e.g., increased or decreased) to maintain normal values. These mechanisms maintain the concentration of hydrogen ions ($[H^+]$) within a narrow range, thereby maintaining the arterial pH within a "normal" range.

The Henderson-Hasselbalch equation expresses the relationship between pH, pK, and the concentrations of an acid and its conjugate base. From the Henderson-Hasselbalch equation, the following relationship among $[H^+]$, P_{CO_2}, and $[HCO_3^-]$ can be derived:

$$pH = pK_a + \log \left([HCO_3^-] / [CO_2] \right)$$

$$[H^+] = 24 \times PCO_2 / [HCO_3^-]$$

This equation shows that the hydrogen ion concentration, and therefore the pH, is determined by the ratio of PCO_2 and $[HCO_3^-]$.

The kidneys are responsible for regulating the serum bicarbonate concentration; this is accomplished by renal reabsorption of filtered bicarbonate and tubular secretion of hydrogen ions. Bicarbonate is mainly reabsorbed in the proximal tubule, whereas the collecting duct is the main location for hydrogen ion secretion. Bicarbonate reabsorption is increased in the setting of volume depletion ("contraction alkalosis"), hypokalemia, and high P_{CO_2}; it is decreased in the setting of low P_{CO_2}, elevated parathyroid hormone (PTH), certain medications (e.g., acetazolamide), and proximal tubular dysfunction (e.g., renal tubular acidosis [RTA]).

Acid excretion occurs through production of acid ($H_2PO_4^-$, NH_4^+) in the urine, which allows for net reabsorption of newly synthesized HCO_3^-. Acid excretion is regulated mainly by extracellular pH. Low pH causes the secretion of aldosterone, which stimulates acid excretion in the collecting duct.

CLINICAL ASSESSMENT OF ACID-BASE DISORDERS

Acidemia is defined as an arterial $pH < 7.35$, whereas alkalemia is an arterial $pH > 7.45$. Acidosis and alkalosis refer to the pathologic processes that cause an increase or decrease in $[H^+]$, respectively. For example, a child may have a mild metabolic acidosis with a concurrent severe respiratory alkalosis, resulting in net alkalemia.

A simple acid-base disorder refers to a single primary disturbance. The simple acid-base disorders are: (1) metabolic acidosis, (2) metabolic alkalosis, (3) respiratory acidosis, and (4) respiratory alkalosis (Table 32.1). With a metabolic acidosis, the primary disturbance is a low serum $[HCO_3^-]$, whereas with a metabolic alkalosis, the primary disturbance is a high serum $[HCO_3^-]$. With a respiratory acidosis, the primary disturbance is a high P_{CO_2}, and with a respiratory alkalosis, the primary disturbance is a low P_{CO_2}.

At the onset of a simple acid-base disorder, the body begins to predictably compensate (see Table 32.1).

TABLE 32.1   Simple Acid-Base Disorders and Expected Compensation

Simple Acid-Base Disorder	pH	Primary Disturbance	Compensation	Predicted Compensatory Response
Metabolic acidosis	<7.35	↓ [HCO$_3^-$]	↓ P$_{CO_2}$ (↑RR)	$P_{CO_2} = 1.5 \times [HCO_3^-] + 8 \pm 2$
Metabolic alkalosis	>7.45	↑ [HCO$_3^-$]	↑ P$_{CO_2}$ (↓RR)	P$_{CO_2}$ increases by 0.7 mm Hg for every 1 mEq/L increase in [HCO$_3^-$]
Respiratory acidosis				
Acute	<7.35	↑ P$_{CO_2}$	↑ [HCO$_3^-$]	[HCO$_3^-$] increases by 0.1 mEq/L for each 1 mm Hg increase in P$_{CO_2}$
Chronic (>24 hr)	<7.35	↑ P$_{CO_2}$	↑ [HCO$_3^-$]	[HCO$_3^-$] increases by 0.35 mEq/L for each 1 mm Hg increase in P$_{CO_2}$
Respiratory alkalosis				
Acute	>7.45	↓ P$_{CO_2}$	↓ [HCO$_3^-$]	[HCO$_3^-$] falls by 0.2 mEq/L for each 1 mm Hg decrease in P$_{CO_2}$
Chronic	>7.45	↓ P$_{CO_2}$	↓ [HCO$_3^-$]	[HCO$_3^-$] falls by 0.4 mEq/L for each 1 mm Hg decrease in P$_{CO_2}$

RR, Respiratory rate.

Respiratory compensation is rapid and accomplished by increasing P_{CO_2} (e.g., alkalemia) or decreasing P_{CO_2} (e.g., acidemia) by changes in ventilation. Respiratory compensation cannot "overcompensate" for or normalize the pH. Expected metabolic compensation is highly dependent on whether the respiratory process is acute or chronic. It is accomplished through regulation of bicarbonate reabsorption and hydrogen ion excretion. In the acute setting, metabolic compensation can occur within minutes. In the chronic (>24 hours) setting, metabolic compensation at the level of the kidney is much slower, beginning 12 to 24 hours after the onset and continuing for several days.

A mixed acid-base disorder occurs when there is more than 1 primary acid-base disturbance. For example, a child with severe pneumonia and sepsis may have a respiratory acidosis due to respiratory failure as well as a concurrent metabolic acidosis from elevated lactic acid. A mixed disorder is suspected when compensation appears to be greater or less than what is expected or deemed appropriate.

Any acid-base disturbance should be evaluated as a three-step process: (1) determine if acidemia or alkalemia is present; (2) determine a cause of the acidemia or alkalemia; (3) determine whether a mixed disorder is present. This evaluation should be interpreted in the context of the clinical situation (e.g., reported symptoms; acute vs. chronic course). Of note, for step 1, there are two instances in which pH may be normal but an underlying acid-base disturbance is present—a mixed disorder whereby the two processes have opposite effects, and simple chronic respiratory alkalosis with appropriate metabolic compensation.

PRIMARY ACID-BASE DISORDERS

Metabolic Acidosis

The primary disturbance in metabolic acidosis is a low $\left[HCO_3^-\right]$ secondary to depletion as a buffer or gastrointestinal/renal losses. The most common cause of metabolic acidosis is diarrhea. The predictable compensatory response to metabolic acidosis is hyperventilation, leading to a decrease in P_{CO_2}. A mixed acid-base disturbance is present if the respiratory compensation is not appropriate based on the Winter formula (see Table 32.1). If the P_{CO_2} is greater than predicted, a concurrent respiratory acidosis is suspected. If the P_{CO_2} is less than expected, a concurrent respiratory alkalosis is suspected.

After a metabolic acidosis has been identified, the anion gap should be determined.

$$\text{Anion gap} = [Na^+] - \left([Cl^-] + \left[HCO_3^-\right]\right)$$
$$\text{Normal range} = 8 \text{ to } 16\,mEq/L$$

The anion gap is the difference between the unmeasured cations (potassium, magnesium, calcium) and unmeasured anions (albumin, phosphate, urate, sulfate). As bicarbonate is depleted, the concentration of other anions is increased to maintain electroneutrality. The added anion can be Cl^- or an unmeasured anion (phosphate, lactate, formate, β-hydroxybutyrate). A normal anion gap occurs if the concentration of Cl^- is increased; in contrast, an increased anion gap occurs when there is an increase in the unmeasured anions.

Causes

The causes of metabolic acidosis can be divided into those that produce a normal anion gap and those that produce an increased anion gap (Table 32.2).

If the anion gap is normal, either loss of $[HCO_3^-]$ has occurred through the gut or kidneys or there has been rapid dilution of extracellular volume. If the anion gap is increased, acids have been added either endogenously (e.g., lactic acidosis or diabetic ketoacidosis) or exogenously (e.g., ingestion). If the osmolal gap is increased in the setting of anion gap metabolic acidosis, ingestion should be suspected.

TABLE 32.2	Causes of Metabolic Acidosis
Normal Anion Gap (Hyperchloremic)	**Increased Anion Gap (Normochloremic)**
• Diarrhea • Bowel, biliary, or pancreatic tube or fistula drainage • Renal tubular acidosis: distal (type I), proximal (type II), hyperkalemic (type IV) • Urinary tract diversions (through intestinal segments) • Posthypocapnia • Ammonium chloride intake • Adrenal insufficiency	• Poisoning: ethylene glycol, methanol, salicylate, toluene, paraldehyde • Kidney failure (uremia) • Ketoacidosis: diabetic ketoacidosis, starvation ketoacidosis, alcoholic ketoacidosis • Lactic acidosis: shock, hypoxemia, severe anemia, acute heart failure • Liver failure • Inborn errors of metabolism (through excessive production of ketoacids, lactic acid, and/or other organic anions) • Malignancy • Intestinal bacterial overgrowth • Medications: nucleoside reverse transcriptase inhibitors, metformin, propofol

Normal serum $[HCO_3^-]$ is 24 mEq/L (range, 20-28 mEq/L) and arterial blood gas P_{CO_2} is 40 mm Hg (range, 35-45 mm Hg).

From Kliegman R, et al.: Nelson Textbook of Pediatrics, ed 20. Philadelphia, Elsevier, 2016.

$$\text{Osmolal gap} = \text{Measured serum osmolality} \\ - \text{Calculated serum osmolality}$$

$$\text{Calculated serum osmolality} = 2[\text{Na}^+] + (\text{Serum BUN}/2.8) \\ + (\text{Serum glucose}/18)$$

Manifestations

The clinical manifestations of metabolic acidosis are related to the degree of acidemia and underlying disorder. Hyperventilation may be present as the child attempts to eliminate CO_2; it is typically subtle, with worsening respiratory distress potentially indicative of worsening acidemia. Ketotic breath or other odors may be clues to a metabolic cause of the acidosis, such as diabetic ketoacidosis or an inborn error of metabolism. If the acidosis is severe, altered mental status, decreased cardiac contractility, and shock may all occur.

Management

As with other acid-base disorders, treating the underlying cause is essential. For most children, maintaining adequate hydration, maximizing cardiac output and perfusion, correcting other electrolyte abnormalities, removing potential toxins, and providing supportive care prevent progression of the acidemia. Many causes of metabolic acidosis do require specific therapy (e.g., administration of insulin in diabetic ketoacidosis, administration of glucocorticoid and mineralocorticoid in adrenal insufficiency, hemodialysis for renal failure).

Depending upon the cause and chronicity, oral or intravenous bicarbonate therapy may be indicated (e.g., RTA, chronic renal failure, salicylate poisoning). There are inherent risks to bicarbonate administration, including hypernatremia, volume overload, and subsequent alkalemia with impaired cell function. If not directly indicated as treatment for a specific cause, bicarbonate administration is typically reserved for severe acute lactic acidosis and severe diabetic ketoacidosis. In these cases, it is not necessary to return the pH to normal; the goal should be to attain a pH of approximately 7.25. When a rapid response is needed, intravenous sodium bicarbonate may be given.

When administering bicarbonate, careful attention must be paid to the serum potassium concentration. If an acidemic child is normokalemic or hypokalemic, life-threatening hypokalemia may be precipitated by the administration of bicarbonate due to shift of potassium intracellularly. In this situation, bicarbonate should be diluted and administered slowly; rapid infusion may result in dysrhythmias.

Metabolic Alkalosis

The primary disturbance in metabolic alkalosis is a high $\left[HCO_3^-\right]$. In children the most common causes are vomiting and diuretic use. Generation and maintenance of a metabolic alkalosis occurs in the setting of two processes: (1) addition of base to the body and (2) impairment in the kidney's ability to excrete the base. The predictable compensatory response to a metabolic alkalosis is hypoventilation, leading to an increase in P_{CO_2}. A mixed acid-base disturbance is present if the respiratory compensation is not appropriate (see Table 32.1). If the P_{CO_2} is greater than predicted, a concurrent respiratory acidosis is suspected. If the P_{CO_2} is less than expected, a concurrent respiratory alkalosis is suspected. In general, appropriate respiratory compensation never exceeds a P_{CO_2} of 55 to 60 mm Hg.

Causes

The causes of metabolic alkalosis are divided into two groups: (1) chloride responsive and (2) chloride resistant (Table 32.3). The division is based on urinary chloride level. Alkalosis in children with low urinary chloride level is due to volume depletion (with losses of sodium, potassium, and chloride). These children require chloride and fluid repletion to correct their volume depletion and metabolic alkalosis; in other words, they are "chloride

TABLE 32.3	Causes of Metabolic Alkalosis
Chloride-Responsive (Urinary Chloride <15 mEq/L)	**Chloride-Resistant (Urinary Chloride >20 mEq/L)**
• Gastric losses (emesis, nasogastric suction) • Diuretics (loop or thiazide) • Chloride-losing diarrhea • Chloride-deficient formula • Cystic fibrosis • Posthypercapnia	High blood pressure • Hyperaldosteronism (adrenal adenoma or hyperplasia) • Elevated renin (renovascular disease, renin-secreting tumor) • 17β-Hydroxylase deficiency • 11β-Hydroxylase deficiency • Cushing syndrome • Licorice ingestion • Liddle syndrome Normal blood pressure • Gitelman syndrome • Bartter syndrome • Autosomal dominant hypoparathyroidism • Base administration (citrate, lactate, acetate)

responsive." In comparison, alkalosis in a child with an elevated urinary chloride concentration does not respond to volume repletion and is therefore termed "chloride resistant."

The main causes of chloride-responsive metabolic alkalosis include vomiting and diuretic use. Vomiting causes alkalemia due to loss of H^+ in gastric fluid. With net loss of acid, there is net gain of bicarbonate. In the setting of persistent vomiting, volume depletion also occurs, worsening the alkalemia due to increased reabsorption of bicarbonate and hydrogen ion secretion. Diuretics lead to alkalemia through volume depletion, which increases angiotensin II, aldosterone, and adrenergic stimulation of the kidney; contraction alkalosis also occurs, limiting urinary bicarbonate losses. Typically, urinary chloride levels are high (>20 mEq/L) immediately following diuretic administration but later become low with appropriate renal chloride retention in a volume-depleted state.

The chloride-resistant causes are divided based on blood pressure. Hypertensive causes are related to elevated aldosterone, which causes retention of sodium and renal excretion of hydrogen and potassium.

Manifestations

The symptoms are typically related to the underlying disease process, associated electrolyte disturbances, and fluid status. In general, alkalemia increases the risk of arrhythmias and can cause hypoxia and altered mental status.

Management

Metabolic alkalosis associated with volume depletion (low urinary chloride) responds to the administration of normal saline solution. Once the fluid and chloride deficits are repleted, renal excretion of bicarbonate allows for resolution of the alkalemia. Remember that an associated hypokalemia must also be corrected before normal saline solution is effective. As with other acid-base disorders, correcting the underlying cause is usually sufficient.

Respiratory Acidosis

The primary disturbance in respiratory acidosis is high PCO_2 due to impaired removal by the lungs. It is often due to severe pulmonary disease, respiratory muscle fatigue, or central nervous system (CNS) depression. The predictable compensatory response depends on if the process is acute or chronic (see Table 32.1). In acute respiratory acidosis, metabolic compensation can occur within minutes due to cellular buffering mechanisms. With chronic respiratory acidosis (>24 hours), more significant renal compensation is needed and occurs over 3 to 4 days. However, $\left[HCO_3^- \right]$

usually does not rise above 38 mEq/L. A mixed acid-base disturbance is present if the metabolic compensation is not appropriate. If the $\left[HCO_3^-\right]$ is greater than predicted, a concurrent metabolic alkalosis is suspected. If the $\left[HCO_3^-\right]$ is less than expected, a concurrent metabolic acidosis is suspected.

Causes

1. Pulmonary disease: pneumonia, pneumothorax, asthma, bronchiolitis, bronchopulmonary dysplasia, acute respiratory distress syndrome, cystic fibrosis, pulmonary edema, pulmonary hemorrhage, hypoplastic lungs
2. CNS depression: encephalitis, hypoxic brain damage, head trauma, brain tumor, primary pulmonary hypoventilation (Ondine curse), medications (e.g., narcotics, barbiturates, anesthesia, benzodiazepines)
3. Respiratory muscle weakness: muscular dystrophy, malnutrition, hypothyroidism, medications (succinylcholine, corticosteroids)
4. Disorders of spinal cord, peripheral nerves, or neuromuscular junction: diaphragmatic paralysis, Guillain-Barré syndrome, poliomyelitis, spinal muscular atrophies, myasthenia gravis, botulism, multiple sclerosis, spinal cord injury, medications (e.g., vecuronium, aminoglycosides, organophosphates)
5. Upper airway disease: aspiration, laryngospasm, extrinsic tumor, obstructive sleep apnea, angioedema

Manifestations

The clinical manifestations of respiratory acidosis depend on the severity, duration, underlying disease process, and presence or absence of hypoxemia. A rapid increase in P_{CO_2} can lead to anxiety, confusion, and hallucinations and may ultimately end in coma. In chronic hypercapnia, sleep disturbances, loss of memory, and daytime somnolence are possible; in addition, coordination and motor disturbances (e.g., tremor, asterixis, myoclonic jerks) may be present. Most importantly, high P_{CO_2} can lead to CNS symptoms, such as headache, papilledema, abnormal reflexes, and focal muscle weakness, due to cerebral vasodilation.

Management

The treatment of respiratory acidosis depends on its severity and rate of onset (acute vs. chronic). In general, management is directed at the underlying cause. Intubation, mechanical ventilation, and transfer to the intensive care unit may all be necessary for a child with moderate to severe respiratory acidosis. Any child with respiratory acidosis requires frequent monitoring with serial arterial blood gas determinations while you are identifying and treating the underlying cause. Tachypnea, labored breathing, and the use of accessory muscles may initially prevent the development of acidosis, but eventual fatigue may lead to rapid decompensation.

Monitoring oxygen saturation alone with a pulse oximeter is inadequate and may be falsely reassuring because preservation of oxygen saturation may continue despite a decline in ventilation. In addition, patients with chronic respiratory acidosis may actually experience progression of their respiratory acidosis when given oxygen, because ventilation in them is driven more by oxygen pressure versus the normal parameters of P_{CO_2} and pH. In general, correction of chronic respiratory acidosis should be performed gradually, with the aim of restoring P_{CO_2} to baseline levels.

Respiratory Alkalosis

The primary disturbance in respiratory alkalosis is low PCO_2, which is usually due to hyperventilation. Other causes include extracorporeal membrane oxygenation (ECMO) or hemodialysis where CO_2 is lost directly into the circuit. The predictable compensatory response depends on if the process is acute or chronic (see Table 32.1). In acute respiratory alkalosis, metabolic compensation can occur within minutes due to cellular buffering mechanisms. With chronic respiratory acidosis (>24 hours), more significant renal compensation is needed and occurs over 2 to 3 days. Of note, a chronic respiratory alkalosis is the only acid-base disturbance where compensation can normalize the pH. A mixed acid-base disturbance is present if the metabolic compensation is not appropriate. If the $\left[HCO_3^-\right]$ is greater than predicted, a concurrent metabolic alkalosis is suspected. If the $\left[HCO_3^-\right]$ is less than expected, a concurrent metabolic acidosis is suspected.

Causes

1. Hypoxemia or tissue hypoxia: pneumonia, pulmonary edema, congestive heart failure, asthma, severe anemia, aspiration, carbon monoxide poisoning, pulmonary embolism, interstitial lung disease, ECMO
2. Lung receptor stimulation: pneumonia, pulmonary edema, asthma, pulmonary embolism, respiratory distress syndrome, pneumothorax
3. Central stimulation: fever, pain, panic attack, liver failure, sepsis, mechanical ventilation, CNS disease (e.g., subarachnoid hemorrhage, encephalitis, trauma, brain tumor, stroke), medications (e.g., salicylate intoxication, theophylline, exogenous catecholamines, caffeine)

Many different stimuli can increase ventilatory drive, resulting in a respiratory alkalosis. For example, arterial hypoxemia or tissue hypoxia can stimulate peripheral chemoreceptors, which signal to the central respiratory center to increase ventilation. The lung also contains chemoreceptors and mechanoreceptors that respond to irritants and stretching and, when activated, will also signal to the respiratory center to increase ventilation. Finally, direct stimulation of the central respiratory center can occur, such as in the setting of CNS disease (e.g., meningitis, hemorrhage, trauma), or by situations that cause pain, stress, or anxiety.

Manifestations

Acute respiratory alkalosis may cause chest tightness, palpitations, light-headedness, circumoral numbness, or paresthesias; less commonly, it may cause tetany, seizures, muscle cramps, or syncope. The paresthesias, tetany, and seizures may be related to decreased serum ionized calcium due to increased binding of calcium to albumin. Light-headedness and syncope may be related to cerebral hypoperfusion secondary to low P_{CO_2}. In contrast, chronic respiratory acidosis is usually asymptomatic because of metabolic compensation.

Management

Most instances of respiratory alkalosis are mild and short-lived. Management of respiratory alkalosis depends on relieving the underlying cause. In cases of hyperventilation secondary to anxiety, rebreathing into a paper bag may be beneficial.

Anemia, Thrombocytopenia, and Coagulation Abnormalities

Shela Sridhar, MD

Anemia is a common problem in the pediatric age group and is often discovered during hospitalization for an acute illness. Many systemic illnesses are accompanied by mild to moderate anemia and do not require extensive evaluation or specific treatment. Similarly, anemia may be expected to be present with many chronic illnesses, and appropriate management of the underlying illness generally prevents progressive worsening of the anemia. When anemia is severe or a systemic illness has not been identified, further evaluation of the anemia may be required to determine the cause and to initiate appropriate treatment. Treatment of anemia based solely on a specific hemoglobin or hematocrit (Hct) value is not always necessary; however, when the anemia results in symptoms or signs of hemodynamic compromise, or when cardiac or pulmonary disease is present, treating the anemia will likely be beneficial.

Thrombocytopenia and abnormalities in coagulation are much less common than anemia in the pediatric population. These abnormalities require further evaluation and often specific treatment. A low platelet count or abnormal clotting study result generally reflects significant illness; therefore, when notified of such abnormalities, your response should be prompt.

ANEMIA

Causes

The potential causes of anemia can be narrowed by considering the patient's clinical signs and symptoms and by the initial laboratory evaluation. An evaluation of anemia should include hemoglobin, Hct, reticulocyte count, red blood cell (RBC) indices (mean corpuscular volume [MCV], mean corpuscular hemoglobin [MCH], mean corpuscular hemoglobin concentration [MCHC]), and RBC morphology. Further evaluation may be necessary, depending on the results of these initial tests. It is important to remember that normal values for some of these measurements vary with age (Table 33.1).

Anemias can be divided into two large categories by analyzing the reticulocyte count:

1. Low reticulocyte count: Inability of bone marrow to produce RBCs
2. High reticulocyte count: Retained ability of bone marrow to produce RBCs

Low Reticulocyte Count: Inadequate production

This category can be further categorized based on the MCV.

Microcytic Anemias (Low Mean Corpuscular Volume)

1. Iron deficiency
2. Thalassemias
3. Lead toxicity
4. Sideroblastic anemia
5. Chronic disease (infection, inflammation, renal disease)

Normocytic Anemias (Normal Mean Corpuscular Volume)

1. Transient erythroblastopenia of childhood
2. Aplastic anemia (congenital or acquired, e.g., drugs)
3. Pure RBC aplasia
4. Bone marrow suppression or replacement (leukemia, tumors, storage diseases, infections, hemophagocytosis)
5. Chronic disease

Macrocytic Anemias (High Mean Corpuscular Volume)

1. Vitamin B_{12} deficiency
2. Folate deficiency
3. Aplastic anemia
4. Pure RBC aplasia (Diamond-Blackfan syndrome)
5. Hypothyroidism

TABLE 33.1	Estimated Normal Mean Values and Lower Limits of Normal (95% Range) for Hemoglobin, Hematocrit, Mean Corpuscular Volume, and Mean Corpuscular Hemoglobin							
	Hemoglobin (g/L)		Packed Cell Volume (%)		MCV (fL)		MCH (pg)	
Age (Years)	Mean	Lower Limit	Mean	Lower Limit	Mean	Lower Limit	Mean	Lower Limit
0.5-4	125	110	36	32	80	72	28	24
5-10	130	115	38	33	83	75	29	25
11-14, F	135	120	39	34	85	77	29	26
11-14, M	140	120	41	35	85	77	29	26
15-19, F	135	120	40	34	88	79	30	27
15-19, M	150	130	43	37	88	79	30	27
20-44, F	135	120	40	35	90	80	31	27
20-44, M	155	135	45	39	90	80	31	27

MCH, Mean corpuscular hemoglobin; MCV, mean corpuscular volume.

High Reticulocyte Count: Increased Loss or Red Blood Cell Destruction

RBC Losses: Bleeding

1. Trauma
2. Gastrointestinal (GI) bleeding
3. Splenic sequestration
4. Pulmonary hemorrhage
5. Ruptured aneurysm
6. Ruptured ectopic pregnancy
7. Intraventricular hemorrhage (in premature infants)

RBC Destruction: Hemolysis

1. Hemoglobinopathies
   Sickle cell disease
   Hemoglobin SC
2. RBC membrane defects
   Spherocytosis
   Elliptocytosis
   Paroxysmal nocturnal hemoglobinuria
3. Enzymopathies
   Pyruvate kinase deficiency
   Glucose-6-phosphate dehydrogenase
4. Extracellular defects
   Isoimmune hemolysis (Coombs positive)
   Fragmentation (disseminated intravascular coagulopathy [DIC], hemolytic-uremic syndrome [HUS], thrombotic thrombocytopenic purpura [TTP])
   Splenomegaly
   Keep in mind that in children with chronic anemia, exacerbations may develop as a result of another cause (e.g., splenic sequestration or aplastic crisis in those with sickle cell disease) and that a single cause may lead to other causes (e.g., chronic GI blood loss leading to iron deficiency).

CLINICAL MANIFESTATIONS

The manifestations of anemia are those of the underlying cause. Pallor is often the initial clue that an anemia is present. The palpebral conjunctivae, mucous membranes, and nail beds are the most obvious sites to look for pallor. Specific manifestations of the anemia depend on whether the anemia is acute or chronic. Acute and rapid onset of anemia secondary to hemorrhage results in signs and symptoms of hypovolemia and/or shock:

1. Tachycardia, hypotension
2. Cool, clammy extremities

3. Delayed capillary refill
4. Diaphoresis, tachypnea

Acute hemolysis may result in tachycardia, tachypnea, and pallor but does not usually produce the same degree of hypovolemia that is seen with hemorrhage. Jaundice secondary to hyperbilirubinemia, dark urine (hemoglobinuria), and/or splenomegaly may be clues to hemolysis.

Chronic anemia results in less obvious signs and symptoms:
1. Pallor
2. Fatigue, lethargy
3. Dyspnea with exertion
4. Mild tachycardia, tachypnea

Management

Determine the severity. The clinical status of the patient, not the laboratory value, should be used to determine the need for treatment. For example, acute hemorrhage may initially result in a mild decrease or even no decrease in the hemoglobin level. If the patient is dehydrated, hemoconcentration may falsely increase the hemoglobin and Hct despite a significant reduction in RBCs. Conversely, many patients are asymptomatic despite profound anemia, especially if the anemia has developed over time.

A patient who is hypovolemic or in shock due to severe anemia needs prompt intervention with a transfusion of packed RBCs (PRBCs) or whole blood. A patient with normal vital signs and a physical examination that does not indicate hypovolemia may need intervention if (1) the hemoglobin level is very depressed and a further drop is anticipated or (2) the hemoglobin level is very depressed and other factors (heart or lung disease) mandate intervention to improve oxygen-carrying capacity. A child with no symptoms and mild to moderate anemia may need further evaluation but probably does not need immediate intervention.

Hypovolemia

The same principles that apply in other conditions of hypovolemia and shock apply in a patient with hypovolemia and anemia (see Chapter 15, Diarrhea and Dehydration, and Chapter 25, Hypotension and Shock). Rapid expansion of the intravascular space is the initial goal.
1. Make sure that the child has at least one (ideally two) large-bore intravenous (IV) lines placed. "Large bore" is defined as the largest that you can place, usually a 16-gauge line in an older child and an 18-gauge line in a younger child or infant.
2. Send blood to the blood bank for an immediate cross match. Always err on the side of requesting more units. The blood is not wasted if you decide later not to use it.

3. Expand the intravascular space. The ideal fluid in this situation, when acute anemia and hypovolemia coincide, presumably because of massive blood loss (hemorrhage or hemolysis), is cross-matched whole blood. If the situation is critical (ongoing rapid blood loss in a patient in shock), O-negative blood should be given. If blood is not yet available, normal saline or lactated Ringer's solution should be infused, starting at 20 mL/kg and additional boluses administered according to the blood pressure response, heart rate, and clinical signs (pulse, capillary refill). Once blood is available, it should be used in place of crystalloid. After volume has been restored and the child is normotensive, the hemoglobin level and Hct should be determined, with additional infusion of blood or PRBCs dependent on the degree of anemia.

4. Determine the cause of the blood loss. This should be done coincidentally with fluid resuscitation. Search for obvious sites of hemorrhage, as well as occult sources. Periumbilical (Cullen sign) or flank (Grey Turner sign) ecchymoses may indicate abdominal hemorrhage. A careful abdominal and rectal examination with Hemoccult determination is mandatory. A chest radiograph should be obtained if pulmonary hemorrhage is a consideration. Review the child's medication list for anticoagulants and the chart for potential coagulopathies or recent surgery.

5. Surgical consultation may be necessary if intra-abdominal bleeding is suspected.

Euvolemia

A euvolemic child does not require immediate intervention but may need a transfusion if symptomatic or the degree of anemia is profound.

1. Determine the cause of the anemia. As noted earlier, a complete blood count with RBC indices, reticulocyte count, and review of the peripheral smear (Fig. 33.1) should allow you to narrow the possibilities or make a definitive diagnosis. Remember that even though hypovolemia is not present, blood loss may have occurred or may be ongoing and the potential exists for rapid decompensation if the patient is hemorrhaging. As in hypovolemic patients, your physical examination should be directed toward signs of obvious or occult bleeding.

2. If a transfusion is necessary, the amount of cross-matched PRBCs to be transfused can be calculated by using the following formula:

$$\text{Volume of PRBCs(mL)} = \text{Estimated blood volume(mL)} \times (\text{Desired Hct} - \text{Observed Hct})$$

$$/\text{Hct of PRBCs}$$

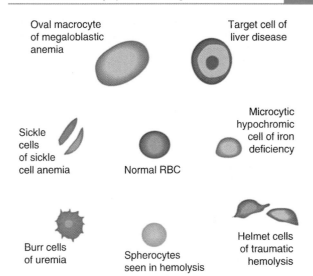

FIGURE 33.1 Examples of blood smears demonstrating helpful diagnostic features associated with specific anemias. *RBC,* Red blood cell. (From Marshall SA, Ruedy J: On Call: Principles and Protocols, 4th ed. Philadelphia, Elsevier, 2004, p 325.)

where the Hct of PRBCs can be estimated to be 65 and blood volume is estimated as follows:

Premature infants	100 mL/kg
Neonates	85 mL/kg
Infants (>1 month)	75 mL/kg
Children	70 mL/kg
Adolescents	65 mL/kg

Alternatively, a transfusion of 10 to 15 mL/kg of PRBCs can be administered. With either approach, rechecking the hemoglobin concentration and Hct in 4 to 6 hours allows you to determine the adequacy of the replacement.

THROMBOCYTOPENIA

Causes

The cause of a low platelet count can be divided into two categories:
1. Inadequate production (bone marrow infiltration or suppression)
2. Increased destruction or sequestration

Inadequate production	Malignancies (e.g., leukemia, neuroblastoma)
	Storage diseases (e.g., Gaucher disease)
	Wiskott-Aldrich syndrome
	Thrombocytopenia absent radius syndrome
	Infections
	Drugs (resulting in marrow suppression)
	Hemophagocytic syndromes (hemophagocytic lymphohistiocytosis [HLH], macrophage activation syndrome [MAS])
Increased destruction	Idiopathic thrombocytopenic purpura
	Systemic lupus erythematosus (SLE)

CLINICAL MANIFESTATIONS

Thrombocytopenia may be asymptomatic, result in petechiae only, or be associated with significant bleeding. The underlying disorder, rather than the specific platelet count, determines the severity of the clinical manifestations. Hemorrhage is generally rare unless the platelet count is less than 20,000/mm^3.

Bleeding secondary to mild or moderate thrombocytopenia tends to involve the skin and mucous membranes rather than deeper internal organs. Petechiae, purpura, bruising, and bleeding from gums or IV sites are seen most often. This is in contrast to bleeding that results from an abnormality in clotting factors, in which deeper bleeding (e.g., hemarthroses) is more common. However, if thrombocytopenia is severe enough, children may be at increased risk for intracranial or other internal bleeding. Purpura secondary to thrombocytopenia is nonpalpable and should be distinguished from palpable purpura, which is more suggestive of vasculitis.

Additional clinical findings and laboratory studies should help you narrow the list of potential causes of a low platelet count. If anemia and/or leukopenia is also present, marrow suppression or SLE should be further considered. Isolated thrombocytopenia is more suggestive of a problem causing increased destruction of platelets (e.g., idiopathic thrombocytopenic purpura [ITP]). The presence of an associated hemolytic anemia increases the likelihood of an autoimmune (SLE, Evans syndrome) or microangiopathic (DIC, HUS, TTP) cause. Reviewing the peripheral smear may suggest a microangiopathy if schistocytes, helmet cells, and other fragmented cells are evident. In such a context, an elevated blood urea nitrogen and/or creatinine level with other signs of renal failure should increase your suspicion for HUS; the additional presence of neurologic symptoms should alert you to the possibility of the much less common diagnosis of TTP. An associated prolongation of the prothrombin time (PT) and partial thromboplastin time (PTT) should raise your suspicion for DIC.

Management

Treatment of thrombocytopenia varies, depending on the underlying cause. In general, platelet transfusions are only beneficial in conditions in which thrombocytopenia is a result of inadequate production. In conditions involving increased destruction, platelet transfusions may temporarily increase the platelet count, but as long as the pathogenic mechanisms leading to increased destruction continue, the platelet count eventually falls again. Nonetheless, if life-threatening hemorrhage is present, platelets should be transfused in these situations, even if it is only a temporary measure.

If a platelet transfusion is necessary, it is customary to transfuse 1 unit of platelets per 10 kg of patient weight. This can be expected to increase the platelet count by approximately 50,000/mm^3. An estimate of the expected increase can also be obtained with the following formula:

$$\text{Platelet count increase } (\text{per mm}^3)$$
$$= 30,000 \times \text{Units transfused}/\text{Total blood volume (L)}$$

The platelet count should be checked 1 hour after transfusion to evaluate the response.

Idiopathic Thrombocytopenic Purpura

Treatment is not required when the patient is asymptomatic and the platelet count is greater than 35,000 mm^3. Treatment options include IV immunoglobulin, anti-Rh D therapy (in patients who are Rh D positive), and corticosteroids. Decisions regarding treatment of ITP should be made in consultation with a pediatric hematologist.

Thrombotic Thrombocytopenic Purpura

Children with TTP are usually quite ill and generally require management in the intensive care setting. Plasmapheresis is usually indicated and other treatments including corticosteroids may be considered. Treatment plans should be undertaken in consultation with a pediatric hematologist.

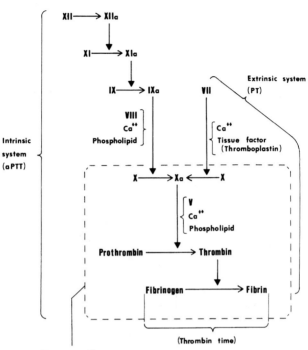

FIGURE 33.2 The coagulation cascade. *aPTT,* Activated partial thromboplastin time. (From Marshall SA, Ruedy J: On Call: Principles and Protocols, 4th ed. Philadelphia, Elsevier, 2004, p 337.)

COAGULATION ABNORMALITIES: PROLONGED PROTHROMBIN TIME AND PARTIAL THROMBOPLASTIN TIME

Causes

The PT tests the extrinsic pathway of the clotting cascade (Fig. 33.2). The PTT tests the intrinsic pathway. The extrinsic pathway is most affected by deficiencies in factors I (fibrinogen), II (prothrombin), V, VII, and X, whereas the intrinsic pathway is most affected by deficiencies in factors VIII, IX, XI, and XII.

Disorders prolonging the   Clotting factor deficiencies
  prothrombin time   (factors I, II, V, VII, X)
                                   Oral anticoagulants (warfarin
                                     sodium [Coumadin])

Disorders prolonging the partial thromboplastin time	Vitamin K deficiency (e.g., hemorrhagic disease of the newborn)
	Liver disease
	Disseminated intravascular coagulopathy
	Heparin (sometimes)
	Clotting factor deficiencies (factors VIII, IX, XI, XII)
	Anticoagulants (heparin; sometimes oral anticoagulants)
	Circulating endogenous anticoagulant (e.g., lupus anticoagulant)
	Disseminated intravascular coagulopathy
	von Willebrand disease (sometimes)

Factor deficiencies can be suspected or excluded by the results of mixing studies, in which normal plasma is mixed 1:1 with the child's plasma. The PT or PTT should "correct" if a deficient factor has been replaced by the addition of normal plasma. Failure to correct is consistent with an anticoagulant.

CLINICAL MANIFESTATIONS

With the exception of lupus anticoagulant, bleeding is the obvious manifestation. Bleeding associated with a prolongation of the PT and/or PTT tends to involve deeper parts of the body, including visceral organs and joints.

Lupus anticoagulant is not associated with bleeding but rather predisposes one to thrombosis. The prolongation of the PTT that is usually (but not always) discovered is the result of in vitro phenomena in which the presence of lupus anticoagulant interferes with the test itself.

Management
Factor Deficiencies
Fresh frozen plasma (10 to 15 mL/kg) or specific factor concentrates can be infused to replace the deficient factor, once identified. Cryoprecipitate (0.2 bag/kg) contains high concentrations of fibrinogen and factor VIII and can also be used when these factors are deficient. If the bleeding is minor, IV or intranasal desmopressin (DDAVP) may be administered to increase plasma factor VIII levels. In children with severe bleeding, the use of

products such as coagulation factor VIIa (recombinant) should be considered. However, these products should not be administered without consulting a hematologist.

von Willebrand Disease

In most cases, bleeding is minor and may be treated with DDAVP, which releases von Willebrand factor (vWF). Less commonly, von Willebrand disease causes major bleeding that may be treated with Humate-P, a factor VIII concentrate that contains high levels of vWF. Cryoprecipitate or fresh frozen plasma is also effective. Use of these products should always be undertaken in consultation with a pediatric hematologist.

Vitamin K Deficiency

Hemorrhagic disease of the newborn occurs during the first week of life when an exaggeration of the normally mild decrease in vitamin K–dependent factors occurs. Prophylactic administration of intramuscular (IM) vitamin K at the time of birth usually prevents hemorrhagic disease but is less effective in premature infants. If bleeding ensues, SC or IM vitamin K, 1 to 2 mg, is effective, and a response should be seen within a few hours.

Intestinal malabsorption and prolonged antibiotic treatment may result in vitamin K deficiency beyond the neonatal period. Vitamin K should be administered orally, subcutaneously, or intravenously (1 mg for infants, 2 to 3 mg for children, 10 mg for adolescents and adults). If vitamin K is ineffective or rapid correction is required, fresh frozen plasma should be administered.

Liver Disease

Liver disease may result in decreased synthesis of clotting factors and subsequent factor deficiencies. For mild bleeding, administration of vitamin K, as outlined previously, may be all that is necessary. If bleeding is severe, fresh frozen plasma (10 to 15 mL/kg) corrects all clotting factor deficiencies except fibrinogen deficiency. Cryoprecipitate (0.2 bag/kg) can be infused to correct the fibrinogen deficiency.

Disseminated Intravascular Coagulopathy

While the underlying cause is being treated, supportive care should include infusions of fresh frozen plasma, cryoprecipitate, and platelets when bleeding, thrombocytopenia, and PT and PTT abnormalities are severe.

Electrolyte Abnormalities

Eric Velazquez, MD

HYPERNATREMIA (SERUM SODIUM >150 MEQ/L)

Causes

Sodium excess
    Improperly mixed formula
    Excessive sodium bicarbonate administration for acidosis
        Ingestion of ocean water
    Hyperaldosteronism
Water deficit
    Inadequate intake
    Renal losses
    Diabetes insipidus (central or nephrogenic)
    Diabetes mellitus
    Osmotic diuresis
    Obstructive uropathy
    Renal dysplasia
Extrarenal losses
    Diarrhea
    Excessive sweating
    Excessive insensible losses (burns, phototherapy)

Manifestations

Hypernatremia is usually the result of abnormal water loss in excess of sodium loss rather than an increase in total body sodium. In children, diarrhea is the most common cause and results in dehydration. With hypernatremic dehydration, the shift of water into the extracellular space tends to preserve intravascular volume; therefore urine output may remain close to normal and such children may initially be less symptomatic than those with other forms of dehydration. Polyuria should suggest diabetes insipidus or diabetes mellitus. In an infant who does not appear dehydrated and has normal urine output, you should carefully determine how the infant is being fed and how the formula has been mixed. Errors in mixing are a common cause of hypernatremia in this age group.

The clinical manifestations of hypernatremia are those that result from the osmotic shift of water from the intracellular compartment to the extracellular compartment. Pulmonary edema may ensue, and its effects on brain cells may result in lethargy, irritability, coma, seizures, hypertonicity, and muscle spasms. Brain hemorrhage is the most serious potential consequence of hypernatremia.

Management

Determine the hydration status of the child and the severity of the hypernatremia. Most infants and children with hypernatremia are dehydrated. Management of a dehydrated patient with hypernatremia is discussed in Chapter 15.

If the patient is normovolemic (or volume overloaded) and hypernatremic, as in instances in which sodium intake has been excessive, diuresis may be useful. Furosemide, 1 mg/kg intravenously (IV) initially with repeated doses at 2- to 4-hour intervals, promotes urinary sodium loss. If a large volume must be diuresed to return the sodium level to normal, urinary losses may be measured and replaced with 5% dextrose in water (D_5W). Frequent monitoring of the patient's hydration status and serum sodium level is mandatory. Remember that serum sodium levels must be corrected slowly (10 to 15 mEq/L per day) because cerebral edema may develop if free water shifts rapidly intracellularly as the extracellular sodium concentration falls.

Severe hypernatremia (>200 mEq/L) may require peritoneal dialysis or hemodialysis and consultation with a pediatric nephrologist.

HYPONATREMIA (SERUM SODIUM <130 MEQ/L)

Causes

The volume status of the patient should guide your differential of potential causes of hyponatremia. An estimate of volume status and the urinary sodium concentration allows you to limit the list of possibilities (Fig. 34.1). A hypovolemic patient is losing sodium (and free water) either through urine or from extrarenal sites. The urinary sodium concentration should allow you to distinguish renal from extrarenal losses. A euvolemic patient may also have urinary sodium losses, but they are lower than in a hypovolemic

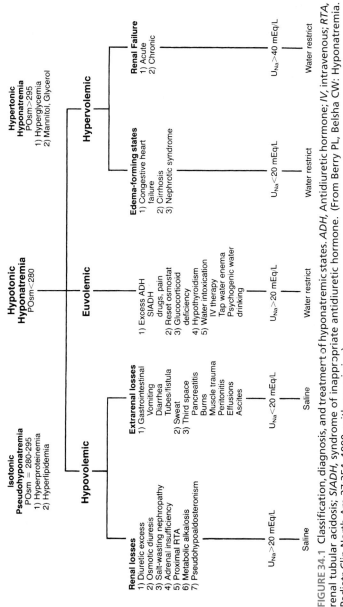

FIGURE 34.1 Classification, diagnosis, and treatment of hyponatremic states. *ADH*, Antidiuretic hormone; *IV*, intravenous; *RTA*, renal tubular acidosis; *SIADH*, syndrome of inappropriate antidiuretic hormone. (From Berry PL, Belsha CW: Hyponatremia. Pediatr Clin North Am 37:354, 1990, with permission)

patient, and water loss is minimal or absent. In some cases (e.g., syndrome of inappropriate antidiuretic hormone [SIADH]), there may be an increase in free water. The urine sodium level in those with euvolemic hyponatremia is concentrated at greater than 20 mEq/L. A hypervolemic patient has edema from heart, liver, or renal disease or overt renal failure. The urinary sodium concentration is usually very high in those with renal failure.

Keep in mind that pseudohyponatremia or factitious hyponatremia may also occur. Pseudohyponatremia is a laboratory measurement error that occurs when excessive protein or lipid is present in plasma. Hyperproteinemia or hyperlipidemia increases plasma volume by decreasing the percentage of plasma that is free water. Some laboratory machines measure and report the sodium concentration in terms of the volume of total plasma rather than plasma water, and therefore the sodium concentration is artificially low. A clue to the presence of pseudohyponatremia is normal plasma osmolality despite a low serum sodium concentration. Factitious hyponatremia is redistribution of water from the intracellular to the extracellular compartment because of excessive extracellular osmolality. Hyperglycemia or the administration of mannitol increases plasma osmolality, thereby resulting in a shift of free water and a fall in the sodium concentration. In general,

$$\text{Decrease in sodium (mEq/L)} = 1.6 \, \text{mEq/L} \infty \text{Increase in blood glucose/100 mg/dL}$$

Manifestations

The clinical manifestations depend in part on the volume status of the child and the underlying cause of the hyponatremia. When hyponatremia develops rapidly (<24 hours) and when it is severe (<120 mEq/L), the following may occur as a result of the intracellular shift of water:
1. Altered mental status
2. Seizures
3. Nausea and vomiting
4. Muscle cramps and weakness
5. Coma

Management

Determine the hydration status of the child and the severity of the hyponatremia.

Hypovolemic Patients

Most children with hyponatremia are dehydrated and hypovolemic, without symptoms such as altered mental status or seizures.

These children can be managed as outlined in the Diarrhea and Dehydration chapter, with gradual replacement of the sodium and water deficit over a 24-hour period.

If altered mental status or seizures are present, more rapid correction of the decreased concentration may be necessary. In this situation, hypertonic saline solution (either 3% or 5%, containing 513 and 855 mEq/L of sodium, respectively) should be administered, with the goal of raising the serum sodium concentration to 125 mEq/L. The following formula can be used to calculate the number of milliequivalents of sodium necessary to achieve this concentration:

$$\text{Sodium (mEq) required} = (125 - \text{Current serum Na}) \times 0.6 \times \text{Weight (kg)}$$

The total required should be infused over a period of approximately 4 hours or at a rate of 5 mEq/kg/hr. Once the serum sodium concentration reaches approximately 125 mEq/L, further corrections of the sodium deficit can proceed as discussed in Chapter 15.

Euvolemic Patients

Euvolemic patients or those with slight increases in extracellular volume usually require water restriction. SIADH production (most often associated with meningitis) or water intoxication are the most likely causes. Restriction to two-thirds of the maintenance fluid requirement is the usual initial treatment; adjustments may be necessary, with frequent monitoring of the serum sodium level. If the child is symptomatic, with seizures or altered mental status, the serum sodium concentration may be increased by combining hypertonic saline solution and diuresis with IV furosemide. In this way, excessive free water is diuresed because a more hypertonic solution is being infused, thereby preventing a further increase in extracellular volume. The same formula discussed for hypovolemic patients may be used to calculate the required amount of sodium to be administered. Serum electrolytes (including potassium) should be measured frequently during such treatment because hypokalemia may ensue during diuresis.

Hypervolemic Patients

Salt and water restriction is required for those with edema-forming states or renal failure. Diuresis with furosemide also helps to decrease extracellular volume. As with hypovolemia and euvolemia, a child with severe, symptomatic hyponatremia may require hypertonic saline solution, which should be combined with diuretics. Dialysis may be necessary for those in renal failure.

HYPERKALEMIA (SERUM POTASSIUM >5.5 MEQ/L)

Causes

Decreased excretion
Renal failure (acute or chronic)
Potassium-sparing diuretics (amiloride, triamterene, spironolactone)
Adrenal insufficiency
Distal tubular dysfunction (type IV renal tubular acidosis)
Impaired extrarenal regulation
    Diabetes mellitus
    Drugs (β-blockers, succinylcholine, angiotensin-converting enzyme inhibitors)
Shift from intracellular to extracellular fluid
    Acidosis
    Tissue destruction (trauma, hemolysis, burns, tumor lysis, rhabdomyolysis)
    Hyperkalemic periodic paralysis
Increased intake
    Potassium supplements (IV or orally)
    Blood transfusions
    Salt substitutes
Factitious
    Difficulty drawing blood (hemolysis, as with a heel puncture)
    Thrombocytosis

Manifestations

The effects of hyperkalemia on the cardiac conduction system are the most significant and may be fatal. The progressive changes that can be seen on an electrocardiogram (ECG) as the serum potassium concentration rises are, in order,

1. Peaked T waves (serum potassium, 6 to 7 mEq/L)
2. Depressed ST segments
3. Decreased R wave amplitude
4. Prolonged PR interval (serum potassium, 7 to 8 mEq/L)
5. Small or absent P waves
6. Wide QRS complexes (serum potassium, 8 to 9 mEq/L)
7. Sine wave pattern
8. Asystole or dysrhythmias

In addition, hyperkalemia may cause paresthesias, muscle weakness, and decreased tendon reflexes as a result of depolarization of muscle cells.

Management

Determine the severity of the hyperkalemia. All patients with hyperkalemia should have an ECG performed immediately to search for the signs just listed. Continuous ECG monitoring is also necessary until the problem is corrected.

Severe Hyperkalemia

If the serum potassium level is greater than 8 mEq/L or ECG changes other than peaked T waves are seen, you should proceed as follows:

1. Notify your supervisor.
2. Remove any potassium from the IV fluids
3. Administer 10% calcium gluconate, 0.5 mL/kg IV over a 2- to 5-minute period. This does not change the serum potassium level but protects the heart from the effects of hyperkalemia. The onset of action is immediate, and effects last approximately 1 hour.
4. Administer sodium bicarbonate, 1 to 2 mEq/kg IV over a 3- to 5-minute period. Make sure to flush the calcium gluconate from the line before giving bicarbonate because the two may be incompatible. The sodium bicarbonate shifts potassium intracellularly; its effect is immediate and lasts for 1 to 2 hours.
5. Administer glucose, 0.5 g/kg, with 0.3 unit of insulin per gram of glucose over a period of 2 hours.
6. Nebulized albuterol will move potassium intracellularly by stimulating β_1-adrenergic receptors.
7. Sodium polystyrene sulfonate (Kayexalate), 1 to 2 g/kg, with 3 mL of sorbitol per gram of resin divided every 6 hours orally or 5 mL of sorbitol per gram of resin as an enema over a period of 4 to 6 hours. This is the only drug treatment that removes potassium from the body. It is estimated that 1 g/kg decreases the serum potassium concentration by 1 mEq/L.
8. If these measures are unsuccessful, hemodialysis is necessary.
9. The serum potassium concentration should be determined every hour until it is less than 6.5 mEq/L.

Moderate Hyperkalemia

If the serum potassium level is between 6.5 and 8 mEq/L and the ECG reveals only peaked T waves, you should proceed as follows:

1. Notify your supervisor.
2. Remove any potassium from the IV fluids.
3. Administer sodium bicarbonate, glucose and insulin, and Kayexalate in the doses outlined earlier.
4. Monitor the serum potassium level every hour until it is less than 6.5 mEq/L.

Mild Hyperkalemia

If the serum potassium level is less than 6.5 mEq/L and the ECG is normal or has peaked T waves only, you should consider correcting other contributing factors (e.g., acidosis), as well as administering Kayexalate as previously outlined. Potassium should again be removed from any IV fluids. If the cause is identified and is not progressive, the serum potassium measurement can be repeated in 4 hours.

HYPOKALEMIA (SERUM POTASSIUM <3.5 MEQ/L)

Causes
Excessive renal losses
    Diuretics
    Antibiotics (penicillins, amphotericin, aminoglycosides)
    Glucocorticoid excess
    Renal tubular acidosis type I
    Hyperaldosteronism
    Vomiting, nasogastric suctioning leading to alkalosis
Extrarenal losses
    Vomiting
    Diarrhea
    Laxative abuse
Shift from extracellular to intracellular space
    Alkalosis
    Insulin
    β-Catecholamines
    Lithium
Inadequate intake

Manifestations
As with hyperkalemia, the cardiac effects are the most significant and include the following:
1. Premature atrial contractions
2. Premature ventricular contractions (PVCs)
3. Flattened T waves
4. Appearance of U waves
5. ST-segment depression
    In addition, neuromuscular symptoms and signs may appear, such as weakness, paresthesias, ileus, and depressed tendon reflexes.

Management
Determine the severity of the hypokalemia. All patients should have an ECG performed and undergo continuous ECG monitoring until the problem is corrected.

Severe Hypokalemia
If the serum potassium level is less than 2.5 mEq/L and there are PVCs, U waves, or ST-segment changes, IV supplementation of

potassium should be considered. Potassium chloride, 0.5 to 1 mEq/kg, up to 10 mEq maximum, can be given IV over a 1-hour period while the patient is continually monitored with cardiac monitor. The serum potassium level should be measured again in 1 hour. Further supplementation can proceed more slowly by adding up to 40 mEq/L of potassium to an IV solution and infusing at the standard maintenance rate.

Moderate or Mild Hypokalemia

In those with a serum potassium level greater than 2.5 mEq/L and no ECG changes, hypokalemia may often respond to correction of the underlying cause, with no need for supplementation. If supplementation is necessary, oral supplements should be sufficient. The serum potassium level should be measured again in 4 to 6 hours to ensure that it does not continue to fall.

HYPERCALCEMIA

Causes

Increased intake
    Vitamin D or A intoxication
    Excessive calcium supplementation
    Milk-alkali syndrome (antacid ingestion)
Increased production or mobilization from bone
    Hyperparathyroidism (primary or tertiary)
    Hyperthyroidism
    Immobilization
    Malignancies (bone metastases, tumor lysis syndrome)
    Sarcoidosis
Decreased excretion
    Thiazide diuretics
    Familial hypocalciuric hypercalcemia
Miscellaneous
    Williams syndrome
    Pheochromocytoma
    Adrenal insufficiency

Manifestations

"Stones, bones, groans, and psychic moans" refer to some of the manifestations of hypercalcemia. Renal stones may develop, and polyuria and polydipsia are also common because hypercalcemia reduces the ability to concentrate urine. Bone pain ("bones") and abdominal symptoms ("groans"), such as pain, nausea, constipation, vomiting, and pancreatitis, may also occur. "Psychic moans" may be manifested as delirium, dementia, psychosis, lethargy, and even coma.

The ECG may reveal a short QT interval and a prolonged PR interval. Dysrhythmias may develop if the hypercalcemia is severe enough.

Management

Determine the severity of the hypercalcemia. Approximately half the total serum calcium is bound to albumin, and the other half is present in a free or ionized form. The clinical effect of hypercalcemia depends on the amount that is unbound or the ionized calcium. Most laboratories routinely report total calcium, which reflects both ionized calcium and calcium that is bound to albumin. Thus, in hypoalbuminemic states, there may be an increase in ionized calcium despite normal serum total calcium. A useful assumption that can allow you to estimate the ionized calcium is that each 1-g/dL decrease in serum albumin decreases bound calcium (and total calcium) by approximately 0.8 mg/dL.

Severe Hypercalcemia

A serum calcium level greater than 14 mg/dL or the presence of symptoms requires immediate treatment. The serum calcium concentration can be reduced by rapid expansion of intravascular volume. Infusing a bolus of 20 mL/kg of normal saline solution results in a reduction in serum calcium concentration as a result of hemodilution and the increase in urinary calcium excretion that accompanies the excess sodium excreted in urine. Urinary calcium excretion can also be promoted with IV furosemide, 1 mg/kg every 2 to 4 hours. While you are monitoring the child's volume status closely, the normal saline boluses and furosemide may be repeated and should result in a fall in the serum calcium concentration. If it does not begin to decrease soon after volume expansion and diuresis, hemodialysis should be considered. Hemodialysis should be considered initially if the serum calcium concentration is greater than 15 mg/dL or the child has severe symptoms (e.g., coma).

Mild or Moderate Hypercalcemia

If the serum calcium concentration is less than 14 mg/dL, you may proceed at a less urgent pace. As with severe hypercalcemia, volume expansion and diuresis help to increase urinary excretion of calcium. Increasing the IV rate to slightly expand intravascular volume after an initial 20-mL/kg bolus of normal saline solution may be sufficient. Likewise, IV furosemide, 1 mg/kg every 3 to 4 hours, should result in a gradual fall in the serum calcium concentration. Prednisone, 1 mg/kg/day, may be helpful because it decreases intestinal absorption of calcium by blocking the effect of 1,25-dihydroxyvitamin D. The effect of prednisone should be apparent within 2 to 3 days. Bisphosphonates and calcitonin are additional potential therapies because they inhibit bone resorption, but they should be used only after consultation with a pediatric endocrinologist.

HYPOCALCEMIA

Causes

Decreased intake
  Vitamin D deficiency (malabsorption, nutritional deficiency, abnormal vitamin D metabolism, lack of sunlight)
  Short bowel syndrome
Decreased production or mobilization
  Hypoparathyroidism
  Pseudohypoparathyroidism
  Vitamin D deficiency
  Hyperphosphatemia
  Magnesium deficiency
  Pancreatitis
  Rhabdomyolysis
  Alkalosis
Increased excretion
  Chronic renal failure
  Drugs (loop diuretics, aminoglycosides)
  Exchange transfusion in neonates

Manifestations

Papilledema, abdominal pain, mental status changes, laryngospasm (stridor), carpopedal spasm, seizures, and paresthesias may all occur. The ECG may reveal a prolonged QT interval. Chvostck sign and Trousseau sign may be present (Figs. 34.2 and 34.3).

Management

Determine the severity of the hypocalcemia by the presence and type of symptoms. An asymptomatic patient does not require urgent correction of the calcium concentration. IV calcium administration entails some special risks (see later); therefore it should be reserved for those who cannot take oral calcium or whose symptoms demand immediate correction.

As with hypercalcemia, first correct for the serum albumin concentration. Hypoalbuminemia is common in hospitalized children, and the ionized calcium concentration may be normal despite a significant reduction in the total serum calcium concentration.

Remember also to check the serum phosphate concentration. If it is markedly elevated, you need to consider correcting the phosphate concentration before administering calcium. Metastatic

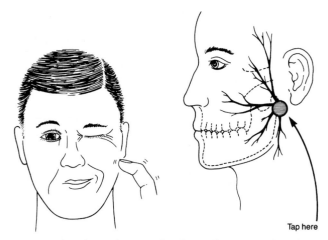

Tap here

FIGURE 34.2 Chvostek sign: facial muscle spasm elicited by tapping the facial nerve anterior to the earlobe and below the zygomatic arch. (From Marshall SA, Ruedy J: On Call: Principles and Protocols, 4th ed. Philadelphia, Elsevier, 2004, p 331.)

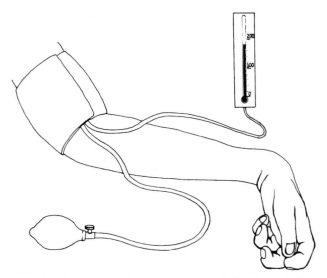

FIGURE 34.3 Trousseau sign: carpal spasm elicited by occluding arterial blood flow to the forearm for 3 to 5 minutes. (From Marshall SA, Ruedy J: On Call: Principles and Protocols, 4th ed. Philadelphia, Elsevier, 2004, p 332.)

calcification may occur if the serum phosphate concentration remains high as calcium is administered.

A symptomatic child should be treated with 10% IV calcium gluconate, 100 to 200 mg/kg over a period of 5 to 10 minutes. Additional doses can be given if necessary. If possible, peripheral infusion of calcium should be avoided. Extravasation of calcium may result in significant tissue necrosis. Scalp veins and other small peripheral veins should be avoided when infusing calcium solutions. Hypotension and bradycardia are also potential effects of calcium infusion; therefore all patients should be monitored while receiving an infusion. Once the symptoms of hypocalcemia have resolved, oral calcium supplementation can be started. Elemental calcium can be given in a dosage of 50 mg/kg/day divided into three to four doses.

An asymptomatic child with hypocalcemia may be treated with oral elemental calcium in the same doses as just listed.

There are several circumstances in which caution is necessary in the treatment of hypocalcemia. In children with abnormal calcium mobilization, such as those with pancreatitis or rhabdomyolysis, care should be taken when correcting the serum calcium concentration because hypercalcemia may eventually result from the release of complexed calcium when the pancreatitis or rhabdomyolysis resolves. In a child with acidosis, the ionized calcium concentration will be increased because of displacement of calcium from albumin. Correction of the acidosis may cause the ionized calcium level to fall even further. Finally, in those with hypomagnesemia, parathyroid hormone release is impaired and the tissue response to parathyroid hormone is also diminished. The magnesium concentration will need to be corrected to treat the hypocalcemia effectively.

REMEMBER

The most important element of the management of any electrolyte problem is close monitoring with repeated measurement of electrolytes to gauge the effect of your treatment plan. The approaches outlined in this chapter allow you to begin thinking about the problem and to initiate a treatment plan, but repeated reevaluation of the patient's clinical status and laboratory studies is essential.

Glucose Disorders

Alison Coren, MD

Glucose is the preferred substrate for most cellular processes. It is particularly important for cerebral metabolism because the brain cannot use free fatty acids and is only partially supported by ketones.

Glucose Homeostasis

Glucose is absorbed in the small intestine and, transported through the bloodstream and into the liver and pancreas via insulin-independent GLUT-2 transporters. Insulin is released by beta cells in the pancreatic islets of Langerhans in response to rising glucose. It stimulates peripheral glucose uptake and glycogen synthesis and inhibits endogenous glucose production and free fatty acid oxidation. Counterregulatory processes maintain euglycemia by suppressing insulin secretion and stimulating glycogenolysis, gluconeogenesis, and lipolysis, most importantly through glucagon, epinephrine, cortisol, and growth hormone.

Hypoglycemia

Symptoms of hypoglycemia stem from the brain's response to glucose deprivation. Neurogenic symptoms (e.g., palpitations, tremor, anxiety, sweating, hunger, parethesias) precede neuroglycopenic symptoms (e.g., confusion, coma, seizures). Symptoms typically occur when the plasma glucose decreases to 50 to 70 mg/dL, although repeated episodes of hypoglycemia blunt awareness and impair hepatic glucose release, perpetuating hypoglycemia. Common causes of hypoglycemia are listed in Table 35.1.

Transient hypoglycemia is expected in the first 24 to 48 hours of life as neonates transition from intrauterine to extrauterine life. Critical labs should be obtained prior to treatment in all neonates >48 hours and children with a blood glucose <60 mg/dL. All point-of-care glucose values should be confirmed using a clinical laboratory method. Bicarbonate, β-hydroxybutarate, lactate, and free

TABLE 35.1	Causes of Hypoglycemia
Inborn errors of metabolism	Glycogen storage diseases
	Gluconeogenesis defects
	Fatty acid oxidation defects
Hyperinsulinism	Infant of a diabetic mother
	Congenital hyperinsulinism
	Insulinoma
	Exogenous administration of insulin
Hormone deficiencies	Hypopituitarism
	Cortisol deficiency
	Growth hormone deficiency
Drugs	Oral hypoglycemics
	Alcohol
	Salicylates
	β-Blockers
Other	Starvation
	Postsurgical dumping syndrome
	Ketotic hypoglycemia

fatty acids are useful for narrowing the differential diagnosis (Fig. 35.1). Consider checking additional labs if a particular diagnosis is suspected.

Treatment should not be delayed if the blood sample cannot be collected quickly. If the child is able to eat, then 15 to 20 g of simple carbohydrate is given. If not, then 2 mL/kg of 10% dextrose is given as an intravenous bolus, followed by 10% dextrose at maintenance with the goal to keep glucose >70 mg/dL. Long-term management depends on the underlying etiology and may include adherence to a particular diet, medication, surgery, and/or consultation with a subspecialist.

Hyperglycemia

Hyperglycemia may be a sign of diabetes mellitus but is also seen in response to stress and some medications (Table 35.2). Symptoms of hypoglycemia may not appear until the concentration of serum glucose exceeds the capacity of the proximal renal tubule to reabsorb glucose, which occurs at approximately 180 mg/dL. Glucosuria drives the classic symptoms of polyuria, polydipsia, polyphagia, and weight loss. The diagnosis of diabetes mellitus is made if the child meets any of the following criteria: random plasma glucose ≥200 mg/dL, plasma glucose ≥126 mg/dL after an eight hour fast on two separate occasions, plasma glucose ≥200 mg/dL two hours after a 75 gram glucose load, or hemoglobin A1C >6.5%. If the diagnosis is unclear, repeat testing should be performed.

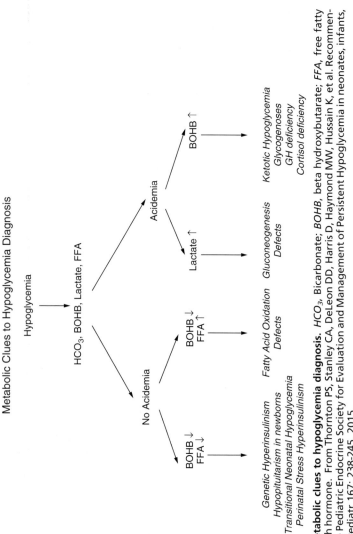

FIGURE 35.1 Metabolic clues to hypoglycemia diagnosis. *HCO₃,* Bicarbonate; *BOHB,* beta hydroxybutarate; *FFA,* free fatty acids; *GH,* growth hormone. From Thornton PS, Stanley CA, DeLeon DD, Harris D, Haymond MW, Hussain K, et al. Recommendations from the Pediatric Endocrine Society for Evaluation and Management of Persistent Hypoglycemia in neonates, infants, and children. J Pediatr 167: 238-245, 2015.

TABLE 35.2	Causes of Hyperglycemia
Stress	Acute illness/sepsis
	Trauma
	Surgery
	Burns
Drugs	Parenteral administration of dextrose
	Atypical antipsychotics
	β-Blockers
	Corticosteroids
	Calcineurin inhibitors
	Protease inhibitors
	Thiazide and thiazide-like diuretics
Diabetes mellitus	Type 1 diabetes mellitus
	Type 2 diabetes mellitus
	Neonatal diabetes
	Maturity-onset diabetes of the young
	Cystic fibrosis—related diabetes

Type 1 Diabetes Mellitus

Type 1 diabetes mellitus (T1DM) is caused by the autoimmune destruction of the insulin-producing pancreatic beta cells. Autoantibodies may be detected in the blood and distinguish T1DM from other types of diabetes mellitus.

Treatment requires insulin replacement. Children with long-standing T1DM typically require between 0.7 and 1 unit/kg/day of insulin. Children with new-onset T1DM may present in "honeymoon," a phase in which they have residual endogenous insulin secretion from remaining beta cells, and require less exogenous insulin. Pubescent children may experience a period of insulin resistance and require more exogenous insulin. Many different insulin analogues and regimens are available (Table 35.3 and Table 35.4). About 1/3 of the total daily insulin dose is given as the basal dose and 2/3 is given as bolus doses with meals.

Approximately 25% of children with T1DM present in diabetic ketoacidosis (DKA). Children with known diabetes may also develop DKA when they deliberately or inadvertently miss insulin or experience illness or trauma that overwhelm homeostatic mechanisms. Signs and symptoms include dehydration, tachycardia, tachypnea, Kussmal respirations, nausea, vomiting, abdominal pain, confusion, drowsiness, and progressive loss of consciousness. Laboratory findings include hyperglycemia, metabolic acidosis (pH <7.30, bicarbonate <15 mmol/L), and ketonemia.

Treatment of DKA starts with fluid resuscitation. A 10 to 20 ml/kg normal saline bolus is given over 1-2 hours and repeated

TABLE 35.3	Types of Insulin
Rapid acting	Lispro (Humalog)
	Aspart (Novolog)
	Glulisine (Apidra)
Short acting	Regular insulin
Intermediate acting	Neutral Protamine Hagedorn (Novolin N, Humalin N)
Long acting	Glargine (Lantus)
	Detemir (Levemir)

TABLE 35.4	Insulin Regimens
Method	**Description**
Basal-bolus	Long-acting insulin is given once daily; rapid-acting insulin is given with meals and snacks
Mixed-split	Intermediate-acting and short-acting insulin are given twice daily with breakfast and dinner
Insulin pump	Continuous subcutaneous rapid acting insulin infusion; boluses are given with meals and snacks

until peripheral perfusion is restored. Subsequent fluid management includes intravenous fluids with a tonicity $\geq 0.45\%$ saline with added potassium, typically 20 mmol/L potassium phosphate and 20 mmol/L potassium chloride or acetate. The goal is to replace the estimated 5% to 10% fluid deficit plus daily maintenance fluid requirements over 48 hours. Usually hyperglycemia resolves before ketoacidosis, so dextrose is added when the plasma glucose drops below 250 to 300 or sooner if the drop is precipitous. An insulin drip infusing at 0.05 to 0.1 unit/kg/hr is started after the initial fluid bolus and continued until the ketoacidosis resolves. Children must be closely monitored with hourly vitals, neurological exams, and point of care glucose checks. Electrolytes are checked every 2-4 hours. Blood urea nitrogen, calcium, magnesium, and phosphorus are often abnormal due to dehydration and urinary losses secondary to DKA. The abnormalities typically resolve with treatment and are followed if abnormal.

Cerebral edema occurs in 0.5% to 1% of children who present in DKA and is associated with a high rate of morbidity and mortality. Risk factors include young age, new onset diabetes, severe DKA, and aggressive initial fluid resuscitation. It usually occurs 4 to 12 hours after starting treatment. Signs and symptoms include headache, vomiting, altered mental status, incontinence, and Cushing triad. Prompt administration of mannitol 1 g/kg or

3% hypertonic saline 5 mL/kg is given over 10 to 15 minutes and repeated if there is no response in 30 minutes.

Type 2 Diabetes Mellitus

Type 2 diabetes mellitus (T2DM) results from insulin resistance and relative insulin deficiency. Some factors that help to distinguish T1DM from T2DM include insidious onset; onset after puberty; association with obesity and other features of metabolic syndrome; presence of acanthosis nigricans; absence of autoantibodies; family history of T2DM; as well as and nonwhite European descent. Many children with T2DM have signs of microvascular and macrovascular complications at the time of diagnosis, including nephropathy, retinopathy, and neuropathy.

All children are encouraged to make lifestyle modifications to promote a healthy diet and exercise. Metformin monotherapy is started in children with a hemoglobin A1C <9. Metformin may cause gastrointestinal upset, so the dose is started at 500 mg daily and increased by 500 mg per week to a maximum dose of 1000 mg twice daily. Insulin is added in children with a hemoglobin A1C ≥9 and those who have not achieved a hemoglobin A1C <6.5 after 6 months of Metformin monotherapy. Other pharmacologic agents may be used but are not U.S. Food and Drug Administration (FDA) approved in children.

Hyperglycemic hyperosmolar state (HHS) is a rare but life-threatening complication of T2DM. Children may present with altered mental status or seizures. Laboratory findings include marked hyperglycemia (plasma glucose >600 mg/dL), hyperosmolality (serum osmolality >330 mOsm/kg), severe dehydration, and little to no ketonuria.

There are no prospective data to guide management of children and adolescents with HHS; however, guidelines have been extrapolated from adult literature. The mainstay of treatment is to replace the fluid deficit, which is estimated to be at least 12% to 15% of body weight. Normal saline boluses are given to restore peripheral perfusion, followed by intravenous fluids with 0.45 to 0.75% NaCl at a rate to replace the fluid deficit over 24 to 48 hours. The goal is to reduce the sodium by 0.5 mmol/L/hr and glucose by 75 to 100 mg/dL/hr. Serum glucose typically drops rapidly with fluid resuscitation. Once the rate of decline is <50 mg/dL/hr, an insulin drip may be added at 0.025 to 0.05 unit/kg/hr to achieve a decrease in serum glucose of 50 to 75 mg/dL/hr.

Monogenic Diabetes

Monogenetic diabetes occurs in 1% to 4% of children with diabetes. Monogenetic forms of diabetes may present similarly to T1DM and T2DM. Neonatal diabetes mellitus should be considered in infants diagnosed with diabetes mellitus at less than 6 months old. Maturity-onset diabetes of the young should be considered in children and adolescents who have a family history of diabetes in multiple successive generations and an absence of autoantibodies and risk factors for T2DM. Genetic testing confirms the diagnosis. Depending on the variant, some monogenic forms of diabetes can be treated with oral hyperglycemic medications, such as sulfonylureas.

Cystic Fibrosis–Related Diabetes

Cystic fibrosis (CF) is caused by a mutation in the CF transmembrane conductance regulator, which is present in the beta cell. Cystic fibrosis–related diabetes (CFRD) primarily results from damage to the islet cells and subsequent insulin insufficiency. It also results from insulin resistance, particularly during acute illnesses and secondary to medications such as glucocorticoids. Children may experience an insidious decline in clinical status in the years leading up to diagnosis. Screening with an oral glucose tolerance test should start at age 10. Insulin replacement is the only recommended medical treatment. Most patients require between 0.5 and 0.8 unit/kg/day when they are at their baseline states of health but may require much higher levels when sick.

Discussion

Physicians should have a high index of suspicion for glucose disorders and be prepared to quickly manage patients with hypoglycemia and hyperglycemia.

CHAPTER 36

Hyperbilirubinemia

Keli Coleman, MD

Hyperbilirubinemia is characterized by excess bilirubin in the blood. An accumulation of bilirubin, a breakdown product of heme, leads to a yellowing of the skin, mucous membranes, and sclerae known as jaundice. Jaundice is not a disease but is a clinical sign of an underlying medical condition associated with hyperbilirubinemia that needs to be investigated further. In adults, jaundice is most often associated with hepatic disorders. In children, although similar potentially severe hepatic illnesses may also be associated with jaundice, most cases of jaundice are transient and without significant consequences. The pediatrician must complete an evaluation to determine the etiology of hyperbilirubinemia and then plan the appropriate intervention. Jaundice in a hospitalized child rarely has an acute onset. The pediatrician on call may be the first to be notified of hyperbilirubinemia, and it is most commonly identified in the newborn nursery.

PHONE CALL

Questions

1. What is the child's age?
2. What are the child's vital signs?
3. Does the child appear ill?
4. What is the child's admitting diagnosis?
5. Has the child ever been jaundiced before?
6. Is the child receiving any medications?

Orders

Obtain the following laboratory tests as soon as possible:
1. Total and direct serum bilirubin level
2. Alkaline phosphatase (ALP), alanine transaminase (ALT), aspartate transaminase (AST), γ-glutamyltransferase (GGT), and lactate dehydrogenase (LDH)

3. Complete blood count, reticulocyte count, and peripheral blood smear
4. In a newborn the mother's and infant's blood types and a Coombs' test will also be helpful

Inform RN

Tell the RN, "I will arrive at the bedside in ... minutes."

Hyperbilirubinemia is rarely life threatening, but in younger children it deserves timely evaluation. In neonates the evaluation should be immediate because in some instances the rise in bilirubin may be rapid and severe and accompanied by life-threatening anemia or place the newborn at risk for kernicterus.

ELEVATOR THOUGHTS

The differential diagnosis of jaundice is extensive. Jaundice in a neonate usually has different potential causes than jaundice in an older child. Direct (conjugated) hyperbilirubinemia and indirect (unconjugated) hyperbilirubinemia are also associated with different causes (Fig. 36.1 and Tables 36.1 and 36.2).

MAJOR THREAT TO LIFE

- Hemolytic anemia–mediated shock, heart failure, or nephropathy
- Kernicterus
- Liver Failure

Hyperbilirubinemia is generally most threatening when its onset is rapid and the bilirubin is unconjugated. In the relatively immature central nervous system of a neonate, especially if premature, unconjugated bilirubin may be deposited in the basal ganglia, hippocampus, and subthalamic nuclei of the brain and can result in severe brain damage and hearing loss.

BEDSIDE

Quick-Look Test

Does the patient appear well (comfortable), sick (uncomfortable or distressed), or critical?

A general rule to follow in estimating the serum bilirubin level in a neonate is that the sclerae become icteric at a bilirubin level of 2 to 4 mg/dL, the face and mucous membrane at a level of 4 to 7, the chest and abdomen at a level of 8 to 10, the legs at levels greater than 12, and the soles of the feet at levels greater than 15. Remember, this is a very rough estimate, and a serum level must be obtained to accurately assess the magnitude of the jaundice. Does the patient exhibit any signs of hemodynamic instability or neurologic deficits?

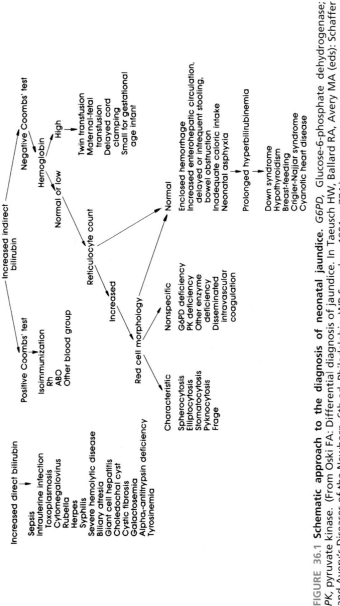

FIGURE 36.1 **Schematic approach to the diagnosis of neonatal jaundice.** *G6PD,* Glucose-6-phosphate dehydrogenase; *PK,* pyruvate kinase. (From Oski FA: Differential diagnosis of jaundice. In Taeusch HW, Ballard RA, Avery MA (eds): Schaffer and Avery's Diseases of the Newborn, 6th ed. Philadelphia, WB Saunders, 1991, p 774.)

TABLE 36.1   Diagnostic Features of the Various Types of Neonatal Jaundice

Diagnosis	Nature of van den Bergh Reaction	Jaundice Appears	Jaundice Disappears	Peak Bilirubin Concentration mg/dL	Age (days)	Bilirubin Rate of Accumulation (mg/dL/day)	Remarks
"Physiologic jaundice"							Usually related to degree of maturity
Full-term	Indirect	2-3 days	4-5 days	10-12	2-3	<5	
Preterm	Indirect	3-4 days	7-9 days	15	6-8	<5	
Hyperbilirubinemia as a result of metabolic factors							Metabolic factors: hypoxia, respiratory distress, lack of carbohydrate
Full-term	Indirect	2-3 days	Variable	<2	1st wk	<5	Thyroid
Premature	Indirect	3-4 days	Variable	<15	1st wk	<5	Genetic factors Drugs
Hemolytic states and hematoma	Indirect	May appear in 1st 24 hr	Variable	Unlimited	Variable	Usually >5	Drugs
Mixed hemolytic and hepatotoxic factors	Indirect and direct	May appear in 1st 24 hr	Variable	Unlimited	Variable	Usually >5	Infection
Hepatocellular damage	Indirect and direct	Usually 2-3 days	Variable	Unlimited	Variable	Variable, can be >5	

From Brown AK: Neonatal jaundice. Pediatr Clin North Am 9:589, 1962.

TABLE 36.2 Differential Diagnosis of Jaundice in Childhood

| Unconjugated Hyperbilirubinemia | | | Conjugated Hyperbilirubinemia | | | | | |
| Hemolysis and Reticulocytosis | | No Hemolysis | Obstructive | Infectious | Metabolic | Toxic | Idiopathic | Autoimmune |
Positive Coombs' Test	Negative Coombs' Test							
ABO and Rh incompatibility	RBC enzyme defect (G6PD deficiency)	Gilbert syndrome	Biliary atresia	Hepatitis A, B, C, D, E	Wilson disease	Total parenteral nutrition	Idiopathic neonatal hepatitis	Autoimmune chronic hepatitis
Autoimmune, systemic lupus erythematosus	Hemoglobinopathy (sickle cell anemia)	Physiologic jaundice of the newborn	Choledochal cyst	Cytomegalovirus	α_1-Antitrypsin deficiency	Acetaminophen	Alagille syndrome	Sclerosing cholangitis
Drug-induced and idiopathic acquired hemolytic anemia	RBC membrane defect (hereditary spherocytosis)	Breast milk jaundice	Cholelithiasis	Herpes simplex 1, 2, 6	Galactosemia	Ethanol	Nonsyndromic paucity of intrahepatic bile ducts	Graft-versus-host disease
	Hemolytic-uremic syndrome	Crigler-Najjar syndrome	Tumor/neoplasia	Epstein-Barr virus	Tyrosinemia	Salicylates	Progressive familial intrahepatic cholestasis	
	Wilson disease	Hypothyroidism	Bile duct stenosis	Coxsackievirus	Fructosemia	Iron	Familial benign recurrent cholestasis	
		Pyloric stenosis	Spontaneous bile duct perforation	Echovirus	Niemann-Pick disease	Halothane	Cholestasis with lymphedema (Aagenaes syndrome)	
		Internal hemorrhage	Bile-mucous plug	Measles	Gaucher disease	Isoniazid	Cholestasis with hypopituitarism	
				Varicella	Zellweger syndrome	Valproic acid	Familial erythrophagocytic lymphohistiocytosis	
				Syncytial giant cell (paramyxovirus)	Wolman disease	Venoocclusive disease		
				Toxoplasmosis	Cystic fibrosis			
				Syphilis	Neonatal iron storage disease			
				Leptospirosis	Indian childhood cirrhosis			
				Bacterial sepsis/urinary tract infection (especially gram negative)	Trihydroxypro stanic acidemia			
				Cholecystitis				
				Fitz-Hugh–Curtis syndrome				

G6PD, Glucose-6-phosphate dehydrogenase; *RBC*, red blood cell.

From Behrman RE, Kliegman RM: Nelson Essentials of Pediatrics, 2nd ed. Philadelphia, WB Saunders, 1994.

Airway and Vital Signs

Tachycardia, pallor, respiratory distress, and poor perfusion can be seen with severe hemolytic processes that can cause heart failure. Fever may represent systemic infection such as sepsis. Children with severe hepatic dysfunction usually appear quite ill.

Selective Physical Examination

HEENT	The sclerae and mucous membranes (especially under the tongue) are very good places to assess jaundice, particularly in darker pigmented children; cephalohematoma or excessive bruising
Cardiovascular	Heart rate, pulse volume, blood pressure, perfusion, jugular venous distention
Abdomen	Distention, hepatosplenomegaly, masses, tenderness, ascites (fluid wave), caput medusa, incision scars
Neurologic	Mental status, tone (axial as well as segmental in infants), cranial nerves, quality of cry, primitive reflexes (Moro, grasp, suck, tonic-neck), motor function

HEENT, Head, Eyes, Ears, Nose, Throat.

Acute cardiac failure can occur with severe hemolytic processes. A change in color of the urine would also be expected with severe hemolysis.

Management

Diagnostic investigation depends largely on the age of the child and the presence of associated findings besides jaundice. The two most common scenarios are discussed in this chapter: (1) a neonate in the nursery or on the inpatient floor whose laboratory results indicate a high bilirubin level is brought to the attention of the on-call pediatrician and (2) a child in whom jaundice develops acutely during a hospitalization.

Neonatal Hyperbilirubinemia

Neonatal hyperbilirubinemia is defined as a total serum or plasma bilirubin greater than 95th percentile on the hour-specific nomogram in a 35-week gestational age or older infant or a total serum concentration of bilirubin greater than 5 mg/dL (86 μmol/L) (Fig. 36.2). Infants at risk for developing neonatal hyperbilirubinemia include premature babies, and infants admitted to rule out sepsis immediately after birth due to prolonged rupture of membranes, maternal chorioamnionitis, or respiratory distress.

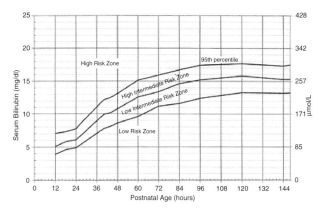

FIGURE 36.2 **Nomogram to determine the risk of specific elevations in serum bilirubin.** (From American Academy of Pediatrics Subcommittee on Hyperbilirubinemia: Management of hyperbilirubinemia in the newborn infant 35 or more weeks of gestation. Pediatrics 114:297-316, 2004.)

Hyperbilirubinemia within the first 24 hours of birth is worrisome. A rapid rise in unconjugated bilirubin in the first 24 hours is common in hemolytic processes involving ABO incompatibility between the infant and the mother, concealed hematoma or hemorrhage, cytomegalovirus infection, sepsis, congenital rubella, or congenital toxoplasmosis. Laboratory evaluation should be initiated immediately and include a complete blood count and peripheral smear, reticulocyte count, ABO type and screen, direct and indirect Coombs' tests, total and direct bilirubin, and serum albumin. Acute hemolytic anemia in a newborn may require not only simple transfusion but also partial or complete exchange transfusion. A cord hemoglobin level of 10 g/dL, a bilirubin level of 5 mg/dL or greater on the first day of life, and a reticulocyte count of 15% or more suggest severe hemolytic anemia and may require at least partial exchange transfusion.

Exchange transfusions require experience and advanced planning to coordinate safely. It is a treatment option reserved for symptomatic infants with severe hyperbilirubinemia that does not decrease adequately with phototherapy. It is prudent to contact an experienced provider to assist with this procedure. Blood for exchange transfusion should be as fresh as possible and be completely cross matched if possible. In acute settings, type O-negative blood may be used. The blood should be warmed to 37 degrees C and should be continuously mixed or gently agitated during the transfusion. The exchange requires large intravenous lines, which in a newborn generally means umbilical venous catheterization (see Chapter 26, Lines, Tubes, and Drains, for the details of umbilical catheterization). When proper positioning of the umbilical line or lines has been confirmed by radiograph, 10- to 20-mL aliquots of blood are withdrawn, alternating with equal volumes of donor blood. Calculation of the total volume of the exchange is based on an estimated total circulating blood volume of 85 mL/kg body weight.

Phototherapy is the treatment of choice for mild indirect hyperbilirubinemia. The infant is placed in a diaper only, or a surgical mask may be used to create a "bikini diaper" so that the maximal amount of skin surface area can be bathed in blue (420- to 470-nm wavelength) light. Bilirubin in the skin absorbs this wavelength, and photoisomerization converts toxic 4Z, 15Z-bilirubin into the unconjugated, configurational isomer 4Z, 15E-bilirubin, which can be excreted without the need for conjugation. One must be conscientious about shielding the eyes of newborn infants from this intense light exposure and monitoring the infant's temperature, regardless of their gestational age. Remember that phototherapy increases the infant's insensible water loss by as much as 20%, and therefore the maintenance fluid requirements of the baby must be adjusted to maintain adequate hydration and ensure good urine output to adequately excrete bilirubin.

The risk to the infant of specific serum bilirubin levels relative to age can be determined by using a nomogram (see Fig. 36.2). Risk factors for the development of severe hyperbilirubinemia are shown in Box 36.1.

In an infant who is 2 to 3 days of age, hyperbilirubinemia may be physiologic and require no intervention if the level remains reasonable. Table 36.1 details several types of jaundice and their onset, along with ranges of bilirubin levels and some of their causes. Levels of 15 mg/dL or less total bilirubin in a full-term infant rarely require intervention. So-called physiologic jaundice, or icterus neonatorum, may be influenced by maternal diabetes, polycythemia, race, male sex, trisomy 21, bruising or cephalohematoma, delayed stooling, oxytocin induction, breastfeeding, and other nonspecific factors.

The diagnosis of physiologic jaundice in term or preterm infants can be established by excluding known causes of neonatal jaundice by history and clinical and laboratory findings, as in Table 36.2. The cause of jaundice should be pursued if (1) hyperbilirubinemia occurs within 24 hours of birth, (2) the level exceeds 12 mg/dL in the absence of risk factors, (3) the level rises at a rate greater than 5 mg/dL/24 hr, or (4) the jaundice persists for longer than 2 weeks.

If the percentage of direct to total bilirubin rises, one must suspect a cholestatic process, hepatocellular damage, or a metabolic disorder (galactosemia, tyrosinemia, α_1-antitrypsin deficiency).

BOX 36.1	Risk Factors for the Development of Severe Hyperbilirubinemia in Infants of 35 or More Weeks' Gestation (in Approximate Order of Importance)

Major Risk Factors

Predischarge TSB or TcB level in the high-risk zone (see Fig. 36.2)

Jaundice observed in the first 24 hr

Blood group incompatibility with a positive direct antiglobulin test, other known hemolytic disease (e.g., G6PD deficiency)

Gestational age of 35-36 weeks

Previous sibling received phototherapy

Cephalohematoma or significant bruising

Exclusive breastfeeding, particularly if nursing is not going well and weight loss is excessive

East Asian race

Minor Risk Factors

Predischarge TSB or TcB level in the high intermediate-risk zone (see Fig. 36.2)

Gestational age of 37-38 weeks

Jaundice observed before discharge

Previous sibling with jaundice

Macrosomic infant of a diabetic mother

Maternal age ≥25 years

Male gender

Decreased Risk[a]

TSB or TcB level in the low-risk zone (see Fig. 36.2)

Gestational age ≥41 weeks

Exclusive bottle feeding

Black race[b]

Discharge from hospital after 72 hr

From American Academy of Pediatrics Subcommittee on Hyperbilirubinemia: Management of hyperbilirubinemia in the newborn infant 35 or more weeks of gestation. Pediatrics 114:297-316, 2004, with permission.

[a]Factors associated with a decreased risk for significant jaundice, listed in order of decreasing importance.

[b]Race as defined by mother's description.

G6PD, Glucose-6-phosphate dehydrogenase; *TcB,* transcutaneous bilirubin; *TSB,* total serum bilirubin.

Direct hyperbilirubinemia is always considered pathologic. Further laboratory testing is necessary, including a prothrombin time (PT) and partial thromboplastin time (PTT) to assess hepatic synthetic function, as well as measurement of the transaminases AST (also known as serum glutamic-oxaloacetic transaminase [SGOT]), ALT (also known as serum glutamate pyruvate transaminase [SGPT]), LDH, ALP, and GGT to assess hepatocellular damage. Testing for cystic fibrosis is indicated, as are abdominal ultrasound studies to determine the integrity of the biliary tree (screening for biliary atresia or a choledochal cyst). Diagnoses such as the latter are also suggested by persistent jaundice in the face of acholic stools and poor weight gain.

Figs. 36.3 and 36.4 present nomograms for the treatment of indirect hyperbilirubinemia in healthy and at-risk term infants with phototherapy and exchange transfusion, respectively.

Acute Jaundice in Children

Jaundice beyond the neonatal period is much less common and is often indicative of an acute, chronic, or critical condition. In this age group, it is important to distinguish between mild, self-limiting conditions and serious liver or hematologic diseases. Acute jaundice in children, especially conjugated hyperbilirubinemia, is almost always a manifestation of severe hepatocellular damage from a hypoxic-ischemic insult, accumulation of a hepatotoxin (acetaminophen ingestion), or acute hepatitis. Because conjugated hyperbilirubinemia is usually a consequence of liver and biliary disease, the initial differential will focus on conditions affecting the liver and biliary tree. These children will benefit from early consultation with a pediatric hepatologist to assist in evaluation and management. As in neonates, accumulation of unconjugated bilirubin in children is usually due to hemolysis of red blood cells with release of bilirubin into the blood. Hemoglobinopathies, erythrocyte enzyme defects, and erythrocyte membrane defects may all cause hemolysis. Conditions that impair the hepatic uptake of bilirubin or conjugation (i.e., Gilbert syndrome and Crigler-Najjar syndrome types I and II) can also increase the level of unconjugated bilirubin in children. Diagnostic evaluation in children is much the same as for neonates. Synthetic hepatic function, as well as hepatocellular injury, must be investigated, as should cholestasis. Acute hepatocellular injury is manifested by an elevation in aminotransferases (AST, ALT), LDH, and GGT regardless of the cause. The most marked transaminase elevations are seen with acute viral hepatitis, hypoxic-ischemic injury, hepatotoxin exposure, and Reye syndrome. A differential rise in ALT or AST can suggest a variety of processes, but usually the two are elevated similarly. Elevation of ALP, 5′-nucleotidases, cholesterol, and conjugated bilirubin suggests obstruction and/or inflammation of the hepatobiliary tract.

Assessment of the synthetic function of the liver is important. The PT and PTT are important functional assays for the various serum globulins manufactured in the liver, particularly vitamin K–dependent clotting factors (II, VII, IX, X). Information regarding the patient's recent travel, dietary history, and family history may provide clues to the underlying cause of potential hemolysis or liver disease. For the on-call physician, little in the way of

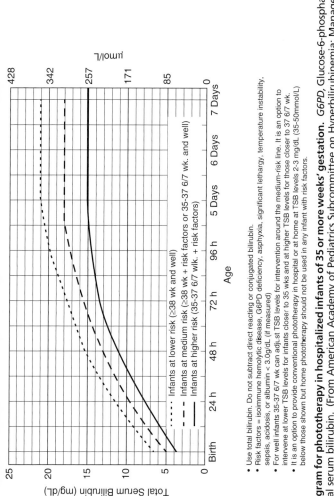

- Use total bilirubin. Do not subtract direct reacting or conjugated bilirubin.
- Risk factors = isoimmune hemolytic disease, G6PD deficiency, asphyxia, significant lethargy, temperature instability, sepsis, acidosis, or albumin < 3.0g/dL (if measured)
- For well infants 35-37 6/7 wk can adjust TSB levels for intervention around the medium-risk line. It is an option to intervene at lower TSB levels for infants closer to 35 wks and at higher TSB levels for those closer to 37 6/7 wk.
- It is an option to provide conventional phototherapy in hospital or at home at TSB levels 2-3 mg/dL (35-50mmol/L) below those shown but home phototherapy should not be used in any infant with risk factors.

FIGURE 36.3 **Nomogram for phototherapy in hospitalized infants of 35 or more weeks' gestation.** *G6PD,* Glucose-6-phosphate dehydrogenase; *TSB,* total serum bilirubin. (From American Academy of Pediatrics Subcommittee on Hyperbilirubinemia: Management of hyperbilirubinemia in the newborn infant 35 or more weeks of gestation. Pediatrics 114:297-316, 2004.)

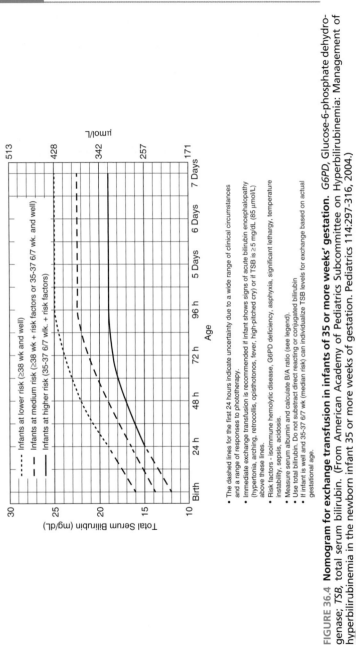

FIGURE 36.4 **Nomogram for exchange transfusion in infants of 35 or more weeks' gestation.** *G6PD,* Glucose-6-phosphate dehydrogenase; *TSB,* total serum bilirubin. (From American Academy of Pediatrics Subcommittee on Hyperbilirubinemia: Management of hyperbilirubinemia in the newborn infant 35 or more weeks of gestation. Pediatrics 114:297-316, 2004.)

intervention can be done in an older child with acute jaundice other than supportive care and initiation of the diagnostic evaluation. Children who have suffered hepatocellular damage are subject to shock and disseminated intravascular coagulation, which may need to be aggressively supported early in their disease while you are completing the diagnostic evaluation.

Summary

Hyperbilirubinemia in a newborn may be physiologic, but a wide variety of pathologic conditions must be considered and ruled out by history, physical examination, and laboratory evaluation. Although rarely life threatening, hyperbilirubinemia may have serious consequences. Management goals include initiating prompt, appropriate therapy (i.e., phototherapy or exchange transfusion) when indicated. A systematic evaluation of the risks of developing severe hyperbilirubinemia is based on the total bilirubin level, gestational age, presence or absence of risk factors, and health of the infant and is facilitated by using an hour-specific bilirubin nomogram. In older children, hepatocellular injury from infection, toxins, or a hypoxic-ischemic event must be ruled out and aggressive supportive treatment instituted at once to allow time to make the diagnosis and initiate more definitive therapy.

Appendices

Pediatric Procedures

James J. Nocton, MD and Rainer G. Gedeit, MD

Procedures are a great source of anxiety for the house officer or medical student. As a pediatric house officer, you may have limited opportunities to perform some procedures; consequently, it may be difficult to feel a sense of competence when you find yourself in the position of needing to obtain intravenous (IV) access or intubate a child. However, if you take advantage of every opportunity to try procedures, you will increase your chances of becoming proficient at such techniques as peripheral IV line placement, venipuncture, arterial blood gas sampling, lumbar puncture, intubation, umbilical line placement, joint aspiration, interosseous line placement, femoral line placement, and peripheral arterial line placement.

The key to success with any procedure involving a sharp object (e.g., a needle) is comfort of the person holding the sharp object. Set up for every procedure in the same way so that the routine is comfortable and automatic. Know the supplies that you will need and prepare them in advance, whether they are blood tubes, culture bottles, slides, or swabs.

For almost every procedure involving needles, there is a choice regarding the use of local anesthesia. Obviously, this is not a consideration in a dire emergency, but that is the exception, not the rule. Small children are fearful and move and resist, thereby reducing the likelihood of success. If properly anesthetized, the child resists and moves less, and you will be a hero when the IV goes in on the first try!

Topical anesthetics can be used for any procedure in which numbing of the skin will be helpful. Many different types of topical anesthetics are available, from creams to aerosols. Learn what is available to you and learn the indications and contraindications for each. Topical anesthetics are ideal for lumbar puncture or joint aspiration, especially in older children. Remember to consider the child's comfort during every procedure; the child's comfort may increase your own.

INTRAVENOUS ACCESS

IV access is an important ingredient in intervention and stabilization of any patient in the hospital. The following is a brief overview of the options available, some helpful technical tips, and a general approach to this procedure in pediatrics.

The legendary house officers who can get an IV line into anyone always have a routine that they follow with every patient, regardless of age. First, try to perform all procedures in a treatment or procedure room. All the supplies are there, and it maintains the patient's room as a sanctuary where the child is free from harm. Second, make sure that all your favorite supplies are set up before bringing the patient into the room. Third, get help to hold the child during the procedure. Do not ever ask a parent to hold a child for a procedure. First, they might faint, whereupon you will have two patients. Second, the parents should "rescue" their child from you afterward, not assist you. Regarding whether parents should observe procedures, if you are not comfortable having the parents in the room, tell them that honestly and explain that you are more likely to be successful if they are not present. Most parents respond favorably if you express your desire to make the procedure easier for their child.

The person holding the patient is as important to this process as the person holding the needle! Give the assistant clear instructions about how to restrain the child and assist you best. This is true in both a dire emergency and routine replacement of a peripheral IV line. Apply a rubber tourniquet above the potential site tight enough to occlude the veins but not so tight that you cannot palpate a pulse distally. Look and feel for the veins in the same places that you have veins, starting at the most distal point. Veins feel hollow, like a straw. Tendons are tense and cordlike. Arteries are firm and deep and should be pulsatile. Look at several different sites before making an attempt. It pays to shop around a little. Remove the tourniquet until you are ready to make your attempt.

The sites that should be explored in any patient include the dorsal hand veins, the radial vein of the wrist, the anterior ulnar vein of the forearm, the median cephalic vein in the lateral antecubital fossa, the median basilic vein in the medial antecubital fossa, the superficial veins of the dorsum of the foot, and the saphenous vein anterior and superior to the medial malleolus of the ankle and along its proximal length on the medial aspect of the foreleg. Next, the external jugular should be considered. Remember, neck lines in any child and scalp IV lines in infants are very distressing to parents and should be choices of last resort. IV line placement is not a benign intervention. Children suffer more complications from IV lines than from any other medical intervention in the hospital.

Selecting the catheter for a peripheral IV line is very important, not only to the success of your attempt but also to the longevity of the line that you place. Whatever size you originally think of, choose one size larger. Larger IV catheters will go in easier and last longer. In most full-term infants, regardless of hydration status, a 22-gauge catheter can be placed in any vein. Frequently in infants, a 20-gauge catheter or even an 18-gauge catheter can be placed in the antecubital, distal saphenous, or external jugular veins. Save the 24-gauge catheters for preterm infants. Smaller IV catheters do not advance into veins easily, cannot handle high flow rates, and cause a jetlike stream within the vessel that damages endothelium and causes infiltration into the surrounding tissues. The bigger needle may appear to hurt more, but it also goes in better and lasts longer, which means fewer IV attempts and less discomfort for your patient.

After you have selected the site, put on your gloves and prepare the site with povidone-iodine scrub and alcohol. Apply the tourniquet again and confirm that this is a good site. Then ask your assistant to gently but firmly hold the child. The IV starter should hold the extremity to ensure its position. Make the attempt boldly to get through the skin in one quick stab. Anticipate the withdrawal reaction and then advance into the vessel.

An IV catheter is a needle within a plastic tube. When you see blood return in the needle, you know that the lumen of the needle is within the lumen of the vessel; it does not necessarily mean that the catheter is within the lumen of the vessel. Because the needle tip extends 2 to 3 mm beyond the catheter, you must advance the needle and catheter a bit more before the catheter can be advanced into the vessel as you withdraw the needle. The blood return in the catheter should remind you to release the tourniquet and place the needle in a safe place away from the field and the child. Instruct your assistant to maintain control over the child until the IV line is safely and securely taped into place. Be meticulous about how you tape the IV line, and do it the same way every time. This ensures that the nurse will not be calling you again in 30 minutes to replace the same IV line.

In conclusion, do not approach placement of an IV line timidly. Confidence begets success. Be systematic, consistent, methodical, and caring, and pick a larger catheter. In addition, know your limitations. If you are not successful, call someone else to attempt the line placement. Rather than leave once help arrives, stay and observe "the master" at work. You may learn more than you expect. Remember that you want to help the patient to be healed and be comfortable. "Getting" a difficult IV line is a big confidence boost, but it should not come at the expense of causing more discomfort to the patient than is acceptable.

If a peripheral IV line cannot be established, a deep or central line may be required. Again, know your limitations. Central lines require experience, time, sterile technique, and sedation and are not to be pursued casually or without supervision. In an extreme emergency, an intraosseous line can be life saving and should be considered within 90 seconds, even in a hospitalized patient. There are many options for insertion of an intraosseous needle. Become familiar with what is available at each institution. In children younger than 3 years, the anterior tibial plateau is prepared with povidone-iodine and alcohol, chlorhexidine, or alcohol. The needle is directed 1 to 3 cm below the tibial tuberosity at a 30-degree angle caudally to avoid the epiphyseal growth plate. Insertion requires firm, steady pressure with a twisting motion through the bone. Less resistance is felt as the marrow cavity is entered. Other options are available for intraosseous placement, including needles that screw into the bone with or without an accompanying "drill." After needle placement, attempt to aspirate, but frequently, no marrow is aspirated. Infusion with a syringe should be free of resistance or soft tissue swelling. In older children the distal end of the femur can be used, with the needle angled 30 degrees cephalad. Once in place, the needle must be secured and the extremity restrained. Again, medical students or house officers must know their own limitations, be willing to learn, and be concerned for the welfare and comfort of the patient.

Lumbar Puncture

A lumbar puncture, or spinal tap, is likely to be the most common procedure performed by a pediatric house officer. Obtaining cerebrospinal fluid (CSF) for culture, microscopy, and biochemical analysis is an essential part of every work-up for sepsis.

For a right-handed person performing a lumbar puncture, the patient's head should be positioned to the left, with the supply kit to the right. This allows you to position your left hand so that your fingers are on the iliac crest and your thumb is on the desired interspace. The right hand is then free to insert the needle and fill the tubes.

The person holding the child is equally important. This person must also monitor the child's condition, especially the respiratory pattern in infants. Infants can be held quite effectively in the left lateral decubitus position or in the upright sitting position (Fig. A.1). Older children, if uncooperative, may require a second holder. Remember, never attempt a lumbar puncture without adequate help.

After you have set up the supply tray and have given your holder or holders their instructions, put on gloves in sterile fashion. With the child in the desired position, prepare the lower part of the back vigorously with povidone-iodine or chlorhexidine. Place the cover drape, and find the anatomic landmarks by positioning your left fingers on the iliac crest and feeling for the posterior iliac spines with your left thumb. The level of the crest should be L2-3, and the

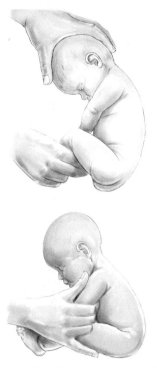

FIGURE A.1 Sitting position for restraining an infant for lumbar puncture. Lateral view.

level of the posterior spine should be L5. Feel for the L3-4 interspace, and keep your left thumb at that level. Using a prefilled 3-mL syringe, inject a small amount of 1% lidocaine subcutaneously. Be prepared for the child to move, and make sure that your holder is also prepared. Once the child settles, advance the needle, aspirate, and inject approximately 0.5 mL of lidocaine. There is no good reason to not use local anesthesia for a lumbar puncture. It will help immensely in avoiding a traumatic or bloody tap because of movement of the child. Return the lidocaine syringe to your sterile tray and insert the spinal needle at a 15- to 20-degree angle cephalad to avoid the posterior vertebral spines (Fig. A.2). If resistance is met, withdraw and angle more cephalad. In a term infant, the needle will advance 1 to 1.5 cm, and then resistance will be felt before the "pop" as the needle penetrates the dura (Fig. A.3). Withdraw the stylet, and watch for CSF backflow. If an opening pressure is

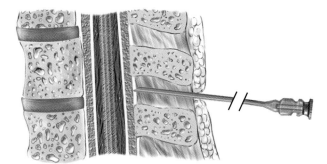

FIGURE A.2 The needle should be inserted in a slightly cephalad direction to avoid the vertebral bodies.

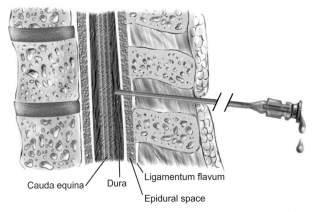

Cauda equina / Dura / Ligamentum flavum / Epidural space

FIGURE A.3 Once the needle has penetrated the dura, the stylet is withdrawn to allow spinal fluid to flow freely.

desired, attach the manometer via the three-way stopcock and determine the CSF level in centimeters. Then proceed to collect approximately 5 mL of CSF in sterile test tubes. Replace the stylet, withdraw the needle, and apply pressure on the site with the left thumb. The holder should allow the child to straighten and relax. A small bandage should be placed and the date written on it.

As with every procedure, a succinct procedural note should be written immediately to document the indications for the lumbar puncture, the technique, the results, and any complications.

Resuscitation Calculations

James J. Nocton, MD and Rainer G. Gedeit, MD

Intubation Equipment

Age/Weight	Endotracheal Tube Size	Laryngoscope Blade
Newborn/3-5 kg	2.5-3.5 mm	0-1 straight
Infant/6-9 kg	3.5 mm uncuffed	1 straight
Toddler/10-11 kg	4.0 mm uncuffed	1 straight
Small child/12-14 kg	4.5 mm uncuffed	2 straight
Child/15-18 kg	5.0 mm uncuffed	2 straight or curved
Child/19-22 kg	5.5 mm uncuffed	2 straight or curved
Large child/24-28 kg	6.0 mm cuffed	2-3 straight or curved
Adult/30 kg	6.5 mm cuffed	3 straight or curved

Resuscitation Medications

Drug	Dosage
Epinephrine	First dose IV/Intraosseous (IO): 0.01 mg/kg (1:10,000, 0.1 mL/kg) Endotracheal tube (ETT): 0.1 mg/kg (1:1000, 0.1 mL/kg) Subsequent doses Repeat every 3-5 minutes during cardiopulmonary resuscitation (CPR)
Atropine	0.02 mg/kg/dose; minimum dose: 0.1 mg; Maximum dose 1 mg
Glucose	IV/IO: 0.5-1 g/kg (1-2 mL/kg of 50% solution)

Calculation of Creatinine Clearance

James J. Nocton, MD

$$\text{CrCl (mL/min)} = U_{Cr}(\text{mg/mL}) \times V(\text{mL/min})/P_{Cr}(\text{mg/mL})$$

$\text{CrCl} =$ creatinine clearance
$U_{Cr} =$ urinary concentration of creatinine
$V =$ urinary flow rate
$P_{Cr} =$ plasma concentration of creatinine
To correct clearance for body surface area (BSA):

$$\text{Corrected CrCl} = \text{CrCl (mL/min)} \times 1.73/\text{BSA}\,(\text{m}^2)$$

Calculation of Alveolar-Arterial Oxygen Gradient

James J. Nocton, MD

The alveolar-arterial oxygen gradient, or $P(A-a)O_2$, can be calculated easily from the arterial blood gas (ABG) results. It is useful for confirming the presence of a shunt.

$$P(A-a)O_2 = PAO_2 - PaO_2$$

- $PAO_2 =$ alveolar oxygen tension calculated as shown subsequently
- $PaO_2 =$ arterial oxygen tension measured by ABG determination
  PAO_2 can be calculated by the following formula:

$$PAO_2 = (PB - PH_2O)(FIO_2) - PaCO_2/R$$

- $PB =$ barometric pressure (760 mm Hg at sea level)
- $PH_2O = 47$ mm Hg
- $FIO_2 =$ fraction of O_2 in inspired gas
- $PaCO_2 =$ arterial CO_2 tension measured by ABG determination
- $R =$ respiratory quotient (0.8)
  Normal $P(A-a)O_2$ ranges from 12 mm Hg or less for infants, children, and adolescents.

In pure ventilatory failure, $P(A-a)O_2$ will remain 12 to 20 mm Hg. In oxygenation failure, *it will increase*.

Adapted from Marshall SA, Ruedy J: On Call: Principles and Protocols, 4th ed. Philadelphia, WB Saunders, 2004, p 425.

Index

Note: Page numbers followed by "*f*" refer to illustrations; page numbers
followed by "*t*" refer to tables; page numbers followed by "*b*" refer to boxes.